Women's medicine

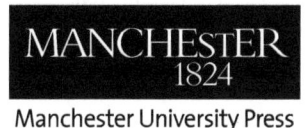
Manchester University Press

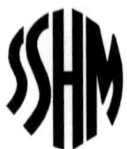

SOCIAL HISTORIES OF MEDICINE

Series editors: *David Cantor, Elaine Leong* and *Keir Waddington*

Social Histories of Medicine is concerned with all aspects of health, illness and medicine, from prehistory to the present, in every part of the world. The series covers the circumstances that promote health or illness, the ways in which people experience and explain such conditions, and what, practically, they do about them. Practitioners of all approaches to health and healing come within its scope, as do their ideas, beliefs, and practices, and the social, economic and cultural contexts in which they operate. Methodologically, the series welcomes relevant studies in social, economic, cultural, and intellectual history, as well as approaches derived from other disciplines in the arts, sciences, social sciences and humanities. The series is a collaboration between Manchester University Press and the Society for the Social History of Medicine.

Previously published

Migrant architects of the NHS *Julian M. Simpson*

Mediterranean quarantines, 1750–1914 *Edited by John Chircop and Francisco Javier Martínez*

Sickness, medical welfare and the English poor, 1750–1834 *Steven King*

Medical societies and scientific culture in nineteenth-century Belgium *Joris Vandendriessche*

Vaccinating Britain *Gareth Millward*

Madness on trial *James E. Moran*

Early Modern Ireland and the world of medicine *Edited by John Cunningham*

Feeling the strain *Jill Kirby*

Rhinoplasty and the nose in early modern British medicine and culture *Emily Cock*

Communicating the history of medicine *Edited by Solveig Jülich and Sven Widmalm*

Progress and pathology *Edited by Melissa Dickson, Emilie Taylor-Brown and Sally Shuttleworth*

Balancing the self *Edited by Mark Jackson and Martin D. Moore*

Accounting for health: Calculation, paperwork and medicine, 1500–2000 *Edited by Oliver Falk and Axel C. Hüntelmann*

Women's medicine

Sex, family planning and British female doctors
in transnational perspective, 1920–70

Caroline Rusterholz

Manchester University Press

Copyright © Caroline Rusterholz 2020

The right of Caroline Rusterholz to be identified as the author of this work has been asserted by her in accordance with the Copyright, Designs and Patents Act 1988.

An electronic version of this book is also available under a Creative Commons (CC-BY-NC-ND) licence, thanks to the support of the Swiss National Science Foundation, which permits non-commercial use, distribution and reproduction provided the author(s) and Manchester University Press are fully cited and no modifications or adaptations are made. Details of the licence can be viewed at https://creativecommons.org/licenses/by-nc-nd/3.0/

Published with the support of the Swiss National Science Foundation

Published by Manchester University Press
Altrincham Street, Manchester M1 7JA

www.manchesteruniversitypress.co.uk

British Library Cataloguing-in-Publication Data
A catalogue record for this book is available from the British Library

ISBN   978 1 5261 4912 1   hardback

First published 2020

The publisher has no responsibility for the persistence or accuracy of URLs for any external or third-party internet websites referred to in this book, and does not guarantee that any content on such websites is, or will remain, accurate or appropriate.

Typeset by
New Best-set Typesetters Ltd

Contents

List of figures	*page* vi
Acknowledgements	vii
List of abbreviations	x
Short biographies of the main characters	xi
Introduction	1
1 Giving birth control medical credentials in Britain: 1920–70	37
2 Sexual disorders and infertility: expanding the work of the clinics	85
3 Medicalising birth control at the international conferences (1920–37): a British–French comparison	137
4 Building a transnational movement for family planning: 1928–70	169
5 Testing IUDs: a transnational journey of expertise	196
Conclusion	224
References	232
Index	255

Figures

1 Pytram Pelvic model: demonstration pelvic front view. Source: 'Demonstration model of the teaching of contraceptive techniques, designed to the specification of Dr Helena Wright, approved by the FPA. Produced exclusively by Pytram Ltd', Wellcome Library, London, SA/FPA/A19/9. *page* 54
2 Pytram Pelvic model: top view showing the interior cavity, with the removal wall. Source: Wellcome Library, London, SA/FPA/A19/9. 55

Acknowledgements

The research for this project was generously funded by the Swiss National Science Foundation, who also provided the funding to make this book open access. I am indebted to many people who actively contributed to making this research possible. First, I would like to thank Simon Szreter, who warmly welcomed me in Cambridge for a six-month visiting fellowship, and provided institutional support, food for thought and friendship through this journey. In Cambridge, I was also lucky enough to count Jesse Olszynko-Gryn as a friend. Both Simon and Jesse read many parts of this book. I am also deeply grateful to Joanna Bourke, Sean Brady and Matt Cook who supported my application for an honorary position at Birkbeck College. There, I met wonderful people and colleagues. Particular thanks to David Byrdan, Marcia Holmes, Simon Jarret, Carmen Mangion, Sarah Marks, Francesca Piana, Kathryn Schoefert, Dora Vargha and Mark Volovici.

A special thank you to Lesley Hall, who has been invaluably kind and helpful during this research by sharing her knowledge, insights and sources. Yuliya Hilevych also deserves a special mention as she has been there for me from my first year as a PhD student to my current position. Her support, friendship, stimulating brain and encouragement, as well as the time she spent reading my work and commenting on earlier drafts of this book, have been essential for me. Special thanks also go to Laura Kelly and Agata Ignaciuk for their friendship, detailed and useful comments and proofreading drafts of this manuscript.

For encouragement, advice, proofreading and feedback at different stages, and in different contexts, many thanks to Laura Beers, Nicole Bourbonnais, Jessica Borge, Sandra Bree, Fabrice Cahen, Sylvie Chaperon, Charlotte Cree, Chris Crenner, Ivan Crozier, Donna Drucker,

Kate Fisher, Alana Harris, Claire Jones, Wendy Kline, Tracey Laughran, Virginie de Luca Barrusse, Helen McCarthy, Ben Mechen, Pauline Milani, Bibia Pavard, Anne-Françoise Praz, Stéphanie Roulin, Tiphaine Robert, Gabrielle Storey and Dawn Wibberley.

I have presented parts of this research at different international conferences and seminars, including the American Association for the History of Medicine; European Society of Historical Demography; Graduate Institute, Geneva (Gender Seminar); University of Exeter (Sexpertise Conference); Society for the Social History of Medicine; University of Brussels (European Sexology Conference); University of Cambridge (Gender Research Seminar); Leuwen University (Social History Seminar); Institute of Historical Research, London (Women's History Seminar); University of Cambridge (Reproductive Politics in France and the UK Conference). I am grateful for the comments I received from members of the audience.

I am very grateful for the assistance of the librarians and archivists at the Wellcome Library, Archives du Planning Familial in Paris, and the Butler Library, Columbia University.

Thank you to Thomas Dark, to Anthony Mercer and to Keir Waddington for support and advice during the publication process at Manchester University Press, and to the anonymous peer reviewers who provided such thoughtful and constructive advice.

Friendship has also helped me to survive long hours of solitary work at the library and moments of doubt. Thank you to Paz Irarrazabal, Ermioni Xanthopoulou, Guillermo Jimenez, Alberto Coddou, Antonia Asenjo, Cathy Herbrand, Claire Horn, Katie Dow and Natalia Delgado.

Portions of this research were originally published as Caroline Rusterholz, 'English women doctors, contraception and family planning in transnational perspective (1930s–70s)', *Medical History*, 63:2 (2019), pp. 153–72 (reprinted by permission of Cambridge University Press), Caroline Rusterholz, 'English and French women doctors in international debates on contraception (1920–1935)', *Social History of Medicine*, 31:2 (2018), pp. 328–47 (reprinted by permission of Oxford University Press), and Caroline Rusterholz, 'Testing the Gräfenberg ring in interwar Britain: Norman Haire, Helena Wright, and the debate over statistical evidence, side effects, and intra-uterine contraception', *Journal of the History of Medicine and Allied Sciences*, 72:4 (2017), pp. 448–67 (reprinted by permission of Oxford University Press).

Acknowledgements

For the support and love over the years, thank you to my parents, siblings, in-laws, colleagues at the University of Fribourg and my closest friends.

I am grateful to my husband Matthieu, who has read and commented on countless drafts of articles and chapters, emotionally supported me through this journey, cheered me up and helped me to get my confidence back when I thought this project was going nowhere. Thank you for your love and patience. I finished the revisions of the book while on maternity leave. A big thank you to my son Louis, who, though he did not nap for long, still allowed me to find time to revise this manuscript. I love you both.

Finally, this book is for all the women doctors and individuals who fought for our reproductive rights and are still fighting to treat women's bodies with the respect and care they deserve.

Abbreviations

AID	artificial insemination by donor
ALRA	Abortion Law Reform Association
BCIC	Birth Control Investigation Committee
BCIIC	Birth Control International Information Centre
BMJ	*British Medical Journal*
BS	Bachelor of Science
CIFC	Council for the Investigation of Fertility Control
FAO	UN Food and Agriculture Organization
FPA	Family Planning Association
ICPP	International Committee on Planned Parenthood
IPPF	International Planned Parenthood Federation
IUD	intrauterine device
MB	Bachelor of Medicine
MD	Doctor of Medicine
MFPF	Mouvement Français pour le Planning Familial
MGC	Marriage Guidance Council
MRC	Medical Research Council
MWF	Medical Women's Federation
MWIA	Medical Women's International Association
NBCA	National Birth Control Association
RF	Rockefeller Foundation
SCBCRP	Society for Constructive Birth Control and Racial Progress
SPBCC	Society for the Provision of Birth Control Clinics
WLSR	World League for Sexual Reform
WPC	World Population Congress

Short biographies of the main characters

Gladys Cox: Born in 1892. Medical officer at the Walworth Women's Welfare Centre. Member of the National Birth Control Association, the Society for the Study and Promotion of Family Hygiene, and the Birth Control Investigation Committee. Author of *Clinical Contraception*.

Sylvia Dawkins: Born in 1904 and qualified in 1929. She left general practice to work in a family planning clinic in 1948. Medical officer of the Islington Family Planning Clinic and clinical assistant at the dyspareunia and fertility clinic, University College Hospital, London. Became a group leader in psychosexual counselling. She died in 1995.

Frances Huxley: Born in 1885 and qualified in 1908. She was a gynaecological surgeon at the Marie Curie Hospital and founding member of the Medical Women's Federation (MWF), serving as the London president in 1928. In 1929, she was elected as a Foundation Fellow of the Royal College of Obstetricians and Gynaecologists. She participated in the Fifth International Neo-Malthusian and Birth Control Conference in 1922, and was the first British woman doctor to present her work on contraception.

Dr Margaret Jackson: Born in 1898. Founding member and medical officer of the Exeter and District Women's Welfare Centre. Member of the medical committee of the Family Planning Association (FPA). She specialised in infertility and artificial insemination, and helped many couples to have children. She wrote extensively on the subject. Jackson also carried out clinical trials on intrauterine devices (IUDs), and her centre became one of the four international centres collecting data on this form of contraception.

Dr Mary Macaulay: Mary Macaulay was medical officer of the Liverpool branch of the FPA between 1930 and 1956, and a marriage guidance counsellor. She wrote *The Art of Marriage*.

Joan Malleson: Born in 1899. Qualified in 1926. She had her own private practice and, alongside it, worked in a family planning clinic. Specialising in contraception and sexual difficulties, she was a member of the executive committee of the National Birth Control Association. For several years, Malleson was in charge of a clinic for difficulties with marital adjustment, which later became a clinic for sexual difficulties, at the North Kensington Women's Welfare Centre. In 1950, she was appointed head of the contraceptive clinic at University College Hospital. A member of the Labour Party and the Eugenics Society, she supported the Abortion Law Reform Association. She also wrote several manuals on contraception and sexual difficulties, and leaflets for the Family Planning Association. Malleson died in 1956.

Prudence Tunnedine: Born in 1928, she studied medicine at Guy's Hospital, qualifying in 1953. She worked in family planning clinics and became specialised in sexual counselling. She was a founding member of the Institute of Psychosexual Medicine.

Helena Wright: Born in 1887. Qualified in 1915. In 1921, she went to China as an associate professor of gynaecology at the Shandong Christian University, returning to England in 1928. She joined the National Birth Control Association and the Birth Control Investigation Committee, and held the post of chief medical officer at the North Kensington Women's Welfare Centre (1930–60). Wright was a founding member of the International Planned Parenthood Federation (IPPF) in 1952, and served as both treasurer and chair on the IPPF's medical committee. She published extensively on the subject of sex in marriage.

Introduction

In 'One Woman's Mission', an article in the *Sunday Times Magazine* in 1973, pioneer birth control activist and female gynaecologist Helena Wright recalled the pivotal moment in her career. In 1928, Wright intrepidly dedicated herself to making contraception both acceptable and accessible. Looking back on this decision, she explained: 'It seemed to me in a prophetic way, that birth control was the single subject that women doctors had to get hold of.'[1] The implications of Wright's vision for women doctors – to 'make contraception respectable' – cannot be overstated. Perhaps more than anyone in her generation, Wright contributed to the spread of birth control at both national and international levels; however, she was not alone in that endeavour. As her crusading remark underlines, women doctors 'got hold' of the subject of birth control from the 1920s onwards.

But how did women doctors undertake this campaign at a time when contraception was a contentious topic that divided the medical profession and, indeed, the broader public? This question has received surprisingly scant attention.[2] I tell this story by exploring the key role that British female doctors played in the production and circulation of contraceptive knowledge and the handling of sexual disorders. I focus first and mostly on Britain and then on the international and transnational levels between the 1920s and the 1970s; I take France as a point of comparison. This study charts the accomplishment of several women doctors as they made their way through the predominantly male-dominated medical landscape. They sought to establish the use of birth control – that is, any practices, methods, and devices that could prevent pregnancy – as a legitimate field of medicine. Alongside their work to medicalise and legitimise birth control, they promoted family planning, or the provision of contraceptive methods to plan and space births, and offered counselling on sexual disorders, fertility and sub-fertility. These areas of practice, which would become a new career path for many women doctors, emerged from women doctors' experiences and encounters with patients in birth control and family planning clinics. Looking at the difficulties experienced by many female patients with planning and spacing births, getting pregnant and having satisfying sexual lives, women doctors tried to address these issues by developing new forms of expertise and practice and thus creating a common professional identity. In so doing, they were especially careful to present these new fields as medical and impart this new knowledge to their colleagues. Their claim to authority was therefore based on their practical experience in the clinics.

These forerunners included Helena Wright (1887–1982), Joan Malleson (1899–1956), Margaret Jackson (1899–1987), Gladys Cox (1892–?, professionally active between the 1920s and 1930s), and Sylvia Dawkins (1904–95). I shed light on the strategies British women doctors used, and the alliances they forged to forward their medical agenda and position themselves as experts and leaders in birth control and family planning research and practice. This book is part of a growing field of research on the medical history of birth control and sexuality.

The medicalisation of birth control is one aspect of the broader history of the medicalisation of the female body, a history that has attracted considerable attention from feminist historians since the 1980s in the context of the feminist health movement.[3] Medicalisation means 'defining a problem in medical terms, using medical language to describe a problem, adopting a medical framework to understand a problem or using a medical intervention to treat it.[4] Feminist critics have identified medicine and gynaecology as central to the oppressive regulation of women's bodies.[5] Historical analysis has often depicted the female body as a site of ideological intervention for numerous actors, be they medical professionals, the Church, traditional healers, the state, or health campaigners.[6] Historians have shown that prior to the Enlightenment, the female body was medically perceived as an inferior version of the male one.[7] More generally, women's bodies were represented as volatile, dangerous, and in need of medical intervention and monitoring.[8] Several scholars have offered a nuanced account of the medicalisation of the female body over the last two centuries. They

Introduction

emphasised the social, medical and political context in which this medicalisation took place and foregrounded the agency of female patients who were not necessarily the passive victims of male doctors.[9] The issue of the medicalisation of birth control in the twentieth century has also been cast in different historical lights. In narratives on the 'long sexual revolution' it has often been presented as an emancipatory process, freeing women from the burden of pregnancies,[10] whereas in feminist criticisms of medicine, this process has been depicted as oppressive, and as part of a more general male-dominated medicalisation of control over women's bodies, symbolised by the use of the stirrups in childbirth or the coerced sterilisations of women.[11]

Hence, the medicalisation process has usually been described as one in which the institution of medicine acted as an agent of social control. However, recent research has challenged this unilateral view. Nikolas Rose went as far as to call 'medicalisation' 'a cliché of critical social analysis'.[12] Nonetheless, Peter Conrad, while acknowledging that 'medicalisation' is too often used in a negative way, suggested that analysing the medicalisation process could be useful if it is done to highlight and articulate the complicated process of medical knowledge construction.[13] Following Conrad's advice, this book moves beyond this dichotomy by re-evaluating the medicalisation process through the contribution of women doctors to the production of medical knowledge on birth control and family planning. I explore the production of medical knowledge in paying attention to the social, medical and cultural setting, but also to the scientific background in which knowledge is produced. In other words, I operate on the cusp of social, cultural and intellectual history. This study focuses on the environment in which women doctors lived, emphasising the opportunities they encountered and the constraints they faced. It examines the contemporary dynamics of scientific controversies around birth control, the way through which scientific practices and procedures around birth control and family planning were implemented and stabilised, and the way that interactions with patients affected women doctors' production of medical knowledge on family planning.

The novelty of this book lies in three key elements. First, the specific focus on female doctors illuminates their agency in the male-dominated field of medicine and reveals their significant role in the medicalisation process. It corrects the narrative of women's reproductive bodies being dominated and controlled by male doctors. The subject of women in medicine has attracted growing interest. Scholars have explored the history of women's entry into the medical profession and into specific medical fields.[14] Clare Debenham's recent study has contributed to the understanding of the relationship between the Society for the Provision of Birth Control Clinics and feminist activism.[15] However, she pays little attention to the contribution of women doctors to family planning centres and to the medicalisation of birth control. While the role of women doctors has not been wholly neglected, the significance of their contribution has been underestimated and obscured by more famous and controversial figures in birth control, such as the British botanist and birth control activist Marie Stopes or the nurse and American birth control activist Margaret Sanger.[16] This book acknowledges women doctors' contributions and examines how they supported, in crucial ways, the medicalisation of birth control and family planning. While particular attention is paid to patients' experiences, this book does not adopt a patient-centred focus but instead offers the first systematic analysis of female doctors' participation in the scientific development of contraception and family planning. Their role in these transformations, which has hitherto been understudied, deserves closer attention since they were at the forefront of the birth control movement, even though they were a minority within the medical field. I argue that they capitalised on the fact that they were assigned to a low-status, feminine field of medicine and turned their practical experience into an asset at both national and international levels. So this book contributes to wider debates about the way female practitioners used particular forms of specialisation – in this case, contraception and family planning – to carve out a territory for themselves and to formulate claims to authority.[17] They medicalised birth control and family planning with a triple agenda in mind: fighting ignorance around contraception in the medical profession and among the public so as to free women from the fear of pregnancy; securing a new expert understanding of the subject that reinforced their authority as doctors; and using this new power to secure job opportunities. Hence, the medicalisation of contraception and family planning was not a dualistic process of good or bad outcomes; rather it encompassed both the notions of emancipation and control. By teaching women how to avoid pregnancy, women doctors empowered them with knowledge. Paradoxically, at the same time, they wielded their medical power over the female body by being the sound voice of knowledge and the main providers of contraceptives.

Second, the transnational perspective allows me to reassess the issue of birth control from a new perspective that emphasises the circulation of scientific knowledge between Britain and France. Taking a transnational perspective on issues related to sexuality and reproduction involves simultaneously considering two levels of analysis, while trying to address their relationships: both national and international.[18] The history of birth control is intrinsically linked with that of population control movements, and has already attracted considerable attention, whether from a eugenic, neo-Malthusian, birth control, or family planning perspective.[19] The focus mainly rests on the national level of analysis, though regional differences were also important and analysed, and the involvement of political, institutional and medical authorities, or activists in debates around these issues, thereby reflecting the 'biopolitics' of Foucault (the power to regulate both individual and social bodies).[20] Recent scholarship has begun to explore the interplay between the aims of these different population control movements.[21] Whereas scholars have identified the transnational networks and actors in associations created before and after the Second World War, and in the circulation of knowledge about sexuality and birth control across national borders, they have mainly focused on the associations that targeted developing countries.[22] Similarly, there is a growing scholarship on internationalism, the history of international health and hygiene and the role of doctors as international experts, as well as that of women as international agents.[23] However, the participation of women doctors as international agents of birth control still deserves a thorough exploration.

Yet much still needs to be done to better understand the reconfiguration of discourses, practices, and scientific knowledge of birth control, family planning and sexuality produced by female medical experts at both national and international levels, targeting the European population. The main focus of this study is Britain, but it takes France as a point of comparison in the last two chapters. While regional differences existed in Britain and France, and in oversea territories, I focus on Britain and France 'at home'. Separated only by the Channel, and yet known for dramatically opposing reproductive policies, Britain and France continue to invite comparison.[24] In the present context, this comparison sheds new light on the way knowledge circulated between the two countries, each with different institutional contexts. This comparative perspective is interesting since Britain and France were pioneers in the fight for birth control, before France became a pronatalist country in the 1920s and enacted a restrictive policy on contraception and abortion. British and French doctors, as well as British and French experts (though some under a pseudonym) were present at international conferences on birth control, and this offers an interesting case study in understanding the impact of reproductive politics on the stances taken by these doctors in two countries which, until then, had a strong Malthusian minority. The study examines the scientific knowledge produced not only at the national level but also at international conferences, as well as the network of actors involved in these conferences; it eventually looks at the mechanisms by which knowledge circulated between countries. This perspective explains why it is difficult to disentangle women doctors' contribution at one specific level without considering their position in another. Their contribution to the medicalisation of birth control and family planning resulted from a dynamic process between their social, political, scientific and medical positions at both the national and international levels. This book argues that there was a constant relationship between the national and international levels that helped women to position themselves as experts. The practical knowledge that women doctors acquired at the national level, which at first was not recognised, was pivotal in making them experts in birth control issues at the international level. While recognising that women doctors worked at both levels, this book considers their contribution separately and does so to ensure the clarity of the argument.

Finally, this research is the first systematic analysis of the production and circulation of scientific knowledge of contraception, family planning, and sexual disorders spanning an important period (1920–70) for each area in terms of legitimisation and institutional stabilisation. Social and cultural historians interested in gender and sexuality have offered fresh narratives on the use of contraception, development in sexual behaviours, norms and mores and the history of intimacy in twentieth-century Britain and France.[25] In particular, the oral history studies of birth control practices by Simon Szreter and Kate Fisher provided insights into the sexuality of ordinary people and their favourite methods of birth control for the period 1920–60.[26] These studies have challenged common assumptions about who oversaw birth control. For the French historiography, Christine Bard and Janine Mossuz-Lavau analysed the history of the development of the Family Planning Association in France, while Bibia Pavard offered an in-depth analysis of the struggles for the provision of contraception and abortion in France. She focused on the actors involved and the strategies they developed to make contraception legally available.[27] However, these historians have mainly focused on one specific aspect of birth control or family planning, analysing, for instance, abortion, contraceptive techniques or practices, infertility or specific sexual disorders.[28] This book extends this body of research by further examining the story of the ways that women doctors shaped the medicalisation of contraception and family planning in Britain and France. It is a much-needed addition to this growing body of research in that it focuses primarily on female medical contributions while avoiding the pitfall of concentrating only on discourses, thanks to a close examination of medical and scientific practices. As a result, it is part of a broader effort to uncover the many different actors and individuals involved in birth control and family planning practices and policy.

The aim of this book is to analyse the overall contribution of women doctors in the broad field of contraceptive methods and family planning which encompasses advice about contraceptives, marital and sexual disorders. This book contributes to recovering a female medical understanding of changing notions of marital sexuality. It argues that women doctors were pivotal in developing a more holistic approach to family planning, playing a more prominent role in shaping scientific and medical knowledge than previously acknowledged. What this book offers, however, is not a narrative of liberation or a Whiggish analysis of scientific discovery from darkness to enlightenment. It is a narrative of struggles, with steps forward and steps back – a story where forming alliances and developing strategies were as important as combatting ignorance around sexuality. It is a narrative that underlines the fact that women doctors' involvement in birth control issues resulted in an increasing 'burden' on women's shoulders, since women had to take responsibility for birth control, though this was at first perceived by these women doctors as empowering.

Women doctors' contribution to the provision and development of modern contraception and scientific knowledge of sexual disorders occurred at a time when the very meanings of reproduction and medicine were being transformed. The half-century covered in this book saw birth control finally becoming widely accepted in the medical profession. The years after the First World War were characterised by the consolidation of modern birth control movements, both in Europe and the United States. This story ends at the point when the Family Planning Act allowed local authorities to provide free birth control to all women (married or single), the Abortion Act legalised abortion by registered practitioners in Britain, and contraception became legally available in France with the enactment of the Neuwirth Law. It was during this shifting context that women doctors' contributions resonated. Therefore, the book locates the productive roles of women doctors within this changing landscape of national and international reproductive politics. It links their involvement in birth control clinics with broader issues surrounding power relationships and expertise within the national and international medical profession. Although this study explores scientific knowledge production and scientific practices around birth control and family planning from 1920 to 1970, the period of 1930 to 1960 is predominant. These were the decades when the medical landscape around birth control and family planning was changing dramatically, and, with the advent of the Family Planning Association (1939), the new focus was on infertility, sexual disorders and new reproductive technologies. Hence, I suggest that the key to understanding women doctors' paths towards birth control and family planning issues lies in the historical relationship between reproductive politics, gendered medical practices, contraceptive culture and the production of scientific knowledge.

Reproductive politics

The subject of birth control has been studied in relation to the history of reproductive politics and has received historical attention for many decades. From 1870 onwards, nearly every European country faced a decline in fertility, known as the 'demographic transition'. While in France the demographic transition started a century earlier than in any other European country, the trend in Britain followed the average pace. From the end of the nineteenth century, an increasing number of

British married couples used birth control, which resulted in a decline in average family size. Many historians and demographers have studied this decrease in fertility and its timing, underlining its diversity across 'communication communities'[29] and its impact on society and family life.[30] In particular, Simon Szreter's comprehensive study of fertility decline in Britain challenged the idea of a unified theory behind the fertility decline across Europe. Several scholars have tried to identify the birth control methods used by ordinary individuals and the extent to which access – or lack of access – to contraceptive information shaped individual behaviour.[31] One of the major research strands resulting from these research questions has been the emphasis on reproductive politics and the role played by experts in campaigning for or opposing birth control.

In Britain and France, this context of declining fertility gave rise to increasing anxieties among contemporary commentators about racial and national degeneracy, and depopulation, though these anxieties were more acute in France.[32] Consequently, the quality and quantity of the future population became a central concern to contemporary experts, including doctors. These anxieties led to different answers in the two countries. Eugenics – a term coined by Francis Galton in his 1883 *Inquiries into Human Faculty* to describe a science 'that focused on manipulating heredity or breeding to produce better people and on eliminating those considered biologically inferior'[33] – was one of the main tendencies before 1920 in Britain, partly due to concerns about colonial expansion. The Eugenics Education Society was formed in 1907, and the majority of its members were recruited from among middle-class professionals.[34] The goal of the society was to improve the quality of the race through two strategies. The first was the implementation of positive eugenic measures aimed at increasing the fertility of people from higher social classes – those considered to be socially valuable. The second was the application of negative eugenic measures designed to prevent the working classes – i.e. the socially worthless or the 'unfits' – from giving birth to too many offspring through birth control or voluntary sterilisation. However, the society achieved limited success in terms of implementing policy since politicians were afraid of alienating part of their parties by supporting a eugenic position, even though eugenic ideas permeated a large part of British society between the wars.³⁵ Researchers have emphasised the different and conflicting connections that eugenics developed with feminism, religion, politicians, and – of particular relevance to this study – medicine.³⁶

In France, pronatalism was the dominant school of thought, though some pronatalists were greatly influenced by eugenics. Pronatalist organisations were created at the turn of the twentieth century, and included the Alliance Nationale pour l'Accroissement de la Population Française (1896), which aimed at raising public awareness of the French demographic deficit and its alleged threat to French military power, and the Groupe Parlementaire pour la Protection de la Natalité et de la Famille (1911), which supported large families.³⁷ French doctors were numerous and actively engaged in the pronatalist movement, 'contributing to pronatalism's symbolic capital', as well as in the eugenics movement.

In both France and Britain, a birth control movement mainly led by neo-Malthusians was active before 1920. Neo-Malthusians were inspired by Thomas Robert Malthus's famous *Essay on the Principle of Population* (1798) in which he argued that population growth, especially among the poor, would outstrip resource growth unless reproduction was contained through 'moral restraint' and postponement of marriage. Neo-Malthusians shared the same motives to limit family size, but advocated different means to achieve them: the use of contraceptive devices. In Britain, the Malthusian League was formed in 1877, following the Bradlaugh-Besant trial, to campaign for information about family limitation. The French educator and scientist Paul Robin had discovered the neo-Malthusian movement during his exile in London, and imported this movement to France. He founded La Ligue de la Régénération Humaine (The League for Human Regeneration) in 1896, and distributed contraceptives until the 1920s.³⁸

In both countries, working-class mothers became the target of increased surveillance by official and voluntary agencies concerned about child welfare.³⁹ For instance, social hygienists – middle-class reformers working in voluntary organisations – promoted education in 'mothercraft', disseminated information on the risks of venereal diseases and encouraged sexuality to be confined within the heterosexual monogamous family. After the First World War, the national landscape around reproductive politics underwent dramatic changes

Introduction

in Britain and France, resulting in two contrasting policies on the two sides of the channel. Campaigns for birth control spread across Britain, and it became a topic of discussion, while a restrictive and pronatalist policy was enacted in France in 1920 that hindered the provision of contraception.

Starting in 1921 in North London with the opening of the first birth control clinic by Marie Stopes,[40] a woman scientist, feminist and ardent eugenicist, several clinics opened across Britain under the auspices of the Society for the Provision of Birth Control Clinics. At the same time, some suffragettes began to fight for sexual equality and fertility control, as did female members of the Labour Party. This happened after women aged over thirty, who met specific qualifications, obtained suffrage in 1918; the right to vote was extended in 1928 to all women on the same terms as men. Raising the topic of birth control before women had the vote might have prevented its introduction. The birth control movement was driven by multiple goals – namely, fighting against poverty, the feminist crusade and eugenic aspirations.[41] Recent work by Stephen Brooke has shown that the birth control movement received limited support from the Labour Party at first, the latter fearing it would alienate its Roman Catholic voters.[42] Arguments drawing on claims about sexual rights or sexual freedom did not fare well within the party. An argument that seemed to have attracted greater backing was that of improving the economic and health condition of working-class mothers – burdened by pregnancies and poverty – through birth control. This argument, as I show in Chapter 1, was also used by women doctors to advocate for the recognition of birth control as a medical field as part of an attempt to reappropriate male narratives.

Richard Soloway has argued that the medical profession was mostly against birth control, with notable exceptions such as the Australian gynaecologist Norman Haire or Lord Dawson of Penn.[43] However, medical stances began to shift as birth control gained in legitimacy after July 1930 when the Ministry of Health (by Memorandum 153/MCW) allowed contraceptive advice to be given in local maternity clinics to married women for whom further pregnancy would be detrimental to health. That same year, Anglican ministers legitimised birth control within Christian marriage at the Lambeth Conference. In 1931, the National Birth Control Council that coordinated the different societies for birth control became the National Birth Control Association

(NBCA). By 1932, eighteen voluntary birth control clinics were operational in Britain.[44]

Fears over population decline in the late 1930s saw the NBCA change its name to the Family Planning Association (FPA) in order to emphasise the positive side of its work. Priority was given to family spacing instead of the limitation of births, and emphasis was put on the 'wanted' child. The outbreak of war in 1939 prompted a slowing down of FPA activities; it created a shortage of rubber, among other issues. During the war, key initiatives began, such as the setting up of the sterility clinics that would define the new orientation of the work of the FPA. By the end of the war, the coalition government had set up the Royal Commission on Population for investigating the fertility of the British population in order to plan for the postwar situation. Based on the work of the Population Investigation Committee, and under the supervision of the Royal College of Obstetricians and Gynaecologists, the survey revealed a growing use of appliance methods of birth control by married women. In 1946, the National Health Service was implemented, but because the legislation made no mention of family planning, the provision of contraception was still being directed by Memorandum 153/MCW. After the war, Britain, like most countries in Europe, experienced a baby boom, which was initially described as temporary. By the start of 1955, the FPA was opening a new clinic at the rate of one every two weeks.[45] The same year, the Conservative Health Minister Iain Macleod visited one of the clinics for the FPA's Silver Jubilee. This visit received great media coverage, precipitating the acceptability of contraception. In 1961, the contraceptive pill arrived on the British market under medical prescription, establishing contraception as the responsibility of the medical profession. In 1967, Labour MP Edwin Brook's Family Planning Act allowed local authorities to provide birth control to all women (married or single), and in the same year the Abortion Act legalised abortion by registered practitioners. In 1974, the National Health Service, some thirty-six years after its founding in 1948, incorporated family planning, and contraception became free to all women regardless of age or marital status.

Meanwhile in France, in 1920, a new law was enacted that forbade the sale, distribution and advertisement of contraceptive devices, making it punishable by fines and imprisonment. Condoms remained permitted since they prevented venereal diseases. This clampdown found its moral expression in Catholic France with the publication of the encyclical *Casti Connubii* in 1931. Natalism inhabited the political centre-ground of interwar France, attracting supporters from both the right and the left, and from all sections of society including the majority of medical professionals.[46] In 1939, the Code de la Famille established a comprehensive system of state support for families, and the 1920 law was strengthened, abortion being now considered a 'crime against the fatherland'. In 1942, in Vichy France, abortion became a crime against the state, on a par with treason. After the war, abortion remained a major issue.[47] Although the birth rate started to increase again from 1942 onwards, demographers remained reluctant to acknowledge the baby boom and maintained pronatalist stances.[48] However, some doctors began actively supporting family planning policies. In 1956, the female gynaecologist Marie-Andrée Lagroua Weill-Hallé created the Association Maternité Heureuse, aimed at spreading information on contraception as a means to avoid abortions. This association became the Mouvement Français pour le Planning Familial (MFPF), a national branch of the International Planned Parenthood Federation. The College des Médecins, the progressive alternative to the conservative Ordre des Médecins, was created in 1962 to gather doctors in favour of the spread of contraceptive knowledge. In conjunction with the left-wing parties, the MFPF led the campaign to abolish the 1920 contraception law, which, in 1967, was superseded by the Neuwirth Law, marking another dramatic change to the political and social landscape of France.[49]

Political campaigners and feminist activists are only one side of the story, and putting women doctors back in the picture allows for a more nuanced account of the supposed success of, and the main actors behind, these birth control and family planning movements. Indeed, focusing on women doctors and the constraints they faced reveal the resistances at play among the medical body. While their work was mainly directed towards their fellow medical colleagues and their potential women patients, and was maybe not as visible as those of their contemporary political campaigners, I argue that British female doctors played a greater pivotal role than previously acknowledged. They helped the birth control movement to shift from a free-thinking radical movement to a professional body that produced knowledge of the requirements of birth control methods and of the handling of sexual disorders in Britain. In addition, British female doctors greatly contributed to spreading the gospel of family planning in France since they became a channel of training and information for French doctors.

Gendered medical practices

British women doctors' involvement in the development of birth control provision and practices took place in a context in which they remained a minority in the male-dominated field of medicine, occupying only a peripheral position. In 1914 there were only 1,000 women on the Medical Register of Britain, but this number increased to 6,300 by 1939, 7,520 by 1951, and 13,271 by 1971.[50] The latter figure represented around 16 per cent of the medical population.[51] The subject of women in medicine has attracted growing interest. We know a lot about the famous women doctor pioneers and their paths towards medicine, and several scholars have investigated the history of British and Irish medical women's entry into the medical profession and subsequent developments, and into specific medical fields, such as surgery. The main narratives from these different stories are about the mountains that women had to climb to gain equal opportunities with their male colleagues.[52] Male doctors fought women's entry into the profession, driven by anxieties about overcrowding and a resistance to working under the supervision of female doctors.[53] For instance, in Britain, between 1870 and 1914, the majority of women doctors were trained in single-sex institutions such as the London School of Medicine for Women. The latter was founded in 1874 by the then soon-to-be woman doctor Sophia Jex-Blake, a leading British campaigner for women's admission to the medical profession who experienced difficulties in obtaining training in Britain and decided to start her own place of training.[54]

The need to protect their gains and promote their interests led these female doctors to create professional associations. The British Medical Women's Federation (MWF) was created in 1916 by a fusion of pre-existing local associations of registered medical women. The MWF sought to defend the position of women in the medical profession, and it published a journal and organised lectures and conferences. As Kaarin Michaelsen has argued, 'The MWF was intended to act as a bridge "between the values of scientific professionalism and those of social feminism", projecting an image of the "woman professional" as "equal but not identical" to male physicians and therefore having "responsibilities and interests that are not exactly the same as men".[55] Its central function was to be a professional body, publicly defending the opinion of medical women on public policy affecting them. In 1924, 700 women were members of the federation, and membership had more than doubled by 1928. In Britain, by 1930, women had overcome a number of obstacles. For example, several hospitals had finally admitted women onto their honorary staff. Significantly, nearly two decades later, all medical schools were opened to women with the inception of the National Health Service in 1948.

Several studies have already shown how women doctors were assigned to fields that were supposedly in line with their 'feminine nature' and to more precarious positions within the medical hierarchy since women graduates had limited access to clinical appointments. There is a body of scholarship on the contribution that women made as women doctors and how their gendered identity was central to their access to medicine and 'constrained' choice of specialties.[56] However, some women also actively chose and exploited these 'constraints' to carve out their own professional space. The argument about the 'feminine nature' was used by the first generation of women doctors in support of their access to medical education. Among them was Sophia Jex-Blake, who drew on the gendered assumptions about women's emotional nature: 'Women have more love of medical work, and are naturally more inclined, and more fitted for it than most men.'[57] Hence, as explained by Laura Kelly, 'those arguing in favour of women's admission to medical schools claimed that there was a demand for women doctors to treat women patients, a role for which they would be eminently suited'.[58] The argument that women doctors were particularly good for women patients and their children was one of the strongest arguments supporting women's access to medical education. Women doctors claimed that their dual experience as women and physicians lent them privileged knowledge to deal with aspects of women's intimate and family lives. It was a way to reconcile the Victorian division of labour – where middle-class women were the guardians of the family's and nation's morality and, as such, had a special role in medicine since they allowed women patients to avoid losing their delicacy and virtue by submitting to male treatment – with women's emancipatory claim to access to education. As a result, women predominantly worked in the less popular fields of welfare provision, public and community health, and in obstetrics and gynaecology in Britain.[59]

Women doctors thus worked in 'feminine fields', and their clinical work focused on children and on women.[60] Their professional orientation was therefore seemingly shaped by their gender. They were developing expertise in neglected and marginalised areas of medicine such as geriatric care and finding effective treatment for the common diseases of slum children.[61] Birth control, mainly aimed at women, was an area that was not yet considered medicine as such and consequently not taught in medical schools. Like obstetrics and gynaecology, birth control was low status. It is not surprising that women doctors were also represented in great numbers in birth control clinics. For instance, in 1932, with the exception of one institution briefly run by Norman Haire, all birth control clinics were headed by women doctors. Yet if, in the late nineteenth century, women doctors used their gendered qualities as a tool to access medical education and to find clinical work, we cannot assume as self-evident the fact that they continued to rely on the argument of their dual experiences as women and doctors to justify their involvement in birth control work. Indeed, as I argue in Chapter 1, women doctors medicalised and colonised birth control in order to make it a field of medicine and more specifically a legitimate one. In so doing, it was not so much their experience as women that they put forward but rather their professional experience as doctors – even if this experience was deeply shaped by their gendered identity within the medical field – appropriating the male medical authority language of 'scientific facts'. By relying on their clinical experience, women doctors created a new form of professional practice and identity where birth control methods were assessed through sound criteria based on statistics and evidence accumulated via first-hand experience. This resort to clinical experience supported their claims to authority. Furthermore, it seems that women doctors were willing to embrace this topic as it could provide them with a new field of work. But women doctors' sympathy and interest in birth control was also a generational issue. Indeed, the women pioneers who fought to access education and make female doctors respectable and legitimate were often initially reluctant to engage with birth control, fearing that it would encourage excessive sexual attention from husbands.[62] Hence, as Lesley Hall has argued, it was younger women doctors who were often in favour of birth control:

'a younger generation of women doctors by contrast were characteristic exponents of the welfare feminism of the era following the achievement of the suffrage. In general practice and maternity welfare work they encountered what they saw as a crying need for reliable and healthy forms of contraception.'[63] As I will show, women doctors mainstreamed the diffusion of information on contraception by publishing sexual and medical manuals and medical articles in medical journals, and campaigned for the better provision of reliable and safe contraceptives. These activities made birth control a legitimate topic within medical circles and increased public discussion on the subject.

Thus, birth control clinics offered important job opportunities for British female doctors, even though the pay was minimal. This was especially true for married female doctors. Usually held in the evening, birth control sessions suited married women doctors seeking to reintegrate into the labour market or to work part-time. This convenience was put forward by several women doctors, such as British doctor Prudence Tunnedine. Born in 1928, she studied medicine at Guy's Hospital, qualifying in 1953. She explained her decision to join a family planning clinic as follows:

> Well by the time my fourth child was born, and married to a country doctor, it was fairly clear that my ambitions to be a hospital obstetrician were getting increasingly unrealistic, and I was just asked if I would start a family planning clinic by a clergyman in the nearby town which wasn't so served then with my gynaecological experience. So it was largely accident in a way. It was evening work, to look after my children myself as far as possible when they were little. [...] You see, we married women with children were virtually regarded as unemployable. We were thought to be sort of a side issue and lots of us did occasional clinic work either in family planning or in child welfare.[64]

I contend that this situation explains why women doctors were so adamant in promoting the spread of scientific knowledge about the subject. Indeed, their active contribution stemmed not only from their will to help and care for women – by ascertaining the efficiency and suitability of contraceptive methods – but also from their lived experiences in the male-dominated field of medicine where they struggled to find clinical work. Women doctors no longer claimed a specific understanding of women's needs due to their common experience as women.

Rather, they relied on their professional experience of working with women patients and framed birth control as a medical and technical field. They established birth control as a new form of medical specialty. The spread of scientific and medical knowledge should also be understood as a strategic move to support the institutionalisation and visibility of this new field of medicine in which many of them had invested their time and expertise.

Contraceptive culture and the production of medical knowledge of birth control

The productive role of women doctors took place in a changing medical context in which laboratory-based medicine was becoming common practice, especially in relation to the testing of birth control methods.[65] With the professionalisation of the birth control movement – from a secularist, free-thinking movement aimed at eradicating poverty with eugenic and feminist aspirations, to an institutionalised movement gathering together doctors and scientists by 1930 – and the expansion of birth control clinics in interwar Britain, efforts to develop better scientific means for contraception grew rapidly.[66] Until the end of the nineteenth century, methods for controlling fertility ranged from coitus interruptus and abstinence, to diverse substances ingested or placed into the vagina, to barrier methods such as the cap, pessary, diaphragm and male condom.[67] Abortion was also widely practiced when contraception failed, despite being illegal except where necessary to save the mother's life. Studies have shown that women did not consider 'bringing their period back' an abortion as such, or a moral fault. Early abortion and contraception were intertwined and understood 'on a fertility regulation continuum'.[68]

The first half of the twentieth century brought the development of chemical contraceptives as well as a number of new intrauterine devices, among them the Gräfenberg ring, which blocked implantation of the egg by inducing a thickening of the uterine lining (endometrial hyperplasia). Despite the development of these new contraceptive technologies, recent studies have underlined that the decrease in marital fertility had more to do with the resort to traditional methods of birth control, such as abstinence and withdrawal, than the adoption of modern methods of contraception. In particular, the landmark study of Simon

Szreter on the decline in fertility in Britain stressed the importance of abstinence as the main method of birth control in Britain up until the 1950s. Kate Fisher's oral history study of birth control behaviours among the working class challenged the common historical assumption that the decline in marital fertility reflected a widespread use of new 'modern' birth control methods as well as the adoption of a 'rational contraceptive behaviour', in which couples discussed and made a 'calculated choice about the number of children they desired'. Couples relied on 'traditional' methods of birth control such as abstinence and withdrawal, and Fisher showed that gender roles were of particular importance to understanding negotiations regarding these issues. She reported that men were deemed responsible for birth control within the marriage because they were typically the initiators of sexual relations; women were expected to be ignorant as a sign of their respectability. Similarly, Szreter and Fisher's comparative study on middle-class and working-class married couples reveals that working-class couples did not discuss birth control together. In practice, this situation made men responsible for contraceptive practices. This type of implicit arrangement was less likely to prevail among middle-class couples, but even so such couples did not necessarily agree on the choice of a particular method; couples regularly reported tensions and disagreements as well as sexual dissatisfaction.[69] Contemporary surveys on contraceptive practices, such as the Lewis-Faning report for the Royal Commission on Population, also noted that as late as 1949 married couples mostly relied on withdrawal or the sheath.[70] The use of traditional birth control methods such as withdrawal or abstinence was also the norm in France during the period covered by the book.[71] Yet, while individuals were reluctant to employ more efficient but more constraining birth control methods, there existed, as early as the 1920s, a strong push towards the spread of information on the advantages of 'modern' and mechanical methods of birth control.

From their opening, the voluntary British birth control clinics favoured female-oriented methods and strongly condemned withdrawal and abstinence, though both were widely practised. Yet tensions developed over the best form of contraception to prescribe. Differences in opinion among members of the voluntary clinic movement about the preferred method soon gave way to open debate. Marie Stopes, who set up the first birth control clinic in London in 1921 and subsequently five others across Britain, recommended use of a greasy suppository in combination with the 'pro-race cap' she had designed. She rejected the diaphragm recommended by the Walworth Women's Welfare Centre, a rival clinic set up by the Malthusian League, on the grounds that it caused cancer, and she was opposed to the sheath.[72] Stopes was looked upon with suspicion by the medical establishment since she was a biologist and did not hold a medical degree. The Australian sexologist Norman Haire also designed his own Haire pessary, a modified version of the vaginal diaphragm that Dr Mensinga had invented in Germany in the 1870s.[73] However, the first inquiry into patients' practices made by the staff of these clinics revealed that the female-oriented methods recommended in birth control clinics – the doctor-fitted diaphragm used with a spermicidal jelly – did not meet with strong enthusiasm on the part of patients, and some women failed to return for follow-up appointments. Hence, the quest for the 'perfect contraceptive' triggered clinical research. Indeed, developing a cheap, easy-to-use, reliable and pleasant contraceptive became a target for birth control activists in the interwar years.[74] In addition, little information was available on the clinical aspect of the methods developed. To examine 'the sociological and medical principles of contraception', certain lay members of the North Kensington Women's Welfare Centre and Cambridge Birth Control Clinic took the initiative of forming the Birth Control Investigation Committee (BCIC) in 1927.[75] An article sent to the *British Medical Journal* (BMJ) presented the aims of the committee: 'The committee serves no propagandist function and desires only to establish facts and to publish these facts as a basis on which a sound public and scientific opinion can be built.'[76] The committee received the financial support of the British Eugenics Society, the Bureau of Social Hygiene – a private body aimed at preventing social problems through scientific research established by the American John Rockefeller, which received contributions from a number of organisations including the Rockefeller Foundation (RF)[77] – and private donors. Sir Humphry Rolleston, physician-in-ordinary to George V and Regius Professor of Physic at Cambridge, acted as the chair, while the psychiatrist, convinced eugenicist and secretary of the Eugenics Society, Carl Paton Blacker, was a founding member. Many other famous male scientists were also members of the committee, such as the British evolutionary biologist and eugenicist Julian Huxley and other members of birth control clinics.

The BCIC functioned as the organ of reference for contraceptive research. It financed clinical research on contraceptive substances and devices carried out in private laboratories and clinics, as well as in birth control clinics. For instance, it supported the work of the Oxford zoologist and eugenicist John Baker on the spermicidal effectiveness of a variety of chemicals.[78] Recent work concentrating on the BCIC has highlighted the prominent role of male scientists in the development and testing of chemical contraception, and in the short-lived distinction the BCIC drew between pure science (the knowledge produced in the laboratory) and applied research (the research confined within clinic and separated from the laboratory)[79]. The book shows that women doctors blurred this distinction between pure and applied research since they liaised between laboratory and patients' needs and conducted clinical trials within birth control clinics.

At around the same time, the International Medical Group for the Investigation of Contraception was set up in London in 1928 by the British suffragette Edith How-Martyn. This organisation aimed to disseminate applied and scientific knowledge of contraception through a network of women physicians, social workers, and birth control activists. In 1930, the office was reorganised into the Birth Control International Information Centre (BCIIC), of which the famous American birth control activist Margaret Sanger was honorary president and How-Martyn was honorary director. The centre published pamphlets, newsletters, bulletins and other information about contraception, new research, and clinic updates. Between 1929 and 1934, five reports were issued by the BCIIC. Blacker, the secretary of BCIC, was in charge of statistical investigations – namely the analysis of data collected in birth control clinics and reviewing the latest progress in contraceptive research.

In 1934, the NBCA set up a medical subcommittee. It functioned as a working subcommittee of practising medical men and women for the 'interchange of ideas and experiences and collection and coordination of the experience of other[s] engaged in the teaching of birth control methods and for the formation and presentation of reports to the executive committee'. Among its members were several women doctors.[80] Dr Cecil Voge, Dr John Baker and Dr Blacker were the consultants on all matters relating to rubber manufacturers, on the spermicidal and chemical properties of contraceptives, on the statistical work, and on the form of leaflets or other literature. The minutes of the committee show that they tested specific brands of contraceptive methods and accordingly wrote to the birth control clinics in order to advise against or in favour of them.

Hence, this book argues that during the emergence of contraceptive methods as a legitimate field of medicine, the imperative for doctors working in this new area, such as women doctors, was to position contraceptive methods as a new specialty and field of research. They did so through careful analysis of statistical evidence from clinical trials and patients' experience with contraceptive methods and family planning. However, I argue that this move towards laboratory-based medicine did not necessarily imply that this new 'scientific' and 'objective' approach meant the loss of the human component of the doctor–patient relationship. Indeed, as I will show, women doctors built on both approaches in order to develop their work in birth control clinics and promote this field of research according to their circumstances and necessities. Patients' individual experiences with birth control and family planning were as determinant as a sound analysis of collected data in choosing a form of birth control. Women doctors heavily relied on their encounters with their patients' sexual needs and tailored their work accordingly. However, women patients were also, to borrow from Nancy Theriot's expression, 'active participants in the process of medicalising women'. They actively sought effective birth control methods, but refused and resisted some forms of birth control that interfered with the sexual act and did not preserve its spontaneity. They also embraced the contraceptive pill, which had become available on the market in 1961.

While taking lived experiences into account, a detailed analysis of the personality and individual attitudes to sexuality, as well as the emotions that guided women doctors' commitment to family planning, is beyond the scope of this book.

*

Based on a qualitative thematic analysis of a diversity of sources that either have been barely exploited or have been analysed for a different purpose, five chapters track the many ways in which British women doctors contributed to the issues of birth control and family planning.

These sources range from medical texts written by and about female doctors (scientific articles, proceedings of international and national conferences, medical and sex manuals, audio recordings of sexual counselling sessions, autobiographies and interviews) to archival material from medical associations in both the UK and France (Eugenics Society, International Planned Parenthood Federation, Family Planning Association, Maternité Heureuse, Mouvement Français pour le Planning Familial, Medical Women's Federation, and Association Française des Femmes Médecins). These chapters are organised thematically and chronologically. In Chapters 1 and 2, I concentrate on women doctors' involvement in birth control at the national level through their work in birth control clinics, the production of scientific knowledge, the carrying out of clinical trials and the setting up of sexual counselling. These chapters build on previous studies on the organisation and aims of birth control clinics, and the motivations behind the birth control movement. Such studies argue that feminist, eugenic and humanitarian motives were often intertwined in the creation and running of the clinics. I do not reject these analyses, but, taking them into account, I argue that by shifting the focus on the role played by women doctors, a different picture appears in which the main imperative was to help other women access reliable contraception. Doing so required a new form of expertise: the service offered in birth control clinics was to be presented as medical, scientific and technical.

In Chapter 1, I focus on the relationship between British reproductive politics and gendered medical practices. I show that while women doctors were being assigned to a peripheral position within the medical hierarchy and to fields that were supposedly in line with their 'feminine nature', they developed their scientific credentials by disseminating scientific knowledge of birth control. This chapter argues that women doctors used the scientific rhetoric from the emerging field of laboratory-based medicine as a strategic move to position both birth control as a legitimate field of medicine and themselves as experts in this domain. They wrote related books based on their extensive personal experience, and engaged in contemporaneous debates on the side effects of birth control. They conducted trials on new methods of contraception and published their results in scientific journals. In so doing, they became a central channel for well-informed, reliable and scientific considerations on contraceptive methods.

In Chapter 2, I explore the way women doctors set up sexual counselling in family planning clinics. I analyse the professional training undertaken by doctors and the kind of knowledge on which they drew to help couples facing sexual disorders. Here, I argue that women doctors developed a holistic approach to family planning, mainly in response to the difficulties faced by their patients. Female sexual pleasure, or the lack thereof, became increasingly important in the advice provided in the clinics. In this way, they helped to challenge what was considered 'abnormal' or pathological in couples' sex lives. I highlight the way women doctors took into account their patients' sexual experiences and desires in order to help redefine the medical understanding of phenomena such as frigidity.

In Chapters 3, 4 and 5 I address the international and transnational dimensions of women doctors' work, and show the setting up of an international movement for birth control and family planning. I analyse British women doctors' influence on French doctors and show the key role played by women doctors in developing the understanding of new contraceptive devices on the international scene.

Chapter 3 turns to women doctors' contribution at the international level between 1920 and 1935 through an explicit comparison between British and French women doctors. In the interwar years, British women doctors, although not numerous, were nevertheless agents of the legitimacy of birth control. Indeed, they were vocal and indispensable in the transnational movement for birth control. Owing to their somewhat peripheral position in the national medical field, they took up the task of the practical aspects of birth control; they opened clinics and fitted individuals. This practical experience paradoxically gave them specific female expertise and power, relative to men, in international associations. While birth control tended to be framed in eugenic/neo-Malthusian terms by male doctors before 1930, it gradually became a medical subject in which scientific vocabulary and concern for individual welfare predominated. Women doctors played a major role in this shift. The international conferences on birth control and population issues positioned women as experts in this medical field, but, as I will show, also revealed national differences between Britain and France. I argue that the two different conceptions of feminism, population policy and reproductive health greatly contributed to positioning British women as comparative leaders in reproductive knowledge.

In Chapter 4, I explore British women doctors' involvement in the transnational movement for family planning. The leading role of British women is not restricted to the interwar years. Indeed, they proved successful in rebuilding a transnational family planning movement after the Second World War. Due to the connections they established before the war, they managed to gather experts on family planning in order to redefine a new 'planned parenthood' movement. Furthermore, British female doctors became a channel of information on family planning training. The last section of Chapter 4 analyses the way in which French female and male doctors used the training provided by British female doctors, such as Helena Wright, to implement family planning services in France. French female doctors eventually supported the family planning movement and learnt from their British colleagues.

Finally, in Chapter 5, I use the case study of the Gräfenberg ring, the first intrauterine device, and later forms of these devices, to exemplify the new expert position acquired by Wright and Jackson in both the international and national spheres. The chapter shows that the social organisation of medicine matters when explaining which voices were heard and who was considered expert in birth control methods during the interwar years and after. It adds to the scholarship on the history of technology by focusing for the first time on the history of the first IUD in Britain and the criteria used to assess a new contraceptive device.

In all, by adopting a comparative and transnational approach with a sustained focus on the role of female doctors over the longer 'mid-century' period, I contribute to the understanding of the role of women doctors in family planning, of the history of family planning (not only in Britain but also in France), of the history of sexual counselling and infertility, and of the professionalisation of women doctors. In so doing, I reinstate the role of some women doctors who have previously been left out of the historical narrative.

Notes

1 S. Raven, 'One woman's mission', *The Sunday Times Magazine* (6 May 1973), p. 28.
2 Lesley Hall and Cornelie Usborne have both focused on the role played by women doctors, but their work mainly opened up new lines of inquiry. See L. A. Hall, 'A suitable job for a woman: women doctors and birth control

to the inception of the NHS' in A. Hardy and L. Conrad (eds), *Women and Modern Medicine*, Clio Medica 61 (Leiden: Brill Rodopi, 2001), pp. 127–47; C. Usborne, 'Women doctors and gender identity in Weimar Germany (1918–1933)' in Hardy and Conrad, *Women and Modern Medicine*, pp. 109–26.

3 For a good introduction to the feminist health movement see W. Kline, *Bodies of Knowledge: Sexuality, Reproduction, and Women's Health in the Second Wave* (Chicago: University of Chicago Press, 2010).

4 P. Conrad, 'Medicalisation and social control', *Annual Review of Sociology*, 18:1 (1992), p. 211.

5 B. Ehrenreich and D. English, *Witches, Midwives and Nurses: A History of Women Healers* (New York: The Feminist Press, 1973).

6 For an excellent review of the scholarship on women, health and medicine see H. Marland, 'Women, health and medicine' in M. Jackson (ed.), *The Oxford Handbook on the History of Medicine* (Oxford: Oxford University Press, 2011), pp. 484–502.

7 T. Laqueur, *Making Sex: Body and Gender from the Greeks to Freud* (Cambridge, MA: Harvard University Press, 1990).

8 A. Bashford, *Purity and Pollution: Gender, Embodiment and Victorian Medicine* (Basingstoke: Macmillan Press Ltd., 1998); L. Gowing, *Common Bodies: Women, Touch and Power in Seventeenth-Century England* (New Haven: Yale University Press, 2003); H. King, *The Disease of Virgins: Green Sickness, Chlorosis and the Problems of Puberty* (London: Routledge, 2004); C. McClive, 'The hidden truths of the belly: the uncertainties of pregnancy in early modern Europe', *Social History of Medicine*, 15:2 (2002), pp. 209–27; N. Oudshoorn, *Beyond the Natural Body: An Archaeology of Sex Hormones* (London: Routledge, 1994); R. Tong, *Feminist Approaches to Bioethics: Theoretical Reflections and Practical Applications* (Boulder: Westview Press, 1997).

9 B. Duden, *The Woman Beneath the Skin: A Doctor's Patients in Eighteenth-Century Germany* (New Haven: Harvard University Press, 1991); O. Moscucci, *The Science of Woman: Gynaecology and Gender in England, 1800–1929* (Cambridge: Cambridge University Press, 1990). Another body of scholarship has focused on the *social* construction of medical knowledge. But some historians have failed to analyse scientific practices and procedures in medicine, or to recognise that male bodies were also pathologised. See in particular C. Benninghaus, 'Beyond constructivism?: Gender, medicine and the early history of sperm analysis, Germany 1870–1900', *Gender & History*, 24:3 (2012), pp. 647–76.

10 H. Cook, *The Long Sexual Revolution: English Women, Sex, and Contraception 1800–1975* (Oxford: Oxford University Press, 2004).

11 A. Oakley, *The Captured Womb: A History of the Medical Care of Pregnant Women* (New York: Basil Blackwell Publisher Ltd., 1984); C. Takeshita, *The Global Biopolitics of the IUD: How Science Constructs Contraceptive Users and Women's Bodies* (Cambridge, MA: MIT Press, 2012); A. Clarke, *Disciplining Reproduction: Modernity, American Life Sciences, and 'the Problems of Sex'* (Berkeley: University of California Press, 1998). On the feminist appropriation of reproduction see M. Murphy, *Seizing the Means of Reproduction: Entanglements of Feminism, Health, and Technoscience* (Durham, NC: Duke University Press, 2012); K. Ratcliff, *Women and Health: Power, Technology, Inequality and Conflict in a Gendered World* (Boston, MA: Allyn and Bacon: 2002).
12 N. Rose, 'Beyond medicalisation', *Lancet*, 369:9562 (2007), p. 700.
13 P. Conrad, *The Medicalisation of Society: On the Transformation of Human Conditions into Treatable Disorders* (Baltimore: Johns Hopkins University Press, 2007); Conrad, 'Medicalisation and social control', pp. 209–32.
14 See for instance L. Kelly, *Irish Women in Medicine, c.1880s–1920s* (Manchester: Manchester University Press, 2013); A. Crowther and M. Dupree, *Medical Lives in the Age of Surgical Revolution* (Cambridge: Cambridge University Press, 2010); C. Brock, *English Women Surgeons and their Patients (1860–1918)* (Cambridge: Cambridge University Press, 2017); E. S. More, E. Fee and M. Parry (eds), *Women Physicians and the Cultures of Medicine* (Baltimore: Johns Hopkins University Press, 2009).
15 C. Debenham, *Birth Control and the Rights of Women: Post-Suffrage Feminism in the Early Twentieth Century* (London: I. B. Tauris, 2014).
16 D. A. Cohen, 'Private lives in public spaces: Marie Stopes, the mothers' clinics and the practice of contraception', *History Workshop Journal*, 35:1 (1993), pp. 95–116; C. Davey, 'Birth control in Britain during the interwar years: evidence from the Stopes correspondence', *Journal of Family History*, 13:3 (1988), pp. 329–45; L. A. Hall, 'Marie Stopes and her correspondents: personalising population decline in an era of demographic change', in R. Peel (ed.), *Marie Stopes, Eugenics and the English Birth Control Movement* (London: Galton Institute, 1997), pp. 27–48; G. Jones, 'Marie Stopes in Ireland. The mother's clinic in Belfast, 1936–47', *Social History of Medicine*, 5:2 (1992), pp. 255–77; R. Soloway, 'The Galton Lecture 1996: Marie Stopes, eugenics, and the birth control movement' in Peel, *Marie Stopes*, pp. 49–76.
17 C. Brock, *English Women Surgeons and their Patients*; A. Digby, *The Evolution of British General Practice 1850–1948* (Oxford: Oxford University Press, 1999).
18 O. Janz and D. Schönpflug (eds), *Gender and History in a Transnational Perspective: Biographies, Networks, Gender Orders* (Oxford: Berghahn, 2014).

For more information on the transnational approach see I. Akira and P. I. Saunier (eds), *The Palgrave Dictionary of Transnational History* (Basingstoke: Palgrave Macmillan, 2009).

19 E. Accampo, *Blessed Motherhood, Bitter Fruit: Nelly Roussel and the Politics of Female Pain in Third Republic France* (Baltimore: Johns Hopkins University Press, 2006); C. Bard and J. Mossuz-Lavau, *Le planning familial: histoire et mémoire, 1956–2006* (Rennes: Presses Universitaires de Rennes, 2007); A. Carol, *Histoire de l'eugénisme en France: Les médecins et la procréation, XIXe-XXe siècle* (Paris: Le Seuil, 1998); A. Drouard, 'Aux origines de l'eugénisme en France: le néo-malthusianisme (1896–1914)', *Population*, 47:2 (1992), pp. 435–59; Hall, 'Marie Stopes and her correspondents'; L. A. Hall, 'Malthusian mutations: the changing politics and moral meanings of birth control in Britain' in B. Dolan, *Malthus, Medicine and Morality*, Clio Medica 59 (Leiden: Brill Rodopi, 2000), pp. 141–63; D. Hodgson and S. Watkins, 'Feminists and neo-Malthusians: past and present alliances', *Population and Development Review*, 23:3 (1997), pp. 469–523; D. J. Kevles, *In the Name of Eugenics: Genetics and the Uses of Human Heredity* (Berkeley: University of California Press, 1986); J. Macnicol, 'Eugenics and the campaign for voluntary sterilisation in Britain between the wars', *Social History of Medicine*, 2:2 (1989), pp. 147–69; P. Mazumdar, *Eugenics, Human Genetics and Human Failings: The Eugenics Society, Its Sources and Its Critics in Britain* (London: Routledge, 2005); K. Offen, 'Depopulation, nationalism, and feminism in fin-de-siècle France', *The American Historical Review*, 89:3 (1984), pp. 648–76; A. H. Reggiani, 'Procreating France: the politics of demography, 1919–45', *French Historical Studies*, 19:3 (1996), pp. 725–54; F. Ronsin, *La grève des ventres: propagande néo-malthusienne et baisse de la natalité française, XIXe–XXe siècles* (Paris: Aubier Montaigne, 1980).

20 A. T. Allen, *Feminism and Motherhood in Western Europe, 1890–1970: The Maternal Dilemma* (New York: Palgrave Macmillan, 2005); E. Chesler, *Woman of Valor: Margaret Sanger and the Birth Control Movement in America* (New York: Simon and Schuster, 2007); Cohen, 'Private lives in public spaces'; Davey, 'Birth control in Britain'; Debenham, *Birth Control*; M. Foucault, *La volonté de savoir: histoire de la sexualité 1* (Paris: Gallimard, 1976); L. Gordon, *The Moral Property of Women: A History of Birth Control Politics in America* (Urbana: University of Illinois Press, 2002); Hall, 'A suitable job for a woman'; E. L. Jones, 'The establishment of voluntary family planning clinics in Liverpool and Bradford, 1926–60: a comparative study', *Social History of Medicine*, 24:2 (2011), pp. 352–69; G. Jones, 'Women and eugenics in Britain: the case of Mary Scharlieb, Elizabeth Sloan Chesser, and Stella Browne', *Annals of Science*, 52: 5 (1995), pp. 481–502; J. Peel, 'Contraception and the medical profession', *Population*

Studies, 18:2 (1964), pp. 133–45; K. Offen, 'Depopulation, nationalism and feminism'.
21 L. Bland and L. Hall, 'Eugenics in Britain: the view from the metropole', in A. Bashford and P. Levine (eds), *The Oxford Handbook of the History of Eugenics* (Oxford: Oxford University Press, 2010), pp. 213–27; P.-A. Rosental, 'L'argument démographique: population et histoire politique au 20e siècle', *Vingtième Siècle: Revue d'histoire*, 95:3 (2007), pp. 3–14; V. De Luca Barrusse and A.-F. Praz, 'Les politiques de population: resituer l'objet de recherche', *Annales de Démographie Historique*, 1:129 (2016), pp. 149–64; S. Klausen and A. Bashford, 'Fertility control: eugenics, neo-Malthusianism, and feminism', in Bashford and Levine, *The Oxford Handbook of the History of Eugenics*, pp. 98–115; A. Bashford, *Global Population: History, Geopolitics, and Life on Earth* (New York: Columbia University Press, 2014).
22 M. Connelly, *Fatal Misconception: The Struggle to Control World Population* (Cambridge: The Belknap Press of Harvard University Press, 2009); P. Tammeveski, 'Repression and incitement: a critical demographic, feminist, and transnational analysis of birth control in Estonia, 1920–39', *The History of the Family*, 16:1 (2011), pp. 13–29; A. Bashford, 'Nation, empire, globe: the spaces of population debate in the interwar years', *Comparative Studies in Society and History*, 49:1 (2007), pp. 170–201.
23 The internalisation of public health began in the mid-nineteenth century. On this history see P. Weindling (ed.), *International Health Organisations and Movements, 1918–39* (Cambridge: Cambridge University Press, 1995); I. Borowy, *Coming to Terms with World Health: The League of Nations Health Organisation 1921–1946* (Frankfurt am Main: Peter Lang, 2009); N. Chorev, *The World Health Organisation between North and South* (Ithaca, NY: Cornell University Press, 2012); A. M. Moulin, 'The Pasteur Institute's international network: scientific innovations and French tropisms' in C. Charle, J. Schriewer and P. Wagner (eds), *Transnational Intellectual Networks: Forms of Academic Knowledge and the Search for Cultural Identities* (Frankfurt: Campus Verlag, 2004), pp. 135–62. Alison Bashford looked at birth control as part of an international interest in population: see Bashford, *Global Population*. A special issue of *Contemporary European History* dealt with the issue of international and transnational experts, see J. Reinish, 'Agents of internationalism', *Contemporary European History*, 25:2 (2016), pp. 195–205. For women as agents in the international sphere see H. McCarthy, *Women of the World: The Rise of the Female Diplomat* (London: Bloomsbury, 2014).
24 M. Latham, *Regulating Reproduction: A Century of Conflict in Britain and France* (Manchester: Manchester University Press, 2002); S. Pedersen,

Family, Dependence, and the Origins of the Welfare State: Britain and France, 1914–1945 (Cambridge: Cambridge University Press, 1995). See also the special issue I co-edited with Jesse Olszynko-Gryn in *Medical History*: J. Olszynko-Gryn and C. Rusterholz (eds), 'Introduction: reproductive politics in Britain and France', *Medical History*, 63:2 (2019), pp. 117–33.

25 Cook, *The Long Sexual Revolution*; M. Cook, *London and the Culture of Homosexuality* (Cambridge: Cambridge University Press, 2003); M. Collins, *Modern Love: An Intimate History of Men and Women in Twentieth-Century Britain* (London: Atlantic Books, 2003); L. Hall, *Sex, Gender and Social Change in Britain since 1880*, 2nd edition (Basingstoke: Palgrave Macmillan, 2012); D. Herzog, *Sexuality in Europe: A Twentieth-Century History* (Cambridge: Cambridge University Press, 2011); M. Houlbrook, *Queer London: Perils and Pleasures in the Sexual Metropolis, 1918–57* (Chicago: University of Chicago Press, 2005); C. Langhamer, *The English in Love: The Intimate Story of an Emotional Revolution* (Oxford: Oxford University Press, 2013); A.-C. Rebreyend, *Intimités amoureuses: France 1920–75* (Toulouse: Presses Universitaires du Mirail, 2008); C. Simmons, *Making Marriage Modern: Women's Sexuality from the Progressive Era to World War II* (Oxford: Oxford University Press, 2009); A.-M. Sohn, *Du premier baiser à l'alcôve: La sexualité des Français au quotidien (1850–1950)* (Paris: Aubier, 1996). There is also a growing scholarship on birth control and family planning in central and eastern countries. See Y. Hilevych, 'Abortion and gender relationships in Ukraine, 1955–1970', *The History of the Family*, 20:1 (2015), pp. 86–105; A. Ignaciuk, 'No Man's Land? Gendering contraception in family planning advice literature in state-Socialist Poland (1950s–80s)', *Social History of Medicine [online]*, hkz007, available at: https://doi.org/10.1093/shm/hkz007 (accessed 25 June 2020); A. Kościańska, 'Sex on equal terms? Polish sexology on women's emancipation and "good sex" from the 1970s to the present', *Sexualities*, 19:1–2 (2016), pp. 236–56; K. Lišková, *Sexual Liberation, Socialist Style: Communist Czechoslovakia and the Science of Desire, 1945–89* (Cambridge: Cambridge University Press, 2018).

26 K. Fisher, *Birth Control, Sex and Marriage in Britain, 1918–60* (Oxford: Oxford University Press, 2006); S. Szreter and K. Fisher, *Sex Before the Sexual Revolution* (Cambridge: Cambridge University Press, 2010).

27 Bard and Mossuz-Lavau, *Le planning familial*; B. Pavard, *'Si je veux, quand je veux': Contraception et avortement dans la société française (1956–79)* (Rennes: Presses Universitaires de Rennes, 2012).

28 See, for instance, B. Brookes, *Abortion in England 1900–67* (Beckenham: Croom Helm, 1988); G. Davis and T. Loughran (eds), *The Palgrave Handbook of Infertility in History: Approaches, Contexts and Perspectives* (London:

Palgrave Macmillan, 2017); S. Franklin and H. Ragoné (eds), *Reproducing Reproduction: Kinship, Power, and Technological Innovation* (Philadelphia: University of Pennsylvania Press, 1998); A. R. Hanley, *Medicine, Knowledge and Venereal Diseases in England, 1886–1916* (London: Palgrave Macmillan, 2017); L. Marks, *Sexual Chemistry: A History of the Contraceptive Pill* (New Haven: Yale University Press, 2001); Fisher, *Birth Control*.
29 S. Szreter, *Fertility, Class and Gender in Britain, 1860–1940* (Cambridge: Cambridge University Press, 2002).
30 S. Szreter, 'The idea of demographic transition and the study of fertility change: a critical intellectual history', *Population and Development Review*, 19:4 (1993), pp. 659–701; M. S. Teitelbaum, *The British Fertility Decline: Demographic Transition in the Crucible of the Industrial Revolution* (Princeton: Princeton University Press, 2014); J. R. Gillis, L. A. Tilly and D. Levine (eds), *The European Experience of Declining Fertility: A Quiet Revolution 1850–1970* (Cambridge: Blackwell, 1992).
31 Cook, *The Long Sexual Revolution*; Fisher, *Birth Control*; Szreter and Fisher, *Sex Before the Sexual Revolution*.
32 For a detailed analysis of the similarities and differences between these countries see my co-edited introduction for *Medical History*: Olszynko-Gryn and Rusterholz, 'Introduction'. More generally see R. A. Soloway, *Demography and Degeneration: Eugenics and the Declining Birthrate in Twentieth-Century Britain* (Chapel Hill: University of North Carolina Press, 1990); Szreter, *Fertility, Class and Gender in Britain*; W. H. Schneider, *Quality and Quantity: The Quest for Biological Regeneration in Twentieth-Century France* (Cambridge: Cambridge University Press, 2002); Klausen and Bashford, 'Fertility Control'; M.-M. Huss, 'Pronatalism in the interwar period in France', *Journal of Contemporary History*, 25:1 (1990), pp. 39–68; J. E. Pedersen, 'Regulating abortion and birth control: gender, medicine, and republican politics in France, 1870–1920', *French Historical Studies*, 19:3 (1996), 673–98; V. De Luca Barrusse, *Les familles nombreuses: une question démographique, un enjeu politique: France, 1880–1940* (Rennes: Presses Universitaires de Rennes, 2008).
33 This definition has evolved over time.
34 Bashford and Levine, *The Oxford Handbook of the History of Eugenics*.
35 This large diffusion of eugenic ideas and their adaptability to the social context has led the historian Soloway to define eugenics as 'a product of the culture of the time rather than a viable science or social sciences. As the times changed so did eugenics.' Kevles distinguishes two different inclinations in the eugenics movement, namely 'mainline eugenics', which prevailed before and during the First World War, and 'reform eugenics', which dominated the interwar years. The first focused on class and race

while the second acknowledged the advances in genetics and the impact of environment on population issues. See Kevles, *In the Name of Eugenics*. See also M. Freeden, 'Eugenics and progressive thought: a study in ideological affinity', *The Historical Journal*, 22:3 (1979), pp. 645–71; Macnicol, 'Eugenics and the campaign'; Mazumdar, *Eugenics*; R. A. Soloway, 'The "perfect contraceptive"': eugenics and birth control research in Britain and America in the interwar years', *Journal of Contemporary History*, 30:4 (1995), pp. 637–64. For the relationship between eugenics and demography but in the US see E. Ramsden, 'Social demography and eugenics in the interwar United States', *Population and Development Review*, 29:4 (2003), pp. 547–93.

36 A. T. Allen, 'Feminism and eugenics in Germany and Britain, 1900–40: a comparative perspective', *German Studies Review*, 23:3 (2000), pp. 477–505; Debenham, *Birth Control*; Jones, 'Women and Eugenics in Britain'; J. Grier, 'Eugenics and birth control: contraceptive provision in North Wales, 1918–1939', *Social History of Medicine*, 11:3 (1998), pp. 443–8.

37 F. Cahen, *Gouverner les moeurs: la lutte contre l'avortement en France, 1890–1950* (Paris: Institut National d'Etudes Démographiques, 2016); J. Cole, *The Power of Large Numbers: Population, Politics, and Gender in Nineteenth-Century France* (Ithaca, NY: Cornell University Press, 2000); De Luca Barrusse, *Les familles nombreuses*; Pedersen, 'Regulating abortion'; Schneider, *Quality and Quantity*.

38 Ronsin, *La grève des ventres*.

39 V. De Luca Barrusse, 'Pro-natalism and hygienism in France, 1900–40. The example of the fight against venereal disease', *Population*, 64:3 (2009), pp. 477–506; A. Davin, 'Imperialism and motherhood', *History Workshop Journal*, 5:1 (1978), pp. 9–65: L. Marks, *Metropolitan Maternity: Maternal and Infant Welfare Services in Early Twentieth Century London* (Amsterdam: Rodopi, 1996).

40 She was the author of *Married Love*, which sold half a million copies in its first seven years and was translated into fifteen languages, and *Wise Parenthood*, published in 1918. N. Hopwood et al., 'Introduction: communicating reproduction', *Bulletin of the History of Medicine*, 89:3 (2015), pp. 379–404.

41 Several studies have assessed the interconnections of these elements: see C. Makepeace, 'To what extent was the relationship between feminists and the eugenics movement a "marriage of convenience" in the interwar years?', *Journal of International Women's Studies*, 11:3 (2009), pp. 66–80; Mazumdar, *Eugenics*; Grier, 'Eugenics and birth control'; J. Carey, 'The racial imperatives of sex: birth control and eugenics in Britain, the United States and Australia in the interwar years', *Women's History Review*, 21:5 (2012), pp. 733–52.

42 S. Brooke, *Sexual Politics: Sexuality, Family Planning, and the British Left from the 1880s to the Present Day* (Oxford: Oxford University Press, 2011).
43 R. Soloway, *Birth Control and the Population Question in Britain, 1870–1930* (Chapel Hill: University of North Carolina Press, 1982), pp. 259–60; A. McLaren, *Birth Control in Nineteenth-Century England* (London: Croom Helm, 1978); A. McLaren, *Twentieth-Century Sexuality: A History* (Oxford: Oxford University Press, 1999).
44 Fisher, *Birth Control*, p. 29.
45 There were 179 clinics in 1955. For more information see A. Leathard, *The Fight for Family Planning: The Development of Family Planning Services in Britain, 1921–74* (London: Macmillan Press, 1980).
46 For more information on this experiment see H. Gruber, 'French women in the crossfire of class, sex, maternity and citizenship' in H. Gruber and P. Graves (eds), *Women and Socialism, Socialism and Women: Europe between the Two World Wars* (New York: Berghahn Books, 1998), pp. 307–8. For other information on natalism and this radical minority see Huss, 'Pronatalism'; P. E. Ogden and M.-M. Huss, 'Demography and pronatalism in France in the nineteenth and twentieth centuries', *Journal of Historical Geography*, 8:3 (1982), pp. 283–98; C. A. Koos, 'Gender, anti-individualism, and nationalism: the Alliance Nationale and the pronatalist backlash against the femme moderne, 1933–40', *French Historical Studies*, 19:3 (1996), pp. 699–723; R. D. Sonn, '"Your body is yours": anarchism, birth control, and eugenics in interwar France', *Journal of the History of Sexuality*, 14:4 (2005), pp. 415–32; Cole, *The Power of Large Numbers*; F. Gordon, *The Integral Feminist: Madeleine Pelletier, 1874–1939* (Minneapolis: University of Minnesota Press, 1991).
47 F. Cahen and C. Capuano, 'La poursuite de la répression anti-avortement après Vichy', *Vingtième Siècle Revue d'Histoire*, 111:3 (2011), pp. 119–31.
48 P.-A. Rosental, *L'Intelligence démographique: Sciences et politiques des populations en France (1930–1960)* (Paris: Odile Jacob, 2003).
49 Pavard, 'Si je veux, quand je veux'.
50 C. Dyhouse, 'Women students and the London medical schools, 1914–39: the anatomy of a masculine culture', *Gender & History*, 10:1 (1998), pp. 110–32; Wellcome Collection, London, SA/MWF/ J4/3, 'Total of women doctors on register in 1971'.
51 M. A. C. Elston, 'Women Doctors in the British Health Services: A Sociological Study of Their Careers and Opportunities'. PhD dissertation, University of Leeds, 1986.
52 Brock, *English Women Surgeons and their Patients*; Crowther and Dupree, *Medical Lives*; Elston, *Women Doctors*; J. Fette, 'Pride and prejudice in the

professions: women doctors and lawyers in Third Republic France', *Journal of Women's History*, 19:3 (2007), pp. 60–86; Kelly, *Irish Women in Medicine*.
53 C. Dyhouse, 'Driving ambitions: women in pursuit of a medical education, 1890–1939', *Women's History Review*, 7:3 (1998), pp. 321–43; Y. Knibiehler, *Accoucher: Femmes, sages-femmes et médecins depuis le milieu du 20e siècle* (Rennes: Editions de l'Ecole des Hautes Etudes en Santé Publique, 2007); A. Digby, 'Women practitioners' in *The Evolution of British General Practice*, pp. 154–86.
54 L. Kelly, '"Fascinating scalpel-wielders and fair dissectors": women's experience of Irish medical education c.1880s–1920s', *Medical History*, 54:4 (2010), p. 506.
55 K. Michaelsen, 'Union is strength: the Medical Women's Federation and the politics of professionalism, 1917–30' in K. Cowman and L. Jackson (eds), *Women and Work Culture, Britain c.1850–1950* (Aldershot: Ashgate, 2005), p. 165.
56 Digby, 'Women practitioners'; Elston, *Women Doctors*.
57 S. Jex-Blake (1874), 'The medical education of women', a paper read at the Social Science Congress, Norwich, October 1873 (London), p. 3, quoted in L. Kelly, '"The turning point in the whole struggle": the admission of women to the King and Queen's College of Physicians in Ireland', *Women's History Review*, 22:1 (2013), pp. 97–125.
58 *Ibid.*
59 The pioneering female doctor, Dr Elizabeth Garrett Anderson, opened a general hospital staffed by medical women for women in 1866. This hospital was renamed the Elizabeth Garrett Anderson Hospital (EGA) in 1917. Digby, *The Evolution of British General Practice*; see also M. A. Elston, '"Run by women, (mainly) for women": medical women's hospitals in Britain, 1866–1948' in Hardy and Conrad, *Women and Modern Medicine*, pp. 73–107.
60 Digby, *The Evolution of British General Practice*, p. 174.
61 On this issue see 'Women in medicine' [online], available at: www.lesleyahall.net/wmdrs.htm (accessed 4 July 2018).
62 Hall, 'A Suitable Job for a Woman'.
63 *Ibid.*, p. 135.
64 Wellcome Collection, London, GC/105/41, 'In the Club', Interview with Dr Prudence Tunnadine.
65 A. Cunningham and P. Williams, *The Laboratory Revolution in Medicine* (Cambridge: Cambridge University Press, 2002); D. Cox-Maksimov, 'The Making of the Clinical Trial in Britain, 1910–45: Expertise, the State and the Public', PhD thesis, University of Cambridge, 1997; B. Toth, 'Clinical

Trials in British Medicine 1858–1948, With Special Reference to the Development of the Randomised Controlled Trial'. PhD thesis, University of Bristol, 1998.
66 On the birth control movement see Debenham, *Birth Control*; Hall, 'Marie Stopes and her correspondents'; Leathard, *The Fight for Family Planning*; Cohen, 'Private lives in public spaces'; P. Dale and K. Fisher, 'Contrasting municipal responses to the provision of birth control services in Halifax and Exeter before 1948', *Social History of Medicine*, 23:3 (2010), pp. 567–85; Soloway, *Birth Control*; Soloway, *Demography and Degeneration*.
67 For an overview of these different methods see J. Olszynko-Gryn, 'Technologies of contraception and abortion' in N. Hopwood, R. Flemming and L. Kassell (eds), *Reproduction: Antiquity to the Present* (Cambridge: Cambridge University Press, 2018), pp. 535–51; H. Cook, 'The English sexual revolution: technology and social change', *History Workshop Journal*, 59:1 (2005), pp. 109–28.
68 G. Davis, 'Health and sexuality' in M. Jackson (ed.), *Oxford Handbook on the History of Medicine* (Oxford: Oxford University Press, 2011), pp. 504–23.
69 Fisher, *Birth Control*; Szreter and Fisher, *Sex Before the Sexual Revolution*, pp. 229–67.
70 E. Lewis-Faning, 'Report of an enquiry into family limitation and its influence on human fertility during the past fifty years' in *The Royal Commission on Population*, Papers Vol. 1 (London: HM Stationery Office, 1949).
71 Rebreyend, *Intimités amoureuses*.
72 Fisher, *Birth Control*.
73 D. Wyndham, *Norman Haire and the Study of Sex* (Sydney: Sydney University Press, 2012).
74 I. Löwy, '"Sexual chemistry" before the pill: science, industry and chemical contraceptives, 1920–1960', *British Journal for the History of Science*, 44:2 (2011), pp. 245–74; Soloway, 'The "perfect contraceptive"'; Marks, *Sexual Chemistry*.
75 Wellcome Library, London, FPA/A/13/5/9, 'Memorandum on work on the Birth Control Investigation Committee, 1927'.
76 H. Rolleston, 'Birth Control Investigation Committee', *British Medical Journal*, 2:3486 (1927), p. 805.
77 On the Bureau of Social Hygiene see Soloway, 'The "perfect contraceptive"'.
78 For detailed information on contraceptive research financed by the BCIC, see Wellcome Library, London, SA/FPA/A13/5, 'Birth Control Investigation Committee'.

79 See in particular N. Szuhan, 'Sex in the laboratory: the Family Planning Association and contraceptive science in Britain, 1929–1959', *The British Journal for the History of Science*, 51:3 (2018), pp. 1–24.
80 Dr Edward Griffith, Dr Helena Wright, Dr Cecile Booysen, Dr Hilop, Dr Margaret Jackson, Dr Marjorie Edwards, Dr Gladys Cox, Dr Olive Gimson, Dr Evelyne Fisher, Dr Mary Macaulay, Dr Sinton See in Wellcome Library, London, PP/EFG/A 2, 'Letter from Holland secretary of the NBCA to Griffith, 16th July 1934'.

1

Giving birth control medical credentials in Britain: 1920–70

[W]omen clients came to us because we were all women. Women doctors, women nurses, women running clinics.[1]

Helena Wright

From the opening of birth control clinics in the early 1920s to the Family Planning Act in 1967, women have been central actors in the campaign for birth control and contraception in Britain.[2] Female doctors, in particular, played a unique role in the practicalities of birth control. They introduced birth control as a field of medical research and practice because they wanted to give their female patients power over their reproductive bodies and because birth control clinics provided them with job opportunities. Indeed, women were disproportionately represented among doctors interested in birth control, and they dominated this field due to their active participation in birth control clinics, the development of training in contraception and the production of medical and scientific knowledge on birth control and contraception. In a nutshell, they colonised birth control and contraception.

This chapter sheds new light on some well-known aspects of the history of birth control and the Family Planning Association, with a focus on the medicalisation process and the initiatives and strategies women doctors used to position themselves as respectable experts in the new field. They developed a specific form of communication with colleagues that relied heavily on specialised medical vocabulary; this discourse was aimed at improving their status and securing new job opportunities within the medical field. When addressing lay audiences, women doctors conveyed a narrative that emphasised the benefits of birth control for society and the family. They made birth control a medical service by offering a detailed description of contraceptives available on the market, providing women with the knowledge to avoid unwanted pregnancies.

While historical analysis of the establishment of birth control clinics in Britain has focused on the discourses of the birth control movement, the production of medical knowledge by those engaged in the movement has attracted little scholarly interest.[3] The most valuable work on this subject is a short article by Lesley Hall which has analysed women doctors' engagement in public debates on birth control. Kate Fisher and Hera Cook have researched sex manuals to identify the public discourses around sexuality and the gendered norms prevailing between 1920 and 1970.[4] They have mentioned the role played by some women doctors, especially Helena Wright and Joan Malleson; however, they have referred to them mainly as sex manual writers rather than as experts who published scientific and medical knowledge of modern birth control methods. This aspect is central to the following section. I examine sex and medical manuals in order to show the type and nature of knowledge that women doctors conveyed, rather than the extent to which the information provided in these manuals was widely available to working- or middle-class readers. While successive editions of a manual might testify to its success with the lay public, this chapter is not concerned with the reception of these books. Rather, what is of interest here is the fact that women doctors took the time to write books to spread scientific information about birth control, and the way they framed this knowledge. These sources are contrasted with other scientific publications in the *British Medical Journal* and the *Lancet*, as well as the archives of the Medical Women's Federation and the Family Planning Association to better understand how women doctors framed contraception when they talked to their professional colleagues.

First, this chapter briefly provides a historical overview of the rationales and common features of women doctors' participation in the birth control movement and birth control clinics. I then move on to exploring the strategies that female doctors developed for medicalising birth control.

Women doctors' involvement with birth control

Until the First World War, and with the exception of doctors involved in the neo-Malthusian and eugenics movements, scholars have shown that many doctors were still ignorant about contraception; some were reluctant to recommend contraception to their patients because they were afraid of undermining their scientific credentials given the enduring Victorian distaste for sex. These doctors thought that their role was to cure illnesses, and they believed that abstinence was the best way to limit family size.[5] Historian Richard Soloway has argued that the medical profession in Britain 'reacted to the early birth control movement with avoidance, animosity, moral injunction and dubious scientific pronouncements'.[6] He has underlined that, until the mid-1920s, there were diverging opinions in the medical profession between opponents of birth control, who condemned it based on moral considerations, and supporters of the dissemination of birth control. While medical journals opposed birth control, the population census of 1911 revealed that doctors had the smallest families of all occupational categories. During, and after, the war, a few high-profile medical figures started to endorse birth control publicly – such as Charles Killick Millard, medical officer for health in Leicester, who called for his colleagues to examine birth control scientifically and leave aside 'moral considerations',[7] and Lord Dawson of Penn in his 1921 address to the Church Congress in Birmingham.[8] Meanwhile, the paleobotanist Marie Stopes, who was not a doctor, opened the first Mothers' Clinic for Constructive Birth Control, in Holloway Road, London, which was run by midwives with the help of consulting doctors. She also founded the Society for Constructive Birth Control and Racial Progress (SCBCRP) to campaign for birth control. This clinic was quickly followed by others opening across London and the rest of Britain. In November 1921, members of the Malthusian League opened the Walworth Women's Welfare Centre behind the Elephant and Castle public house in one of London's poorest neighbourhoods. In 1924, the Society for the Provision of Birth Control Clinics (SPBCC) was created to campaign for municipal clinics, and won its first battle in July 1930 when the Ministry of Health, through Memorandum 153/MCW, allowed contraceptive advice to be given in local maternity clinics to married women for whom further pregnancy would be detrimental to health.

In 1926, a compilation titled *Medical Views on Birth Control* was published in which most of the authors repeated their moral reluctance to accept birth control and affirmed that its use caused sterility. This publication, Soloway explains, marked a turning point within the medical profession; in response to their elders' objections, younger physicians stated that 'opposition to birth control had become counterproductive', making the profession appear 'reactionary or inhuman'.[9] Conflicting stances linked to a generational gap within the medical community characterised the first decade of the expansion of birth control clinics.

In this controversial context, a limited group of vocal female doctors, drawing on their own experience in birth control clinics, alongside male doctors such as Lord Dawson of Penn, Norman Haire and C. P. Blacker, tried to convince their medical colleagues that birth control was a legitimate, effective and medically harmless means for preventing conception in order to fight poverty and reduce the incidence of abortion. Albeit a minority in the medical field, British women doctors engaged with birth control issues in relatively high numbers.[10] The fact that birth control could become a female medical specialty was recognised by male doctors as early as 1923. For instance, in a special issue of *The Practitioner* dedicated to birth control, the editor explained that medical schools did not teach birth control, and he suspected that this situation would not change for male doctors; however, he predicted that for women doctors, training would take place, thus placing birth control under their responsibility.[11]

Clinics set up by the SPBCC were all headed by medical officers who were women. Female lay activists and women doctors were thus pivotal in the creation and running of the birth control clinics,[12] as Helena Wright, a female gynaecologist at the North Kensington Women's Welfare Centre and an important birth control activist and central figure of this book, explains in the quotation opening the chapter. This quote implied that there was a common and obvious understanding that female patients would turn to female doctors for birth control advice more easily than to male doctors. Wright, who was born Lowenfeld, came from a wealthy London family and graduated as a medical doctor from the London Royal Free Hospital School of Medicine for Women in 1915, where she had been trained by Winifred Cullis, Professor of Physiology at the University of London and a future member of the Birth Control Investigation Committee. During the war, although a pacifist, Wright worked in a military hospital in Bethnal Green, where she met the captain and surgeon Henry Wright. They were married in 1917, and Wright soon found herself pregnant. In 1918, Henry Wright was invalided from the army due to possible tuberculosis of the lungs. To help Henry recover from the disease, the couple and their firstborn, Henry Beric, went to Cornwall. Staying in the same hotel were Marie Stopes and her husband, Humphrey Verdon Roe. The two couples got along well, and Wright and Stopes had long discussions while walking along the beach together. Wright had previously read Stopes' notorious book, *Married Love*. Stopes had the manuscript of her forthcoming book, *Wise Parenthood*, with her, and asked Wright to review it. Wright accepted, provided that she could 'point out anything that she thought was rubbish'. Wright recalled the horrified look on Stopes' face, but the latter eventually agreed.[13] That was her first formal encounter with birth control. In 1919, along with her husband and their two sons, Wright left for China, where she would serve as Associate Professor of Gynaecology at the Shantung Christian University Hospital. There, Wright witnessed and treated the dramatic consequences of repeated and consecutive pregnancies, gaining intimate knowledge and experience of the subject. In 1927, the family, now with four sons, returned from China for what Wright thought would be a short period, as their plan was to return. However, due to the Japanese invasion of the north of China, Wright's family was forced to stay in the UK. At this stage, she had to figure out what she wanted to do and where she wanted to work. As she explained in an interview in 1978, she thought: 'birth control is under the horizon. It's time it came up. I'm going to do it.'[14] This decision was undoubtedly influenced by her previous experience in China.

One of the many reasons underpinning women doctors' commitment to the provision of birth control was the desire to improve women's health. During the first quarter of the twentieth century, as explained in the introduction, women doctors were primarily working in community health, in the voluntary state-sponsored welfare centres, or in the field of gynaecology and obstetrics, where they witnessed the difficulties faced by overburdened working-class mothers.[15] The hostility female doctors met within the male-dominated field of medicine, as explained in the introduction, meant that they specialised in 'feminine areas of work' where they had greater and closer contact with working-class women than their male colleagues. As a result, many female doctors joined the birth control movement aimed at providing information about, and access to, birth control to every poverty-stricken married woman via maternal welfare centres. Indeed, their own experience of witnessing working-class mothers' poverty, social misery and difficulties drove their strong commitment to provide safe contraceptives. Their commitment to birth control originated from humanitarian motives to help other women in need. This particular experience might explain why female doctors outnumbered male doctors in their support for birth control, the latter being less in contact with working-class women's struggles.

There was a clear influence from feminism here, as women setting up and working in birth control clinics were also members of feminist associations.[16] Many important feminist activists who were committed to suffrage activity were also involved in the birth control movement; for example, Eva Hubback was a founding member of the National Birth Control Association, Dora Russell was involved in setting up the Worker's Birth Control Group,[17] Mary Stocks and Charis Frankenburg founded the Manchester, Salford and District Mothers' Clinic, and Stella Browne actively campaigned for birth control and was a co-founder of the Abortion Law Reform Association.[18] Clare Debenham has argued that the SPBCC should be considered as a feminist organisation founded by women for the good of women[19]. Moreover, the birth control clinics favoured female-oriented methods and strongly condemned withdrawal and abstinence, which were not only unreliable but detrimental to the sexual happiness of married couples. To gain acceptability, birth control had to be presented as supporting the stability of the institution of the family. Therefore, an important argument was to explain how birth control contributed to the sexual happiness of a couple by relieving the fear of pregnancy, allowing spouses to enjoy each other, which in turn strengthened their union. Women patients attending the clinics were fitted with devices that, according to the female staff that populated the clinics, gave them control and power over their own reproductive bodies. The feminist orientation of the birth control movement was also acknowledged by contemporary male medical colleagues. For instance, C. P. Blacker, honorary secretary of the Birth Control Investigation Committee, wrote an article on methods of birth control published in *The Practitioner* in 1933. He explained that the sheath was the method commonly used, despite its lack of support from the birth control movement. The unfavourable disposition towards the method, in his view, rested on the fact that 'among the most vigorous of the proponents of birth control are to be found women with strong feminist convictions who regard the male sex collectively as lacking in consideration for the feelings of their womenfolk and therefore as incapable of taking the primary responsibility in the matter of controlling reproduction.'[20]

The goal of the birth control movement was to reduce the suffering of working-class women and improve their health and living conditions through the provision of efficient female-controlled birth control methods via welfare centres. It is not surprising then that a fair number of these women doctors were on the left side of the political spectrum, since they were in favour of state involvement in the provision of birth control.[21] For instance, Joan Malleson wrote an open letter in 1924 with other Labour members in *Labour Woman*, 'appealing to all party members who realise the need for [contraceptive] knowledge among the workers, to raise the matter for discussion at their branch of meeting; to send resolutions to our Labour Minister of Health, and to the forthcoming Party Conferences, and to sign a petition that such information should be given.'[22] The same year the Workers' Birth Control Group was set up by women from the Labour Party. The group campaigned for the provision of information about birth control by local authorities through maternity and child welfare centres. They specifically framed birth control as a working-class issue and argued that birth control methods would improve the health of working-class mothers. The Labour women promoted a feminism that valued marriage and motherhood and, as a result, tried to raise the status of these occupations.[23]

Eugenic rhetoric was also part of the narrative supporting female doctors' participation in birth control clinics, since the main targets of birth control were overburdened working-class mothers who had too many children.[24] For instance, Stopes was a convinced eugenicist. In her famous sex manuals, *Married Love*, *Wise Parenthood*, and *Radiant Motherhood*, she presented birth control as a way of creating a 'new and irradiated race'. There were also clear connections between members of the Eugenics Society and the SPBCC and SCBCRP. The Eugenics Society formally promoted birth control as a negative eugenic measure, primarily targeting the poor, from 1926. Eugenicists were afraid that working-class people were reproducing at far greater rates than their middle- and upper-middle-class counterparts. Members of the Eugenics Society were involved with the governing boards of SPBCC and SCBCRP. The Eugenics Society also financially supported the BCIC.

Moreover, the Eugenics Society and the FPA shared headquarters on Eccleston Square, London, from 1938 to 1949. Despite the official endorsement of birth control by the Eugenics Society, and the fact that several members of the society, such as Joan Malleson, were also members of the SPBCC, studies have shown that daily practice at the clinics tended to marginalise eugenic ideas; women patients came from both the working and middle classes, and every woman was welcome in the clinic.[25] Nevertheless, eugenics considerations around differential fertility were used to support women's efforts to campaign for improving the health of working-class mothers. Reminiscences of eugenic rhetoric, while uncommon, were sometimes found in the archives, especially when it came to explaining the failure of some contraceptive methods – there sometimes existed a class bias against the inability of working-class women to follow instructions and commit themselves to one method[26]. In fact the majority of women doctors working in the clinics came from the upper middle class. These 'lady doctors' were sometimes disconnected from the living conditions of working-class women; living in overcrowded housing with a lack of privacy and sanitation, many poor and working-class women found it difficult to use contraceptive methods that needed to be inserted, removed and washed every day. Kate Fisher has argued that the clinics therefore failed to encourage working-class women to successfully use female methods of birth control, but that, despite this, they did not tailor their service to better consider patients' individual preferences.[27] As Fisher has convincingly demonstrated, working-class women considered that it was their husband's responsibility to take care of birth control, and they valued ignorance and spontaneity in the sexual act. As a result, taking the lead and responsibility for birth control, as well as undertaking some form of preparation such as putting in a cap, ran counter to their expected gender and marital role of being sexually passive and ignorant. This discrepancy between female doctors' views on the suitability of female contraceptives and the lived experiences of working-class women remained a contentious issue before the advent of the pill, and might account for the long-lasting use of traditional methods of birth control. As I will show, this situation could be explained by the belief that the cap or diaphragm, combined with spermicide jelly, met the medical criteria developed by female doctors to assess birth control methods at a time when birth control became a field of medical research. In addition, while these middle- and upper-middle-class doctors might have sometimes been more concerned with prescribing efficient means of birth control than ascertaining that the methods could be successfully used, this did not mean that they did not take their patients' experiences into account. Indeed, in their views, reliable and efficient methods were key to limiting births and, as I will show in Chapter 2, they also developed sexual counselling as an answer to their patients' needs.

Many of the women doctors working in birth control clinics were also members of the Medical Women's Federation, such as the above-mentioned Joan Malleson, who worked as a psychosexual counsellor at the Telford Clinic; Dr Olive Gimson, medical officer for the Manchester, Salford and District Mothers' Clinic; and Dr Phoebe Bigland, founding doctor of the Mothers' Welfare Centre in Liverpool. Membership of the MWF also shows that women doctors were aware of their marginal position and actively developed ways of supporting each other. Although several individual members of the MWF increasingly backed birth control, especially from the mid-1920s onwards, this was not the case for all members. The main opponents of birth control were doctors who had started practising at the end of the nineteenth century and were 'strongly influenced by turn-of-the-century eugenicist anxieties and social purity feminism'. The female doctors in favour of birth control were 'characteristic exponents of the welfare feminism of the era following the achievement of the suffrage'.[28] For instance, conflicting stances were expressed in the first meeting on birth control organised by the MWF in 1921, during which three contributions were made. The first, a eugenic plea for state birth control, was offered by Dr Elizabeth Wilks, who had qualified in 1894 and was a committed suffragette and member of the Women's Tax Resistance League. Indeed, she underscored that the 'classes superior in intelligence and capacity practised birth control whereas the less intelligent and the degraded had neither the prudence nor the initiative to take any measure for limiting their offspring'.[29] The second contribution was that of Dr Mary Scharlieb, born in 1845 in London, who belonged to the first generation of women doctors to obtain medical degrees. Scharlieb first went to Madras, then came back to London in 1878 and entered the London School of Medicine for Women, where she obtained her Bachelor of Medicine (MB) in 1881 and a gold medal for obstetrics. She then was appointed senior surgeon at the New Hospital for Women and later at the Royal Free Hospital. Scharlieb was a convinced eugenicist and Anglo-Catholic who was 'highly conventional in her moral attitude', since she was part of what historians call social purity feminism.[30] As such, during her speech in front of the MWF, she clearly laid out her reluctance about birth control based on the fear that it would encourage husbands towards 'too frequent sexual intercourse' by removing the 'fear of consequences'.[31] Florence Barrett (Lady Barrett), a distinguished obstetric and gynaecological surgeon, was the third contributor to this conference. She was also one of the first women to graduate in medicine. Lady Barrett acknowledged that 'medical women should think out their own views'.[32] A resolution was passed that strongly disapproved of 'the public propaganda now being carried on in favour of Birth Control'. This disapproval was plausibly targeting Marie Stopes and the launch of her Society for Constructive Birth Control and Racial Progress. This was the only conference on birth control by the MWF before the Medical Women's International Association organised an international conference on the subject in 1934, as we shall see in Chapter 3. In October 1921, the president of the MWF, Louisa Martindale, gave her presidential address on 'Birth Control' to the London association of the federation. She shared the same concern as Scharlieb about the excessive sex drive of men. Martindale recognised that the legitimate aim of the birth control movement was to improve the conditions of women's lives, but held the opinion that there were 'worthier ways' to achieve this aim.[33]

Scharlieb reaffirmed her reluctance to support birth control at the session on 'Medical Women and Public Health Problems' during the 1922 Congress of the Royal Institute of Public Health. She explained that 'artificial prevention of conception was injurious both physically and morally'.[34] While Scharlieb's condemnation was based on social purity feminism, Barrett's concerns about birth control drew on eugenics rhetoric. At the same session, as well as during her presidential address to the MWF in November 1922, she urged that it should be left up to individual medical practitioners to decide whether birth control should be recommended to a patient. She stressed the need to discourage 'normal healthy individuals'[35] from using birth control while encouraging 'the unfit – not by propaganda, because that would not touch them – but by state interference' to use it. However, during the

1922 congress, others supported the birth control movement provided that patients were already parents.

Training of doctors, nurses and medical students

Valuable tactics in medicalising birth control and making it a legitimate field of medicine were to teach it as such and to emphasise that, as in other medical fields, contraception required medical competences that could only be acquired through specific training. Women doctors proved successful in doing this, and they trained doctors, nurses and medical students at women's welfare centres. The initial decision to offer classes on contraceptive methods represented an attempt to fill a perceived gap in medical knowledge, as well as to make birth control a specialty for which doctors needed particular training. In Britain, contraception was not part of the medical curriculum during the period under study. As Sylvia Dawkins, a family planning doctor from the end of the Second World War onwards, recalled in an interview for Television History Workshop in 1988, 'contraception just was not regarded as a medical subject' during her training at the London Hospital School of Medicine at the end of the 1920s. She stressed her lack of knowledge: 'I did not know anything about it and it was only when patients began to ask about it later that I realised the need [...]. So the demand of the patient made me, forced me eventually into learning, so I went to North Kensington and I was taught by Helena Wright.'[36]

In 1922, the MWF advocated that women doctors and students receive improved training of 'sex hygiene and the methods commonly in use for control of conception'[37] while condemning any public propaganda on the subject. As a result, the MWF decided to publish leaflets on the issue, while denying any responsibility for the content expressed in such leaflets. Three publications were issued by members of the federation. *The Eugenic Aspect of Conception Control*, by Elizabeth Wilks, was a eugenic appeal 'for the limitation of the family in the case of its inferior stocks and greater productiveness among those of superior quality'. However, no mention was made of the methods to be used to limit the size of the family. The second leaflet, by Lady Barrett, a distinguished obstetric and gynaecological surgeon who feared that contraception might encourage sexual excesses on the part of the husband, was entitled *General Questions of Sex and Marriage*, and omitted any mention of contraception. The third leaflet, by Rhoda H. Adamson, was designed for doctors. *Methods of Conception Control* presented the reader with a brief overview of the pros and cons of available methods of birth control: 'Medical practitioners today are compelled by their patients to consider the question of control of conception and are expected by them to be acquainted with the main facts of its practice.' However, the leaflet offered minimal practical description of the fitting of birth control devices. As a result, the only way for women doctors to gain practical information, before the setting up of lectures by the women's welfare clinics, was to write to the birth control activist Marie Stopes.[38] By 1930, the MWF seemed to have reached an agreement on the need for medical training in contraception, as shown by the following resolution that was accepted in 1931: 'That instruction in birth control methods with the medical reasons for and against be included in the ordinary gynaecological curriculum.'[39]

In 1932, the NBCA carried out a survey on training in contraception among London's twelve hospitals. The poor results encouraged the NBCA to offer its own training programmes at birth control clinics. It was not until 1936 that the first medical school, the British Postgraduate Medical School, provided an annual lecture on contraception. The inaugural speech was given by Wright.[40] Hence, given the lack of training, women doctors proactively taught the basics of contraception to medical students, doctors and nurses. From 1929, training sessions for doctors (at first just women doctors) and nurses were provided at the North Kensington and Walworth Women's Welfare Centres on Wright's initiative. Indeed, when Wright returned to London after her five years as a missionary in China, she decided that she would work in birth control. To do so, she 'tried to find out what was already on' in London by visiting the three clinics that were open at that time. In the Marie Stopes clinic, she discovered that Stopes had been altered by years of struggle with the Catholic Church, who had warned her that the caps used by the Walworth and North Kensington clinics were causing cancer. 'It was paranoid nonsense', remembered Wright. She then went to visit the Walworth clinic, headed by a female general practitioner, who told her: 'Dr Wright, you must be very careful. You must only use this kind of cap. We have heard that Marie Stopes uses another one and she is causing cancer of the uterus.' Wright described this moment as the point when she made a 'far-reaching conclusion', which was that birth control work 'could not be done by general practitioners, only by specialists. It had to be a specialty which was specially trained for and which gained its own respect.'[41]

Since medical schools refused to teach birth control, Wright, who was the medical officer in charge of North Kensington Women's Welfare Centre, took the issue into her own hands and taught birth control to medical students and doctors. The centre soon became a hub for training,[42] and in 1933 it wrote to postgraduate colleges[43] and deans of medical schools to offer help in the matter. To Wright, training medical and postgraduate students was an 'urgent necessity' in a context of 'growing demand amongst the public for scientific advice'.[44]

In 1934, medical students from Guy's Hospital, King's College Hospital, London Hospital, St Thomas' Hospital, Royal Free Hospital, St Mary's Paddington Hospital, and Charing Cross Hospital received training at the North Kensington and Walworth Women's Welfare Centres.[45] An anecdote illustrates the public attitude that prevailed at that time. A young gynaecologist, William Nixon – who would become Professor of Obstetrics and Gynaecology at University College Hospital and would open the first family planning clinic in the outpatient department of a London teaching hospital in 1948 – brought his students to the session held at the North Kensington centre. However, he did this during the evening, 'under the cover of darkness', as coming to the birth control clinic in daylight was too adventurous. Women doctors also appealed to the nursing profession and taught them on the subject. Wright, Malleson, Dr Gladys Cox, Dr Greta Graff, Dr Cecile Booysen and Dr Mary Redding, all members of the Society for the Provision of Birth Control Clinics and the MWF, taught medical students who had completed their gynaecological courses, medical practitioners, and nurses between 1933 and 1939. Dr Mary Macaulay, who was the medical officer for the Liverpool branch of the FPA, also trained doctors at the Liverpool clinic who were willing to teach birth control in private practice, and those who wished to become medical officers for voluntary or municipal clinics.[46]

The requirements for training sessions were listed in a memorandum issued in 1934 by the medical committee of the North Kensington centre, headed by Helena Wright. This memorandum resulted from the observation that methods recommended and taught in the clinics varied from clinic to clinic and from one medical officer to another. In an attempt to overcome this problem and harmonise the information given at birth control clinics, close cooperation was sought between clinics and the laboratories where birth control methods were tested. This cooperation was believed to guarantee that the lectures provided in clinics were at the forefront of contraceptive knowledge. Lecturers were expected to be au fait with the latest clinical updates to birth control methods that informed clinical practice: 'it is essential that only up-to-date methods should be used and that these should have been as thoroughly tested as possible both clinically and in the laboratory to ensure that they are both effective and harmless'.[47] This aspect was significant, as it ascertained that contraceptive methods were to be considered from a scientific and medical angle, placing the issue under the scope of a new field of medicine and research that was quickly developing and improving. Moreover, this requirement also reflected the female doctors' intense commitment to improving the effectiveness of birth control. The objective of this training was to familiarise students with birth control techniques and to introduce them to the placement of contraceptive devices. The memorandum was meant to encourage the National Birth Control Association to set up a 'small working medical sub-committee'[48] to shape the work done in various clinics based on the guidelines devised by the memorandum.

The teaching syllabus developed by Wright in 1939 for the British Postgraduate Medical School, based at Hammersmith Hospital, explains the theoretical content of the training. She started her lecture by presenting the three elements through which to assess contraceptive methods, which were based on the criteria put forward by the BCIC: the mechanical dimension, which should be a protection of *os uteri* against direct insemination during ejaculation; the chemical aspect – that is, the need for the method to kill the sperm; and the psychological dimension, which requires that the method advised should be acceptable for both parties. She stressed the necessary characteristics of all good methods: 'effective, easy-to-learn, harmless and cheap'.[49] The patient's preferences and subjective experiences were therefore central to the prescription of a 'good birth control method'. She then displayed the methods that were used at the time and provided a short description of how they worked. The training was not only theoretical, but also applied and practical. Students were required to bring along rubber gloves – a clear indication they were not to remain passive while acquiring scientific knowledge of birth control, but to be engaged in active learning. Demonstrations were initially carried out on the patients who happened to be there seeking contraceptive advice. However, it quickly became clear that this solution was not ideal, even with the careful selection and consent of the patient beforehand. The instructing doctors felt that they were violating 'the personal confidence and the purely disinterested charity which animated the clinics'.[50] Hence, it was decided to pay each patient five shillings for her help. The training session, therefore, helped to define the women's welfare centre as a centre of expertise, making it the first and primary source of systematised medical knowledge of contraception. While the onset of war might have slowed the teaching process, Wright continued to give lectures on birth control in the North Kensington Women's Welfare Centre.

Female doctors pursued this engagement after the Second World War. Wright, Dr Redding and Dr Jackson, as members of the medical subcommittee of the FPA, drafted a memorandum for training clinics in 1950. Indeed, developing the methods of teaching contraception and family planning to medical personnel remained a key objective for the FPA and for female doctors who wanted to enhance their working conditions by making contraception and family planning a recognised specialty. Female doctors developed the requirements for a training clinic and, more specifically, set the qualification standards for both the medical officer in charge of teaching and the trainee. The medical officer in charge should have experience involving at least a hundred clinical sessions, while the trainee should have a pleasant personality and previous gynaecological experience, as assessed by her/his ability to perform a rapid and accurate pelvic examination and to spot any gynaecological abnormalities, and by her/his familiarity with the use of a vaginal speculum. A considerable number of gynaecological ailments could be identified in a thorough gynaecological examination, highlighting the necessity of performing such examinations as a preventive measure. Owing to this procedure, a large number of women who attended the clinics and who suffered from gynaecological disorders were treated, reducing the incidence and severity of their diseases. Wright placed considerable stress on the necessity of using a speculum,[51] an efficient instrument for visually examining and assessing the cervix and the condition of vaginal mucous membranes. 'Fingers and especially fingers in rubber gloves could not accurately detect the same conditions as the eye could see', she argued.[52] The speculum enabled future medical officers to become 'scientific observers with a unique opportunity to collect detailed-facts about the pelves of thousands of healthy women, and this opportunity no other branch of medicine had at the moment. Full and accurate records should be kept as an authoritative source of data about healthy women.' The main strategy used by female doctors is stated in this excerpt: to present themselves as the guardians of sound, objective scientific facts. These facts contributed to the positioning of contraception as a new field of medicine. The emphasis on scientific objectivity echoed the growing importance of data collection in ascertaining medical statistics during the interwar years, as shown in the following section.[53]

In 1953, to complete the 1934 memorandum on training, Wright developed a detailed teaching syllabus to be used in every training clinic. Considerable emphasis was placed on practical skills. She first demanded that the 'pupils' should have read in advance the book she had written for medical students. This element is interesting insofar as it showed how deeply committed Wright was to spreading scientific knowledge of birth control within the medical community. Not only did she provide training, but she also wrote a practical manual aimed at educating medical students on the subject. For the first visit, Wright recommended the display of different caps and pessaries. Following this, the students were taught the characteristics demanded of each type of cap. The students should therefore deduce which method would be the best suited to each individual patient. Medical students were next instructed to undertake a full manual pelvic examination for every new patient, followed by one carried out with the help of the speculum. While practising this examination, the students were enjoined to describe – in words and out loud, to the medical officer – the position, size, and any other characteristics of the cervix and the fundus, and their relationship to one another, as well as the condition of the ovaries.[54] The pupil was advised to mentally review what contraindication existed for each type of cap. While examining a patient who had come for a second visit, the trainee should make sure that the patient had inserted the cap correctly, that the size of the cap was adequate, and that the patient understood how to wash and care for the cap. For routine patient visits, the students were instructed to check whether the patient had inserted the cap properly and whether there were any alterations of the vaginal conditions; they were also told to perform a full pelvic examination. After having completed the training sessions, the pupil would be able 'to do at least one correct fitting of all the types of caps and understand the doses and functions of the various types of chemical'. Hence, the aim was to provide the student with the best chance of becoming familiar with the practical and theoretical dimensions of the different methods.

Wright's work to ease and reinforce the training of medical students on birth control did not end with the training syllabus. In 1956, she designed a body model on which 'actual caps can be fitted and [that] has a transparent tummy so that trainees and patients can both feel and see how the cap is placed'. In the leaflet presenting this pelvic model, anatomically correct in shape and proportion, it is underlined that its aim was twofold: 'the demonstration and teaching of contraceptive techniques to doctors, medical students and patients, and the teaching of bi-manual palpation of the uterus to medical students'. The central portion of the abdomen can be removed, allowing for detailed observation of the placing of contraceptive appliances. By designing such a model, Wright committed herself not only to the teaching of birth control methods but to the *accurate* teaching of the methods. Indeed, with such a model, medical students could be trained in the placing of contraceptive devices, thus avoiding any harm when done on real female bodies.[55] The use of the body model reflected a change in teaching from passive observation to active participation. With this new technology, students would gain applied and practical experience, mastering their skills.

Meanwhile, from 1948 onwards, members of the medical subcommittee made inspection visits to family planning centres and clinics to control the quality of the service offered, as well as to determine the suitability of these centres for training.[56] In 1955, there were twenty-nine training centres, and 256 doctors and nurses received training during the year.[57] Dr Mary Redding, a member of the medical subcommittee and instructing doctor, set the standard for training centres.[58] She assessed the premises of the centres, and took care to make sure there were enough rooms and spaces to protect the patients' privacy. The medical equipment was specified as follows: vaginal specula, Cheatle forceps, disinfectant, steriliser, and other elements. Cards and a card index cabinet for collecting information about new patients also had

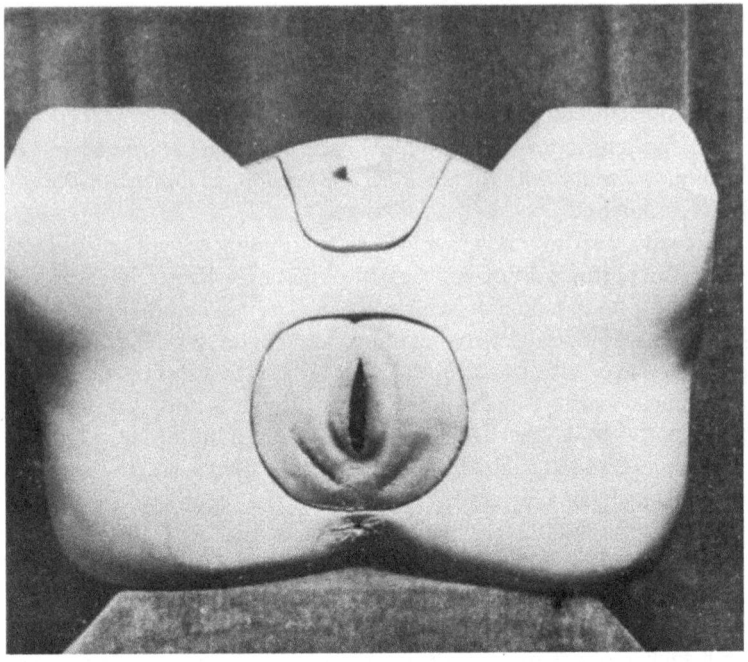

Figure 1 Pytram Pelvic model: demonstration pelvic front view

to be available for lay staff. Besides assessing the premises and interior space of the clinic, Redding scrupulously verified the quality of the professional service and the atmosphere of the clinic. She would take a full professional history of the clinic's members and was sensitive to smoothness in the running of the clinic. The competence of the doctor and the way she instructed the patient and ascertained the latter's gynaecological condition through a thorough gynaecological examination with the use of the speculum was central to good professional practice. Interpersonal skills such as kindness, gentleness and the ability to explain technical principles and methods clearly were essential qualities for creating a 'nice atmosphere' where the patient would feel at ease and could overcome her feelings of shyness or fear about specific methods of birth control.[59] These elements show that women doctors were preoccupied with the well-being of their patients,

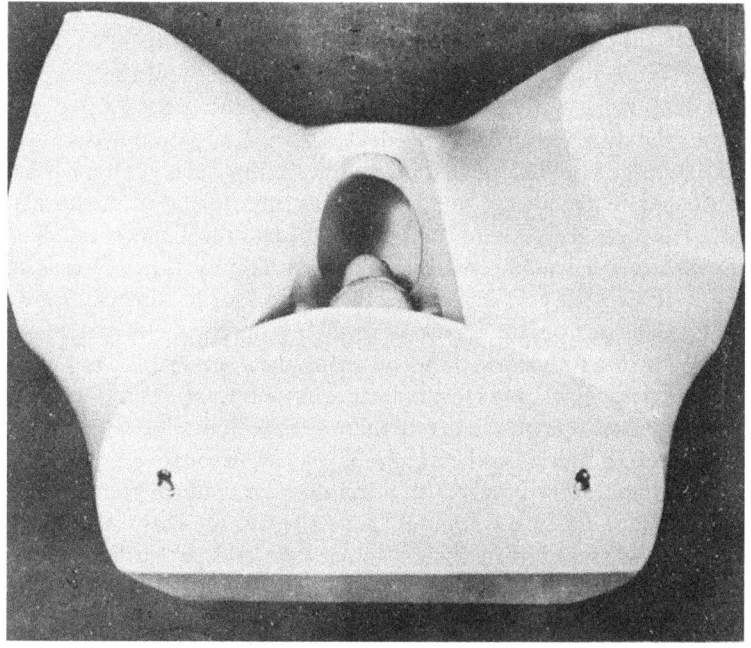

Figure 2 Pytram Pelvic model: top view showing the interior cavity, with the removal wall

as well as with their lived experience and attitudes towards birth control.

Despite the efforts made by birth control clinics to encourage training in contraception, the 'official' training – i.e. that offered by medical schools – did not substantially improve in the years immediately following the Second World War due to the inception of the NHS, which did not integrate contraception within its prerogatives. In 1949, the MWF asked the deans of twenty-seven medical schools whether they provided instruction on contraceptive techniques; their responses revealed that only four schools provided special lectures on this topic, while the majority of schools claimed to give 'some sort of instruction, in the course of ordinary obstetric and gynaecological teaching'.[60] Hence, the need to instruct medical students did not disappear.

This need was recognised by the Royal Commission on Population, appointed in 1943, which reported in 1949 that 'the giving of advice on contraception to married persons who wanted it should be accepted as a duty of the National Health Service (and) the initial duty to give advice should rest with the family doctor'.[61] The Royal Commission also acknowledged the lack of medical training in this field, but hoped that this could be remedied through an adjustment of the medical curriculum. However, there seems to have been a lack of willingness to adjust the medical curriculum – which could be partially explained by the fact the creation of the NHS meant that the medical curriculum was already under pressure from other areas of medicine, since a survey carried out in 1957 by the FPA showed that no change had taken place: 'out of 36 medical schools, 12 gave a formal lecture in contraception and 7 schools arranged clinical instruction, 6 of these at FPA clinics'.[62]

In 1956, Dr Sylvia Dawkins replaced Joan Malleson for a lecture-film demonstration on contraceptive techniques for the final year students of all London medical schools at University College Hospital Medical School. Professor Nixon chaired the session and paid tribute to the pioneering work of Malleson, who had recently died. Sylvia Dawkins then discussed the medical, social and economic indications for contraception and described the methods available and the technique of fitting caps. The class was such a success that 200 students were turned away from the lecture due to a lack of space.[63] Women doctors, therefore, carried on teaching contraception to medical students; however, despite repeated calls to include contraception in the medical curriculum, no compulsory adjustment occurred until the incorporation of family planning into the NHS in 1974.

Expertise and the medicalisation of birth control

In a context in which medical training on contraception was not compulsory and did not fare particularly well in attracting medical students and support from the medical profession, British women doctors were particularly active in disseminating information on the techniques of contraception to their colleagues in order to compensate for this lack of information. The spread of technical knowledge was meant to familiarise doctors with birth control methods, ultimately encouraging them to prescribe these methods in their private practice. Until the 1930s, as the introductory section showed, moral arguments were often invoked in public and medical debates on birth control, and unproven claims were made about the detrimental effect of contraceptives on women's fertility. Women doctors first needed to shift the signification away from the 'moral' to the 'medical' by configuring birth control and contraception as a medical subject and technique. Second, they refuted the unfounded affirmation that contraception led to sterility. As a result, women doctors asserted their authority in this new field of medicine by wrapping themselves in a technical and medical rhetoric and committing themselves to the accuracy of medical knowledge on birth control and contraception. This, in turn, enhanced their credence and credibility, as well as that of the field.

Four books were specifically written for a readership of professionals, aiming to provide doctors with a better understanding of the different methods of birth control. However, to be taken seriously, women doctors first needed to show their expertise in the subject. They proved it on the basis of their extensive private experience in birth control clinics and private practices. Joan Malleson published *The Principles of Contraception: A Handbook for General Practitioners* in 1935. Born in 1899 in Leicestershire, Malleson first undertook medical training at University College London, but soon moved to the Charing Cross Hospital due to the hostility against female students she faced at the first institution. She graduated as MB, BS (Bachelor of Science) in 1926, at which point she was already the mother of two sons with the actor Miles Malleson, whom she had married in 1923. Among her friends were many progressive personalities, such as the philosopher Bertrand Russell, and the author, feminist and socialist campaigner Dora Russell. Malleson was also a close friend of the sexual reformer Havelock Ellis, who seemed to have exercised a great influence on her career. She was later a clinical assistant at the West End Hospital for Nervous Diseases, before becoming the medical officer in charge of the birth control clinic at Ealing Borough Council. She was also a member of the National Birth Control Association, which later became the Family Planning Association. Specifically dedicated to her medical colleagues, her book referred to her private practical experience as a source of scientific legitimacy: 'having considerable experience of contraceptive work, both in birth control clinics and in general practice, I propose, where authorities differ, to offer my own technique, believing it to be fairly representative'.[64] Thus, this experience provided Malleson with the credentials among her colleagues to teach them contraception: 'this is strictly a clinical manual, a work on methods that have proved useful in general practice, and that any practitioner can learn easily, and can equally teach to patients'.[65] Wright similarly drew on her medical experience in her many books on birth control and sexuality. For instance, *Contraceptive Technique* (1950) specifically targeted a medical audience. The second edition of this book was published in 1959 with the subtitle *A Handbook for Medical Practitioners and Senior Students*, and a third edition was published in 1968. In the first edition, she ensured her practical medical experience was central to her argument: 'Every doctor who spends any time teaching patients contraceptive technique develops her own or his own ideas about the choice and type of appliances. This handbook therefore only claims to be the embodiment of the principles and practices I have found effective in my experience over the last twenty years.'[66] These women doctors never relied on their 'shared' experience as women and doctors to justify their writing but rather drew on their professional experience only. They medicalised birth control by placing their expertise at the fore. Their professional credentials in birth control were therefore grounded in real-life clinical experience.

Two women doctors also used the credentials of famous established male individuals to endorse their books and their medical credibility, mirroring the persistent gender dynamic in which women were invisible in the medical field and women doctors struggled to be considered as experts. Thus, making strategic alliances by using the credentials of eminent men who were birth control advocates was a way to shed light on women doctors' scientific work. Furthermore, these alliances attested to women's ability to move in different networks, from all-women associations to groups of high-profile doctors. Dr Gladys Cox published *Clinical Contraception* in 1933; it was re-edited in 1937.[67] Lord Horder, Physician to the Prince of Wales, a 'progressive with impeccable establishment credentials',[68] president of the Eugenics Society from 1935, and future president of the FPA, wrote the introduction. He presented the need to address birth control medically as a key new objective of modern medicine. He also underlined the professional experience of the author, deeming her 'qualification for the task therefore undoubted'.[69] Some thirty years later, this strategy was still used by Mary Pollock, a gynaecologist at the North Kensington Marriage Welfare Centre (the name was changed from North Kensington Women's Welfare Centre in 1953), who edited a book titled *Family Planning: A Handbook for the Doctor* in 1966. Lord Brain, president of the FPA, wrote the foreword, while Norman Morris, Professor of Obstetrics and Gynaecology at the Charing Cross Hospital Medical School, wrote the introduction. Two influential male allies contributed to acknowledging the scientific orientation of the book, illustrating the fact that even after thirty years of female doctors' practical engagement with contraception they still needed the support of male professionals. Norman Morris explained that the book 'includes contributions by many distinguished writers, all of whom are well-known experts in their particular subject'.[70] Out of the sixteen contributors of the book, fourteen were women doctors.[71]

Framing their work within contemporary international debates on birth control and reproduction was another efficient way for women doctors to display their mastery of medical debates. Several women were part of the international movement for birth control that developed in the 1920s and culminated with the 1930 Zurich International Conference on Birth Control (see Chapter 3). In Zurich, they presented their experiences in birth control clinics and learnt the latest developments in birth control methods. They used this new knowledge in their handbook. In her 1933 book, Cox carefully reviewed each method of birth control available at the time and quoted research carried out by other scientists and medical researchers that she had met in Zurich, such as Ernest Gräfenberg and the American gynaecologist and birth control advocate Robert L. Dickinson. She addressed the issues of the time: ovulation, the 'duration of life of the extruded ovum', and the effect of 'orgasm on fertility', a hotly debated issue at that time. Malleson also referred to the work of other foreign practitioners. Moreover, women doctors updated their books according to the latest scientific advances and medical developments in contraceptive methods. For instance, in the third edition of *Contraceptive Technique*, Wright explained how she had integrated two new chapters according to the new advances made since the second edition: 'Notable projects in research have been mainly along two lines: the inhibition of ovarian activity by the administration of synthetic hormones, and the prevention of unwanted conceptions by the introduction into the uterine cavity of various shapes of inert plastic materials. Details of both these methods are new additions for the book.'[72]

Complementing the spread of knowledge through books, women doctors participated in medical conferences in order to share the knowledge they had gained through their experiences in birth control clinics and to assert their command of the subject. In 1932, the National Birth Control Association held a conference in London. Among the speakers were Helena Wright, Dr Gladys Cox, Dr Margaret Jackson, and Mrs Francis Ivan Knowles (the surgeon in charge of the women's clinics in Waltham Town), alongside prominent medical men such as Dr Killick Millard, Dr Lancelot Hogben (professor of social biology at the London School of Economics), Dr John R. Baker, and Dr H. M. Carleton from the University of Oxford. While most of the male doctors and scientists presented their most recent research on developing an effective means of birth control, women doctors mainly presented the work that they carried out in women's welfare centres, based on their practical experience. These medical conferences were integral to contraception being presented and accepted as a medical field. Cox situated contraceptive work within the spectrum of gynaecology by underlining the fact that contraceptive methods were not 'chosen arbitrarily, but [the choices] were based on the patient's medical history and the knowledge obtained as a result of the gynaecological examination'.[73] Meanwhile, Wright presented her results with the Gräfenberg ring, an intrauterine device (see Chapter 4). In 1933, the NBCA organised a second conference on contraception. Wright and Knowles were again in attendance, alongside other women doctors working in welfare centres, such as Dr Lilias Jeffries of Brighton, who qualified as MB in 1908 and MD (Doctor of Medicine) in 1915 at the University of London, and Malleson. They all underlined the need to provide medical birth control advice, and Malleson explained that she approached the subject of birth control in her private practice even when 'she was being consulted on quite different matters'.[74] In addition, they placed the delivery of birth control advice and devices within the scope of preventive medicine by highlighting its benefit to public health. Since prescribing contraception required a gynaecological examination, gynaecological disorders and lesions could therefore be discovered and cured, enabling women to regain 'their health and vitality'.[75]

Their medical colleagues represented one audience that women doctors needed to target in order to medicalise contraception and make it acceptable. The second audience was the lay public. Women doctors imparted practical knowledge of birth control methods to the lay public through the publication of sex manuals. Here, again, they relied on their experience in birth control clinics and family planning centres as a primary source of knowledge. Wright wrote *Sex Factor in Marriage* (1930) and *Birth Control, Advice on Family Spacing and Healthy Sex Life* (1935). The former sold over one million copies and was considered a bestseller from the year of its publication.[76] The latter was published in the Cassell's Health Handbooks series. The jacket presenting the series underlined the fact that 'each of these health handbooks has been specifically written by a qualified physician from personal knowledge and experience. These medical authors have been chosen because they have living, day-by-day contacts with the sick and the well, and are in a position to understand the problems of ordinary men and women when ill-health visits them or their family.'[77] After the Second World War, the need to educate the lay public did not disappear, and three more books were written by female doctors who worked in family planning clinics and relied on this expertise; each of these books contained a small chapter on contraception.[78] In sum, women doctors drew on their clinical experiences as a way of evidencing their expertise to justify the fact that they published on the subject. Women doctors working in birth control clinics therefore shared a similar professional identity based on first-hand accumulated experience.

Producing accurate scientific and medical knowledge on birth control

Once they had asserted their expertise, women doctors further wielded their authority by using highly expert medical language. Fisher and Szreter have shown the inaccessibility of interwar birth control manuals to women (and men) without a secondary school level of literacy. In this section, I argue that this inaccessibility reflects women doctors' will to position birth control as a medical subject, mastered by specialists. Of course, communicating sexual knowledge to wider audiences and discussing birth control were problematic due to the very nature of the subject, which was often associated with taboo and embarrassment;

using scientific and medical rhetoric helped to keep the subject decent and prevented potential charges of obscenity. Consequently, they presented themselves as experts in this new medical field and improved its status by positioning it as a technical specialty. The readership they targeted – their fellow colleagues – explained their emphasis on medical rhetoric. However, simpler leaflets designed for female patients containing basic information on birth control and contraceptive devices were available in the birth control clinics.

Birth control manuals contained technical medical language to describe the female and male genitals and the techniques for inserting contraceptives. These books were real practical manuals for doctors and medical students from which they could obtain medical information and detailed explanations of how to choose and fit the suitable method of birth control, especially for patients suffering from gynaecological conditions. For example, the first page of Cox's book displays a diagram illustrating the types of mechanical contraceptives available and their proper position within the vagina.[79] She presented each method in great detail, elaborating on the methods' advantages, inconveniences and possible harmful effects. The main caps and pessaries available on the market were also presented to the readers. She then offered a thorough explanation of how she taught her patients the correct way to fit the pessary. Patience was, in her view, an essential component of good teaching practice. First, she instructed the patient, already fitted with a pessary, to digitally explore her own vagina and to note the 'loose rubber diaphragm'. Cox continued by explaining to the patient how to remove the pessary by hooking her fingertips under the rim and pulling on it. The patient would then observe the pessary while listening to the description of its place within the vagina. The fourth step, which Cox described as the most important part of the procedure, was the patient's exploration of her own vaginal cavity and the identification of the cervix. Finally, the patient underwent her own fitting of the pessary and the doctor checked that its position was correct. Importantly, this procedure meant that, for some women patients, it was the first time that they had touched their own sexual organs, which empowered them with knowledge of their own bodies, even though some of them found it off-putting.

Following the same type of argumentation, in her book Malleson reviewed each method of birth control and included diagrams that she drew herself – based on her own clinical experience – depicting the right and wrong position of each contraceptive appliance.[80] Similarly, Wright took the reader of her *Contraceptive Technique* step by step through the technique for fitting caps; the position of the patient in the medical office was described, as well as the necessary manual and speculum examinations to ascertain the 'position and size of the fundus, cervix and ovaries'.[81] Finally, Wright provided a practical and detailed outline on the insertion of the device.[82] This explanation was aided by drawings and a clear diagram, which ensured that these explanations were understood by the reader. The common layout of the books, with step-by-step descriptions and visual depictions, was seemingly intended to equip fellow colleagues with basic contraceptive knowledge so that they could advise their own patients. Malleson's and Wright's books were positively reviewed in the *Journal of the Medical Women's Federation*. The reviewers stressed the clarity of practical information that enabled doctors to use contraceptive techniques: 'This book is to be warmly recommended to all general practitioners who wish for reliable information as to the best method of birth control now in use';[83] 'Dr Wright has explained so carefully the method of fitting these contraceptives that it would be possible for doctors unable to attend training for this work, to be confident to fit patients.'[84]

In addition to disseminating medical information on the different contraceptive methods and devices, women doctors played an active role in the medical debates surrounding birth control and contraception that took place in the columns of the main medical journals. Indeed, they responded to other medical stances that they did not find scientifically and medically accurate. Constantly confronted with unfounded claims on the disastrous side effects of contraception, they adopted the rhetoric of laboratory-based medicine to refute these claims, which favoured sound and objective facts. Relying on statistical evidence,[85] a tool from the social sciences that was still new for medical investigation, consequently reinforced and expanded the scientific dimension of their work and was strongly promoted by the BCIC – notably through the publication of Enid Charles's statistical analysis of the results of the practice of contraception.[86] They criticised the position of the medical opponents to birth control by deconstructing their methodology and their lack of scientificity. This strategy seemed to be particularly dictated by their need to position themselves as legitimate and scientific experts of contraception. Of course, this was not the only reason they sought reliable data and results; they also wanted to assure physicians and female patients of the efficacy and harmlessness of available contraceptive products and to support access to reliable contraception.

The following examples illustrate that male doctors who were opponents of birth control tried to undermine the credibility of female doctors by engaging them in debates, but in so doing they paradoxically strengthened the female doctors' credentials because, in the course of the debates, women doctors displayed their expertise. First, as early as 1930, Jackson, who would become a member of the BCIC in 1935, wrote a letter to the *British Medical Journal* entitled 'Birth Control and the Medical Opinion', as an answer to a statement made by a male colleague in the House of Commons in a debate on maternity and child welfare. The male colleague asserted that 'all medical authority was overwhelmingly opposed to birth control'. Jackson called for the avoidance of emotional arguments, breaking with the feminine stereotype of women's emotional reasoning, and instead advocated for a scientific examination of the evidence supporting birth control: 'It is surely time that members of the medical profession should cease to make such rash statements and should weigh this matter from a scientific standpoint unbiased by any personal, ethical or sociological considerations [...] any public utterances emanating from doctors should be supported by reliable statistics based on scientific investigation.'[87]

Similarly, in 1930, Lella Secor Florence, the honorary secretary of the Cambridge Women's Welfare Association, published *Birth Control on Trial*, and presented the book as a 'dispassionate and honest inquiry into the methods of contraception advised'. This study, which she wrote with the help of the medical officer of the clinic, Mrs Robson, relied on the analysis of the first 300 cases at the Cambridge Birth Control Clinic from 1925 to 1927. Humphry Rolleston, Physician in Ordinary to the King and Regius Professor of Physic at the University of Cambridge, wrote the foreword; he presented Florence's work as an 'unbiased investigation into various problems connected with birth control'[88] and praised her study as 'a model example of how the data should be obtained and marshalled'. Here, again, the fact that a high-profile medical man with indisputable credentials endorsed this study provided it with legitimacy. While the search for accurate scientific knowledge of methods of contraception had been a key task for women doctors, this search for objective data was not a straightforward successful enterprise. They acknowledged the limitations of the data they collected, particularly while trying to assess the efficiency of contraceptive methods. For example, Florence warned the reader of *Birth Control on Trial* that her aim was not to undertake 'a conclusive statistical study of the relative merits of contraceptive methods' but rather to 'offer a precise and scrupulous examination, case by case, of the experience of women who have attempted deliberately to limit their families'.[89] Specific statistics were hard to attain, and several factors prevented the adequate statistical analysis of data collected in the clinics.

One issue that limited the use of data collected in clinics was that the term 'failure' in itself seemed to be understood differently across clinics. While carrying out the statistical analysis of the first 300 cases of the Cambridge clinic, Florence referred to failures where 'the appliance was being properly used, or after it had been given up either because the patient's condition was not sufficiently normal to permit of its use, or because the appliance caused pain, or because the patient found it so distasteful that she could not continue, or because she was too nervous and frightened to use it and had no confidence in it, or even because she was too stupid to apply it successfully'[90]. The Manchester clinic, meanwhile, recognised cases where women got pregnant, despite using the method correctly on all occasions, as failures. Stopes' clinic based their percentage of failure on the number of women who returned to the clinic and announced an unwanted pregnancy. Hence, Stopes misleadingly considered women who never came back for a follow-up appointment as successfully practising contraception. Cox, in her 1933 book, shed light on the discrepancy of this definition, which made the comparison of information and data a rather complicated enterprise, especially since the follow-up of the patients was a difficult task and undermined the representativeness of the data collected. She nevertheless quoted data collected in London and Cambridge women's welfare centres to illustrate her argument, as did Malleson.

In 1936, in order to improve the quality of the data and to standardise the information collected, Dr Margaret Jackson designed, with the help of C. P. Blacker, a standard case-card for every women's welfare centre to use to record patients' information. The cards contained space for details relating to 'age, parents, siblings, occupation, education, religion and income of both spouses, date(s) of marriage, details about pregnancy, use of contraceptives, sexual habits and frequency of intercourse, medical history, general and pelvic examination, and records of subsequent visits and progress of the case'.[91] This standard procedure should have permitted the collection of accurate data that was comparable between the various clinics and that eased statistical analysis. This type of data collection was similar to those in venereal disease clinics, with one main difference being that in VD clinics data were anonymised.[92] However, two years later, Helena Wright still acknowledged the difficulty in gathering any reliable statistics due to 'the large numbers of factors concerned; the difficulty of comparison between them and the intractable nature of the material, i.e. patients'.[93] Nonetheless, by ascertaining these limitations, women doctors showed their drive to collect reliable and honest information.

Using statistics and data collected in birth control clinics served to refute negative claims about birth control and contraception, and they positioned the latter as a matter of scientific applied research. Moreover, Jackson and Malleson participated in the debates about fertility, sterility and contraception that took place in the *Lancet* and the *British Medical Journal* in 1938 and 1943. They wrote letters to the two journals to rectify statements made by Dr Green-Armytage at the West London Medico-Chirurgical Society on 7 January 1938; he published in those journals that 'contraceptive measures in the early days of marriage were inimical to pregnancy later'[94] and that chemical contraception 'upsets the physiological pH of the vagina that lead to erosion and endocervicitis'.[95] They also reacted to the reply of George Alabaster, published in the *Lancet*, supporting this statement and adding another charge against birth control related to chronic changes in the cervix uteri. Steering the debate towards medical science, they attacked the lack of evidence for the idea that the use of contraceptives before the first pregnancy increases the incidence of cervicitis:

> Mr Green-Armytage has replied to our remonstrance that statistics can be made to prove anything … and they are naturally biased. But is it not scientific custom to consult statistics and records in the expectation of finding at least as high a degree of dependability as that gained by the personal impression of an observer? Particularly must this be so when the subject is one such as this, which invites prejudices of a social or ethical nature.[96]

They based their rebuttal on the pitfall of Green-Armytage's statistical demonstration: 'without a control series of observations on nulliparous women who have used no contraceptives and an estimate of the percentage of newly married couples, using contraceptives, he is expressing no more than a pious opinion.'[97] In contrast, the data they utilised to support birth control were presented as highly scientific, since they came from 'direct clinical observations of thousands of cases and scientifically conducted experimental work.'[98] They underscored the care with which contraceptive devices were being tested: 'Methods are submitted to controlled clinical trial; rubber appliances and chemical products are subjected to stringent tests for efficiency and harmlessness before they are placed on the list of approved goods.'[99]

In 1943, Malleson wrote to the *BMJ* in support of an article that questioned the assumption that contraception in women who did not yet have a child was liable to cause sterility. She stressed how difficult it is to eradicate this idea since it was deeply rooted in 'people's superstitions.'[100] She then reacted to the statement of Green-Armytage that contraception induced sterility due to lack of semen absorption from the vagina. She urged that scientific data be used to test such a hypothesis: 'Its verification would clearly rest with the research worker and statistician.'[101] Therefore, she suggested using the data collected in birth control clinics: 'Among the contraceptive clinics there are some hundreds of thousands of case records from which part, at least, of the data could be deduced' and offered to carry out 'a statistical inquiry into the advent of pregnancy among couples who have and have not used previous contraceptive measures'. In addition, she also rectified Green-Armytage's quotations of colleagues' textbooks by providing longer excerpts of them which included 'the whole relevant context.'[102] Likewise, Margaret Jackson, as an expert in sterility, responded to a 1943 article published by a male general practitioner, Dr R. H. P. Hick, who reported successfully treating his sterile patients by sending them to one of his local gynaecologist colleagues.[103] Jackson flagged up the vague definition of sterility: 'it might be pointed out that if a couple is by them ranked as sterile "after even a few months" this may account for a proportion of their success', and made a plea for a scientific assessment on treatment that relied on 'accurate recording of observations over a period of many years.'[104] This strategy of discrediting opponents of birth control by resorting only to scientific consideration had already been used by female doctors to contest the hitherto medically dominant paradigm of menstrual illness.[105]

Finally, the last contribution of women doctors in the production of scientific and medical knowledge was their involvement in clinical trials, either as the main investigator of the trials or as a member who liaised with laboratory experts. In the interwar years, trials on contraceptive methods were carried out by the Birth Control Investigation Committee as well as by the medical subcommittee of the National Birth Control Association, of which many women doctors were members. Contemporary surveys and inquiries carried out by members of the NBCA and the Family Planning Association highlighted the reluctance of patients to use the female-controlled contraceptive devices prescribed in the clinics. They shed light on the underlying reasons that made the use of barrier methods difficult, such as the aesthetic disadvantages of the method, the fact that women were shy and uncomfortable touching their own genitals, and the notion that sex should be spontaneous and something for which women did not want to prepare. In addition, learning how to fit a cap was not always easy, since it involved two medical appointments. Sylvia Dawkins, who taught contraception, remembered: 'You see, if you gave a barrier method you had to instruct the people how to use it. You fitted them, say, with a diaphragm, instructed them, asked them to go home and practise putting it in and out, come with it in, so we could ensure they've got it right, you see, and knew what they were doing.'[106] The search for other reliable contraceptives therefore remained a key goal for birth control clinic members. As explained in the introduction, the BCIC specialised in the testing of contraceptive substances and devices within the laboratory; many of its members were scientists, such as Dr John R. Baker of the Department of Zoology and Comparative Anatomy at the University of Oxford, Dr H. M. Carleton of the Department of Physiology at the University of Oxford, and Dr Cecil Voge, a chemist from America. The BCIC established the criteria for the base standards of efficacy, safety and harmlessness that contraceptive devices and products had to meet. They also tried to find the 'ideal chemical contraceptive' and developed the spermicide Volpar.[107] The way such work on contraceptives was allocated within the BCIC was highly gendered: male scientists worked in the laboratory developing new contraceptives and testing spermicides on animals, while female doctors were the intermediate agents liaising between the laboratory experiment and the lived experiences of the patients; female doctors were also key to supporting the provision of contraception. This gendered model of contraceptive science was one in which prestigious positions of highly technical experts belonged to men while the responsibility for applying the research, and conducting clinical trials and their follow-ups, fell on women.

Many women doctors carried out clinical trials in family planning and private practices on new contraceptive products tested by the BCIC to assess their quality, efficacy and safety. Among them were Wright, Dr Cecile Booysen, Jackson, Dr Greta Graff, Dr Eleanor Mears, Dr Mary Peberdy, Dr Denise Pullen and Dr Ellen Grant. For instance, Booysen was tasked with gathering information on quinine, a drug first used to treat malaria but which had been used as a spermicidal jelly. She presented a report based on the collection of results of the original work by various research workers and on her own clinical experience. The recommendation made by Booysen was to give up quinine as a chemical component of spermicide jelly due to its irritating effect, lack of efficiency, difficulty in dissolving and side effects.[108] Dr Jackson did the same type of inquiry into the 'spermicidal power of various proprietary results' in 1935. She underlined the lack of a standard method for testing and stressed the subsequent variability of results.[109] Hence, women doctors participated in informing the medical community about the efficiency and safety of contraceptive methods available on the market. Jackson and Wright conducted many interviews with members of the BCIC and shared with them their requirements, worries, and accounts of problematic encounters with patients and contraceptive methods. Based on the work of the BCIC, Wright and Malleson developed the first 'Approved List of Proprietary Contraceptives' in 1934, which was to be amended 'as clinical evidence accumulates'.[110] This list gained authority and was regarded as the only list of informed medical information regarding contraception and its efficacy.

After the Second World War, a new medical subcommittee was established to coordinate trials on contraceptive products and to collect updates and report on contraception, sub-fertility, training and publications. The committee was made up, mostly, of women doctors. In 1954, trials were carried out on new spermicides soon to be available on the market, and, in 1959, oral contraception was tested. Meanwhile, in 1957, the US Food and Drug Administration approved Enovid for the treatment of menstrual disorders; the same pill was branded Enavid in Britain. Controlled clinical trials of some of the available oral progesterone pills were instituted under the auspices of the Council for the Investigation of Fertility Control (CIFC), established in 1957 by the FPA (chiefly undertaken by Dr G. I. M. Swyer and Jackson) thanks to the financial support of Captain Oliver Bird, a Conservative MP with a strong interest in family planning. The history of the pill and its connection with population issues, the Cold War, and the threat of overpopulation is well known, and the first clinical trials of the pill in Britain have been thoroughly analysed by Lara Marks. One important element to remember is the active role played by women doctors in the British trials. After having ascertained the harmlessness of the pill on rats and mice, large-scale trials were initiated, first in Birmingham, then in Slough, London, Barnet, Exeter, Manchester, Liverpool, Leicester and Brighton.[111] These trials were 'design(ed) to find out how acceptable such a method of birth control is to women in this country, to find the lowest dose which would be effective and reduce costs and side effects and to find the simplest method of administration'. Consent forms were signed by every patient participating in the trials, as well as their husbands. The women doctors carrying out these trials followed a strict experimental methodology and were asked by the CIFC to give feedback every month to help assess the efficiency and possible harmful effects of contraceptive products. They reported any side effects experienced by patients and accordingly updated trial procedures. For instance, urine tests became mandatory when women doctors realised that oral contraceptives could induce a decrease in glucose tolerance. The North Kensington Marriage Welfare Centre also carried out a trial on oral contraceptives under the supervision of Dr Margaret Blair and Dr Eleanor Mears. Besides carrying out clinical trials, several women doctors also sent the methods used by their patients at the time when a failure occurred to be tested in a laboratory. In 1954, Wright received a patient who had a miscarriage, even though she was using a birth control method. Dr Wright sent a batch of three tubes of Volpar paste used by the patient, because 'she was anxious that the tubes of paste used should be tested'. Several similar occurrences were found in the archives which testify to Wright's commitment to determining the efficiency of the methods her patients used.[112] Thus, female doctors functioned as a channel between lived experience of patients, doctors and laboratory experiment.

Women experts in contraception

The extent to which women doctors succeeded in being recognised as experts could be assessed by their growing participation in medical conferences, external committees and working groups appointed by the government. This recognition was intrinsically connected with their ability to construct alliances and utilise negotiation skills. Indeed, to do their work, they needed to be able to reach a consensus and ally with important groups and politicians to gain support for their cause.

In 1930, Wright was asked to speak at a major public conference on 'Birth Control by Public Health Authorities', in the Central Hall, Westminster, on 4 April. The conference was organised by the Society for the Provision of Birth Control Clinics, the Workers' Birth Control Group, the National Union of Societies for Equal Citizenship and the Women's National Liberal Federation. Its aim was the withdrawal of the ban on the provision of birth control advice in public health welfare clinics. Delegates attended from public health authorities, maternity and child welfare centres, Labour Party women's sections, Women's Cooperative Guilds, birth control clinics, and other local bodies. The chairman and chairwoman were Dr Killick Millard, and suffragist, feminist and eugenicist Mrs Eva Hubback, a close friend of Wright. Wright spoke as medical officer for the North Kensington Women's Welfare Centre. She presented her experience with her patients to stress the positive effect of birth control education and training on the health of working-class women, and focused on two recent cases she had handled. The first was a working-class woman, a mother of four children, who was in good health, but who financially could not afford an additional child; she therefore lived in perpetual anxiety due to her ignorance of the means to avoid pregnancy. The second case was a patient who had had six abortions and had eight living children. Wright presented birth control as the best way to help these mothers and improve their well-being:

> What can be hoped for from the dissemination of adequate Birth Control Instruction? We can free mothers entirely from the fear of unwanted

pregnancies. We can free them from the danger of the fact of repeated pregnancies, and so conserve their health to a very large extent. We can free the sex life of these people from the unnatural and bad psychological restrictions that are at present happening. We can produce the state of happiness, stability and normality which we have observed very often in the cases of our patients who have been our patients for two or three years and have had a chance to see what a difference it makes to their lives.'[113]

The chairman, Dr Killick Millard, acknowledged the important role of Wright in the conference: 'In some respects Dr Wright's paper is the most important we have heard this morning. Dr Wright is the officer in the fighting line. She has given us a sort of "Journey's End" story direct from the trenches.'[114] The conference ended with the following resolution sent to the Minister, Arthur Greenwood: 'to call upon the Minister of Health and Public Health Authorities to recognise the desirability of making available medical information on methods of Birth Control to married people who need it'.[115] This was partially effective: the Ministry of Health permitted local health authorities to provide birth control advice for married women, but only for women whose lives would be endangered by a further pregnancy.

Wright also played a decisive role in the outcome of the Lambeth Conference, where she spoke for the newly formed National Birth Control Council. She recalled her contribution at a conference she attended in 1978:

> In 1930, I was summoned to address the bishops at the Lambeth Conference. I went alone, the only woman present, and described to the platform of puzzled elderly gentlemen exactly what we were doing. They listened politely, slowly woke up and had become interested in being told about conditions of which, up till then, they had heard nothing. When I ended by summing up our activities in one sentence, 'We teach poor, overworked mothers how to free themselves from further unwanted pregnancies. Who could possibly object to that?', there was silence.[116]

Wright demonstrated that she had the skills to interest her audience as well as to attract support from these 'elderly gentlemen'. These skills might have been developed through necessity, as women doctors had to make their way in a male-dominated profession and learn how to gain the backing of male peers.

Joan Malleson is another salient example of the growing presence of female doctors in working parties; she was a witness at both the Birkett Committee and the Royal Commission on Population. In 1937, the Birkett Committee was set up by the government to clarify whether doctors could perform an abortion to save a woman's life. Malleson was a member of the Abortion Law Reform Association (ALRA), established in 1936 to campaign for legalisation on abortion.[117] She presented evidence in front of the committee and supported contraception as a preventive measure against abortions. In 1945, Malleson, alongside Margaret Pyke, secretary of the Family Planning Association, was invited to present evidence to the Royal Commission on Population. Prior to this, in 1943, the Ministry of Health had announced the appointment of a commission tasked with the gathering of evidence on the state of the British population and suggestions for measures to be taken in the national interest to influence its future trend. The commission asked several bodies, such as the FPA, the Eugenics Society, and the Population Investigation Committee, to present memoranda and evidence on issues related to population. Malleson's participation revealed the fact that she was held in high esteem by the members of the commission and was regarded as an expert in family planning. The memorandum of the FPA urged the establishment of 'small friendly centres at which married couples could find help in their difficulties and problems' and made the plea for the financial support of the government in the setting up and running of such centres. To a question asked about the possible influence of widespread provision of contraceptives on the decrease in the birth rate, Malleson replied by underlining the long-term positive effect of efficient contraceptive methods: 'I should say there is little doubt if you look over a decade with decent contraception available, you will have young people marrying sooner than they would dare to marry otherwise, and that in itself is generally a good thing for the birth rate taken again another decade because those people have not risked, they have not tried living in celibacy for another five years and risked venereal diseases and abortions and a lot of bad things which arrive from marrying so late.'[118] Therefore, she clearly connected the provision of contraception with the reduction of the incidence of abortion and the improvement of the well-being of the individual, which would ultimately benefit society.

After the war, Margaret Jackson was the keynote speaker for the sixth Oliver Bird lecture in 1962 on 'oral contraception in practice'. The Oliver Bird lecture was inaugurated following Bird's financial donation to the FPA for the development of research in contraception in 1957. Annual lectures were subsequently given by eminent research workers, including Dr Gregory Pincus from the US, father of the contraceptive pill, who spoke on 'Fertility Control with Oral Medication' in 1958; Alan Parkes from the National Institute for Medical Research UK; Albert Tyler from the California Institute of Technology; and Alan F. Guttmacher, an eminent obstetrician-gynaecologist and president of the Planned Parenthood Federation of America. This talk reflected the prominent role Jackson played in the scientific community at that time, and she was well-aware of the importance of the conference as a space for elite research. As she noted, 'My five predecessors have all been high-powered scientists with considerable reputations and academic records.' The aim of her talk was to bring the audience 'up-to-date' with the latest clinical work on oral contraception. She described in detail the components of the diverse contraceptive pills tested and available on the market.

Finally, Sylvia Dawkins, who was trained as a general practitioner and left general practice to work in a family planning clinic in 1948, featured, alongside William Nixon, Professor in Obstetrics and Gynaecology, in the short film *According to Plan*. The film was produced for the London Foundation for Marriage Education by Eothen Films Ltd, a film production company specialising in medical films, and was released in 1964.[119] The short film was aimed at promoting family planning by giving medical information on methods of contraception and means of obtaining contraceptive advice. The fact that both Professor Nixon and Sylvia Dawkins appeared in the film shows that they were held in high esteem and considered experts in contraception.

The film's inaugural scene showcases a family at play; the father laughs and plays with his two children, and the mother reads a book to the youngest before the parents put them to bed. During this scene the narration underlines the benefit of family planning for society and stresses that 'children should be wanted'. An animated diagram then presents the functioning of the reproductive system, providing detail about the different methods of contraception. Sylvia Dawkins then appears in her consultation room at the Royal College Hospital with a female patient. Dawkins is dressed in her medical uniform and is shown asking questions of the patient while carefully taking notes. The voiceover explains that the doctor's role is to help the patient plan her family, and in order to achieve this task successfully she will 'need to get to know all about you and about how you feel about it all; that is very important, your feelings, so don't pretend if you want the best advice'. Dawkins's expression is one of empathetic interest, as she is shown nodding and smiling to the patient. She is then shown performing a thorough pelvic exam and later presenting the patient with the different types of caps. The narrator continues with the description of the pill and stresses that the patient must get a doctor's prescription to obtain it, while Dawkins examines the patient to determine whether she will be suitable for the pill. The voiceover then instructs the viewer to see her doctor regularly for assessment to ensure there are no side effects from the contraceptive pill. This scene not only places contraception under the responsibility of the doctor but also presents Dawkins as a specialist with skills in gynaecology who listens to and advises her patients.

Conclusion

From the early establishment of birth control clinics to the Family Planning Act in 1967, female doctors were at the forefront of medical research on birth control and contraception. Birth control clinics, or women's welfare centres as they were called in the 1920s and 1930s, represented a job opening for women doctors. In a context where female doctors generally held less prestigious positions in the medical hierarchy and where birth control divided the medical profession, women doctors campaigned to make birth control a focus of scientific research and were pivotal in the medicalisation of birth control. These fights had their ups and downs. Women doctors positioned themselves as experts in birth control and contraception by publishing books and articles in highly prestigious journals and by engaging in scientific debates on the side effects of birth control. This expertise was credited, as evidenced by their inclusion as members of committees and working parties. Thus, they greatly contributed to steering the medical debate towards scientific observations of the effects of birth control. They also developed a specific form of communication that relied on expert medical and scientific rhetoric fuelled by terms such as 'objective facts', 'careful observation', 'clinical data' and 'reliable statistics based on scientific investigation'. The adoption of the new tool of statistics not only represented a strategic move to enhance the perception of contraception as a medical field directed by specialists, but also proved successful in allying important scientists to their side, as I demonstrate in Chapter 5. Clinical trials were instituted to test the efficiency and safety of new contraceptive methods, and though women doctors enabled the medicalisation of contraception, their ultimate goal, which was the formal integration of contraception into the medical curriculum, failed. Medical schools and university hospitals proved very resistant and continued to ignore the call for basic training in contraception. Female doctors seemed to lack the formal support of medical schools. Yet this failure was only partial, since they instituted formal training in birth control clinics and family planning centres which medical students and doctors could attend.

A second restraint on their enterprise was how they were paid for their work. Though family planning clinics were populated by women doctors – representing a job opening for them – until 1974, when the NHS took over family planning, they were paid for each session of work. This meant that they had no paid leave and no superannuation arrangement. Furthermore, their travel expenses and travel time were not covered.[120]

A third downside of this struggle rested on the fixation on female methods of contraception, such as the cap with spermicide jelly, which were presented as the only effective methods of birth control until the release of the contraceptive pill. While their efficiency was without doubt highest between the 1920s and 1960s, female patients were reluctant to use these methods, resulting in subsequent nonattendance at follow-up appointments. Women doctors were convinced that teaching the patient how to fit a cap, and explaining the advantages of this method, gave women power over their reproductive health; they expected women patients to happily embrace these new methods. The first generations of women doctors who facilitated the provision of contraceptives and related information believed that contraception, and more specifically female methods, freed women from the burden of involuntary pregnancies. However, what they perceived as empowering would, with the advent of the contraceptive pill and new IUDs, be denounced as a new form of oppression by feminist health activists.

Notes

1. B. Evans, *Freedom to Choose: The Life and Work of Dr Helena Wright, Pioneer of Contraception* (London: The Bodley Head, 1984).
2. Some arguments in this chapter appeared in *Medical History*. See C. Rusterholz, 'English women doctors, contraception and family planning in transnational perspective (1930s–70s)', *Medical History*, 63:2 (2019), pp. 153–72.
3. Soloway has focused on the birth control movement: see Soloway, *Birth Control*; Soloway, *Demography and Degeneration*. See also Hall, *Sex, Gender and Social Change in Britain*; L. A. Hall, *The Life and Times of Stella Browne: Feminist and Free Spirit* (London: I. B. Tauris, 2011).
4. Fisher, *Birth Control*; Cook, *The Long Sexual Revolution*.
5. Soloway, *Birth Control*, pp. 259–60. A. McLaren, *Birth Control in Nineteenth-Century England* (London: Croom Helm, 1978); McLaren, *Twentieth-Century Sexuality*.
6. Soloway, 'The "perfect contraceptive"', p. 639.
7. Charles Killick Millard quoted in Soloway, *Birth Control*, p. 257.
8. Peel, 'Contraception and the medical profession'. Although this article is dated, it remains the reference for a historical overview of doctors' stances on birth control.
9. Soloway, *Birth Control*, p. 275.
10. Hall, 'A Suitable Job for a Woman'.
11. 'Contraception' in *The Practitioner*, 111 (1923), p. 5.
12. Debenham, *Birth Control*; Leathard, *The Fight for Family Planning*.
13. Wellcome Collection, London, PP/HRW/B.21, 'Brian Harrisson, Confidential discussion with Helena Wright, 27 Feb 1977'.
14. *Ibid.*
15. Anne Digby argued that women doctors, when entering the field at the turn of the century, 'operated in [a] semi-detached professional-sphere'. See A. Digby, *The Evolution of British General Practice*, p. 154. For the history of maternal and infant welfare centres see Oakley, *The Captured Womb*. For this history but in London see L. Marks, *Metropolitan Maternity*.
16. Debenham, *Birth Control*.
17. L. Hoggart, 'The campaign for birth control in Britain in the 1920s' in A. Digby and J. Stewart (eds), *Gender, Health and Welfare* (London:

Routledge, 1996), pp. 143–66. She pointed out the role played by working-class women in the campaign for birth control.
18 On Stella Brown see Hall, *The Life and Times of Stella Browne*.
19 Debenham, *Birth Control*.
20 C. P. Blacker, 'The choice of a contraceptive', *The Practitioner*, 131:3 (1933), p. 256.
21 On the interactions between the Labour Party and the issue of sexuality see Brooke, *Sexual Politics*. See also L. Hoggart, 'Socialist feminism, reproductive rights and political action', *Capital and Class*, 24:1 (2012), pp. 95–125.
22 *Labour Woman*, 12:3 (1924) quoted in Brooke, *Sexual Politics*, p. 50.
23 Hoggart, 'Socialist feminism'. On maternalism and socialist feminism see P. Thane, 'Visions of gender in the making of the British welfare state: the case of women in the British Labour Party and social policy, 1906–45' in G. Bock and P. Thane (eds), *Maternity and Gender Policies: Women and the Rise of the European Welfare States 1880s–1950s* (London: Routledge, 1991), pp. 93–118.
24 On the relationship between eugenics and motherhood see Davin, 'Imperialism and motherhood'.
25 Cohen, 'Private lives in public spaces'.
26 Some reports of women's welfare centres emphasised the failure of certain methods due to the inability of women to follow the instructions received at the birth control clinics.
27 K. Fisher, 'Contrasting cultures of contraception: birth control clinics and the working-classes between the wars' in M. Gijswijt-Hofstra, G. M. van Heteren and T. Tansey (eds), *Biographies of Remedies: Drugs, Medicines and Contraceptives in Dutch and Anglo-American Healing Cultures*, Clio Medica 66 (Amsterdam: Rodopi, 2002), pp. 141–57.
28 Hall, 'A Suitable Job for a Woman', p. 135.
29 'Reports of societies', *British Medical Journal*, 2:3157 (1921), p. 11.
30 On her relationship with eugenics see Jones, 'Women and eugenics in Britain'. On the relationship between Mary Scharlieb and religion see J. R. deVries, 'A moralist *and* moderniser: Mary Scharlieb and the creation of gynecological knowledge, ca. 1880–1914', *Social Politics*, 22:3 (2015), pp. 298–318.
31 'Reports of societies', *British Medical Journal*, 2:3157 (1921), p. 11.
32 *Ibid.*
33 *Lancet*, ii (1921), p. 75, quoted in Hall, 'A suitable job for a woman', p. 133; Wellcome Collection, London, SA/MWF/B.2/1, 'Birth Control', *Medical Women's Federation Newsletter* (Dec 1921).
34 Wellcome Collection, London, SA/MWF/B.2/1, *Medical Women's Federation Newsletter* (Jul 1922).

35 Wellcome Collection, London, SA/MWF/B.2/1, *Medical Women's Federation Newsletter* (Nov 1922).
36 Wellcome Collection, London, GC/105/26, 'Transcript of the interview with Sylvia Dawkins', Television History Workshop, 1988.
37 Wellcome Collection, London, SA/MWF/B.2/1, *Medical Women's Federation Newsletter* (Nov 1922).
38 Lesley Hall has shown that several women doctors got in touch with Stopes on this issue. Hall, 'A Suitable Job for a Woman', pp. 139–40.
39 Wellcome Collection, London, CMAL SA/MWF/A 11/4, 'Minutes of the meetings of the Council of the Medical Women's Federation, 8 May 1931'.
40 Helena Wright's private archives, held at the Wellcome Library, show that she gave lectures on contraception to various medical students and nurses at the clinics. For instance she trained nurses on 'Sex hygiene and the family' during a Special Course in Public Health and General Nursing on 12 June 1933 at the College of Nursing. See Wellcome Collection, London PP/HRW/B.13.
41 *Ibid.*
42 The clinics under the supervision of Marie Stopes also provided a practical demonstration for doctors and medical students, and Stopes collaborated with the Royal Institute for Public Health to offer training sessions in 1930 and 1931. On this aspect see C. E. L. Walker, 'Making Birth Control Respectable: The Society for Constructive Birth Control and Racial Progress, and the American Birth Control League, in Comparative Perspective, 1921–38'. PhD dissertation, University of Bristol, 2007.
43 The postgraduate medical institutions were established in the final decade of the nineteenth century and tailored to meet the educational needs of the general practitioners. A. Digby, *Making a Medical Living: Doctors and Patients in the English Market for Medicine, 1720–1911* (Cambridge: Cambridge University Press, 1994), pp. 100–1.
44 Wellcome Collection, London, SA/FPA/NK 41, 'Copy of letter sent to deans of medical school, 5th September 1933'.
45 Wellcome Collection, London, PP/HRW/B13, 'List of training', and Wellcome Collection, London, SA/FPA/NK41, 'List of training'. See also Wellcome Collection, London, MS.9178/3/1, 'Walworth 70th anniversary historical material'; Wellcome Collection, London, SA/FPA/A13/85B, 'Association of Inspectors of Midwives, programme of conference and post-graduate week, May 1936'.
46 Wellcome Collection, London, SA/FPA/A19/1, 'Report of the Second national conference of branches, 1.12.1939'.
47 Wellcome Collection, London, SA/FPA/NK41, 'Memorandum from the North Kensington Women's Welfare Centre to the National Birth Control Association, July 5th 1934'.

48 *Ibid.*
49 Wellcome Collection, London, PP/HRW/B 13, 'British Postgraduate Medical School, birth control by Helena Wright, 22nd of June 1939'.
50 Wellcome Collection, London, PP/MCS/B.2, 'Information for the National Birth Control Association Committee, 1932'.
51 These gynaecological instruments have been widely discussed in gynaecology manuals, such as D. B. Hart and A. H. Freeland Barbour, *Manual of Gynaecology* (Edinburgh: W. & A. K. Johnston, 1890). For information about medical opposition to the speculum, see Moscucci, *The Science of Woman*, pp. 112–30.
52 Wellcome Collection, London, SA/FPA/NK 69, Helena Wright, 'the use of a speculum' in 'Report of a conference of clinical medical officers and nurses, 7th November 1953'.
53 Cunningham and Williams, *The Laboratory Revolution in Medicine*.
54 Wellcome Collection, London, SA/FPA/A14/96.2, 'Teaching syllabus'.
55 On the pelvic model see Wellcome Collection, London, SA/FPA/A14/196, 'Letter from the Secretary of the Clinics Medical Sub-Committee to Dr Evelyn Roberts, 26 January 1956'; SA/FPA/A19/9, 'Demonstration model of the teaching of contraceptive techniques, designed to the specification of Dr Helena Wright, approved by the FPA. Produced exclusively by Pytram LTD'.
56 Wellcome Collection, London, SA/FPA/A5/4, 'The Family Planning Association, Eighteenth Annual Report, 1948–49'.
57 Wellcome Collection, London, SA/FPA/A5/7, 'Family Planning Association Annual Report, 1955–56'.
58 Wellcome Collection, London, SA/FPA/A14/160/2, 'Suggestion for inspection reports, 1952'.
59 For detailed assessments of the different visits see Wellcome Collection, London, SA/FPA/A14/160/2, 'Mary Redding'.
60 'Memorandum on Family Planning with particular reference to contraception', *British Medical Journal*, 1:4758 (1952), p. 595.
61 Royal Commission on Population, Report, Cmd. 7, 1949.
62 Wellcome Collection, London, SA/FPA/A10/10 IPPF, 'Eleanor Mears, "The Medical Student and Sex Education", paper presented to I.P.P.F. Conference at the Hague, 1961'.
63 Wellcome Collection, London, SA/FPA/A16/5/1, *The Journal of Family Planning*, 5:4 (1957), p. 18.
64 J. Malleson, *The Principles of Contraception: A Handbook for General Practitioners* (London: V. Gollancz Limited, 1935), p. 9.
65 *Ibid.*, p. 10.

66 H. Wright and H. B. Wright, *Contraceptive Technique: A Handbook for Medical Practitioners and Senior Students* (London: J&A Churchill Ltd., 1951), p. 5.
67 There was also a long tradition of women doctors using their medical expertise to write manuals of health guidance for laywomen. For instance, Scharlieb wrote *Health and Fitness* in 1921. Lesley Hall has shown that women doctors also wrote many sex education manuals. See L. A. Hall, 'In ignorance and in knowledge: reflections on the history of sex education in Britain' in L. D. H. Sauerteig and R. Davidson (eds), *Shaping Sexual Knowledge: A Cultural History of Sex Education in Twentieth Century Europe* (London: Routledge, 2009), pp. 19–36; L. A. Hall, *Outspoken Women: An Anthology of Women's Writing on Sex, 1870–1969* (London: Routledge, 2014). See also Elston, 'Women Doctors in the British Health Services', p. 249. See also G. Jones, *Social Hygiene in Twentieth Century Britain* (London: Croom Helm, 1986).
68 Hall, 'A suitable job for a woman', p. 109.
69 G. Cox, *Clinical Contraception* (London: Heinemann, 1933). Cox graduated MB, BS in 1923, and then was the medical officer to the Walworth Women's Welfare Centre. She also published *The Woman's Book of Health* in 1933 and was a member of the medical subcommittee appointed by the NBCA in 1934.
70 M. Pollock (ed.), *Family Planning: A Handbook for the Doctor* (London: Tindall & Cassell, 1966).
71 The women doctors contributing to the book were Sylvia Dawkins (medical officer at the Islington Family Planning Clinic), Rosalie Taylor, Eleanor Mears, Josephine Barnes, Margaret Moore White, Margaret Neal-Edwards, Mary Egerton, Margaret Blair, Jean Passmore, Elizabeth Draper, Alison Giles, Margaret Pyke and Helena Wright.
72 H. Wright, *Contraceptive Technique: A Handbook of Practical Instruction*, 3rd edition (London: Churchill, 1968), p. 5.
73 'Medical problems of contraception', *British Medical Journal*, 1:3726 (1932), p. 1047.
74 'Medical problems of contraception', *British Medical Journal*, 2:3784 (1933), p. 120.
75 *Ibid.*
76 Evans, *Freedom to Choose*, p. 154.
77 H. Wright, *Birth Control: Advice on Family Spacing and Healthy Sex Life* (London: Cassell, 1935), p. 3.
78 See in particular: M. Moore White, *Womanhood* (London: Cassell, 1947); M. Macaulay, *The Art of Marriage* (London: Delisle, 1952); S. Dawkins, *Planning your Family* (London: Foyles Health Handbooks, 1959).

79 Cox, *Clinical Contraception*, p. 10.
80 Malleson, *The Principles of Contraception*.
81 Wright and Wright, *Contraceptive Technique*, p. 22.
82 *Ibid.*, p. 31.
83 K. Murphy, 'Joan Malleson, the principles of contraception', *Medical Women's Federation Quarterly Review*, (1935–6), p. 65.
84 E. H. 'Margaret Moore White, *Womanhood*', *Medical Women's Federation Quarterly Review* (1959), p. 37.
85 Donald Mackenzie has shown the relationship between the development of statistics and the eugenics movement. Indeed eugenics was a driver in motivating the development of the discipline. All of its founders – Galton, Pearson, Fisher – were convinced eugenicists. See D. Mackenzie, *Statistics in Britain, 1865–1930: The Social Construction of Scientific Knowledge* (Edinburgh: Edinburgh University Press, 1981).
86 E. Charles, *The Practice of Birth Control: An Analysis of the Birth-Control Experiences of Nine Hundred Women* (London: Williams & Norgate, 1932).
87 M. Jackson, 'Birth control and the medical profession', *British Medical Journal*, 1:3621 (1930), pp. 1022–3.
88 L. Secor Florence, *Birth Control on Trial* (London: George Allen and Inwin Ltd., 1932), p. 3.
89 *Ibid.*, p. 12.
90 *Ibid.*, p. 71.
91 M. Jackson, 'A medical service for the treatment of involuntary sterility', *The Eugenics Review*, 36:4 (1945), p. 117.
92 On this subject see Hanley, *Medicine, Knowledge and Venereal Diseases*. See also A. R. Hanley, '"Sex prejudice" and professional identity: women doctors and their patients in Britain's interwar VD service', *Journal of Social History* [online], shz066, available at: https://doi.org/10.1093/jsh/shz066 (accessed 25 June 2020).
93 *Ibid.*
94 M. A. Pyke, 'Contraception and fertility', *Lancet*, 231:5972 (1938), p. 405.
95 M. Jackson, 'Contraceptives and fertility', *British Medical Journal*, 1:4026 (1938), p. 539.
96 J. Malleson, 'Contraceptives and fertility', *British Medical Journal*, 1:4025 (1938), p. 484.
97 *Ibid.*
98 Jackson, 'Contraceptives and fertility', p. 539.
99 *Ibid.*
100 J. Malleson, 'Contraception and sterility', *British Medical Journal*, 2:4317 (1943), p. 434.
101 *Ibid.*

102 J. Malleson, 'Contraception and sterility', *British Medical Journal*, 2:4328 (1943), pp. 796–7.
103 R. H. P. Hick, 'Advice on sterility', *British Medical Journal*, 1:4300 (1943), p. 707.
104 M. Jackson, 'Advice on sterility', *British Medical Journal*, 1:4303 (1943), p. 803.
105 J. Malleson, 'Contraception and sterility', *British Medical Journal*, 2:4322 (1943), p. 587; J.-M. Strange, 'The assault on ignorance: teaching menstrual etiquette in England, c.1920s to 1960s', *Social History of Medicine*, 14:2 (2001), pp. 247–65.
106 Wellcome Collection, London, GC/105/26, 'Transcript of the interview with Sylvia Dawkins, Television History Workshop, 1988'.
107 See in particular J. R. Baker, 'The spermicidal powers of chemical contraceptives: II. Pure substances', *Journal of Hygiene*, 31:2 (1931), p. 211. On the development of contraceptive research see Löwy, '"Sexual chemistry" before the pill'; Soloway, 'The "perfect contraceptive"'.
108 Wellcome Collection, London, PP/EFG/A.2, 'The national birth control association, medical sub-committee, the present position with regard to the sale and distribution of contraceptives 1936'.
109 Wellcome Collection, London, PP/EFG/A.2, 'Minutes of the Medical sub-committee, 3rd March 1935'.
110 Wellcome Collection, London, SA/FPA/A7/5, 'Approved List, October 1937'.
111 Wellcome Collection, London, SA/FPA/A14/188, 'Letter from the General Secretary of the FPA to Greta Graff, 6 April 1954'; E. Mears, 'Clinical trials of oral contraceptives', *British Medical Journal*, 2:5261 (1961), pp. 1179–83; P. Eckstein et al., 'The Birmingham oral contraceptive trial', *British Medical Journal*, 2:5261 (1961), pp. 1172–9; M. Jackson, 'Oral contraception in practice', *Journal of Reproduction and Fertility*, 6:1 (1963), pp. 153–73. See also Wellcome Collection, London, SA/FPA/A4/A1.3, 'C.I.F.C Trials Branches Barnet'; SA/FPA/A5/158B, 'Minutes of the fourth meeting of doctors conducting Council for the investigation of fertility control, oral contraceptive trial, 30 June 1964'; 'Letter from Eleanor Mears to all medical officers conducting contraceptive trials, 13 January 1965'; E. Mears, 'Oral contraception: the results', *Family Planning*, 10:4 (1962), p. 4.
112 Wellcome Collection, London, SA/FPA/NK/69/638, 'Letter from the Secretary of the North Kensington Women's Welfare Centre to Dr Carruthers, 16th of July, 1954'.
113 Wellcome Collection, London, PP/EPR/B3: Box 2, 'Report of the Conference on the Giving of Information on Birth Control by Public Health Authorities, London, 4.4.1930', pp. 14–15, 17.

114 *Ibid.*, p. 15.
115 Evans, *Freedom to Choose*, pp. 136–7.
116 Wellcome Collection, London, PP/HRW/B.14, H. Wright, 'What women have done through medicine not by medicine, Osler Club, October 12th 1978'. The private papers of Wright held at the Wellcome Collection reveal that, between 1929 and 1958, she spoke at more than 105 conferences on the topics of 'birth control', 'family spacing', 'sex education' and 'sex problems', in many different places such as the Midwife Institute, Presbyterian Church, Kings College, Sheffield City Hall, Marriage Guidance Council etc. She was indefatigable.
117 She was a witness for the defence of Aleck Bourn when he was on trial, in 1938, for having induced a miscarriage in a 14 year-old girl who had been raped by soldiers. Malleson had referred the girl to him.
118 Wellcome Collection, London, SA/FPA/A18/1, 'J. Malleson, "Report of Evidence given to the Royal Commission on Population", 27th of April 1945'.
119 See https://wellcomelibrary.org/item/b2847868x#?c=0&m=0&s=0&cv=0 (accessed 11 November 2017). On the use of mass media to build support for contraception see M. Parry, *Broadcasting Birth Control: Mass Media and Family Planning* (New Brunswick: Rutgers University Press, 2013).
120 Wellcome Collection, London, SA/MWF/H.41/8, 'NHS regulation circular with comments from the MWF'.

2

Sexual disorders and infertility: expanding the work of the clinics

Oh this isn't so boring if you get your climax.

Joan Malleson, 1950s[1]

During the interwar period and onwards, family planning centres expanded their birth control sessions into sexual advice, which became available primarily through the activities of women doctors in Britain. They set up advisory sessions on 'sub-fertility', which were framed as sexual disorders and infertility, and published on these issues.[2] As was the case with the development of medical knowledge of birth control, working in women's welfare centres and birth control clinics provided women doctors with a privileged position from which to observe, learn, acquire and develop new skills. Among these new skills were the handling of sexual difficulties and infertility. Birth control clinics and women's welfare centres therefore constituted spaces for experimentation in these new domains. Paradoxically, it was the specific nature of the clinics and the fact that working there meant occupying a marginal position within the medical hierarchy that allowed scope for exploration and innovation. The constant need to assert the legitimacy of this new field was a driver for developing new medical knowledge and therapeutics. Joan Malleson, Helena Wright and Margaret Jackson played a pivotal role in the development of this field. Their most important contribution was to create and sustain a new holistic approach to family planning where birth control advice (as we saw in Chapter 1), sexual disorders and infertility were treated together. They contributed to the development of the prevention and treatment of sexual disorders and thus participated in the medicalisation of sexuality. Women doctors paved the way for the formal integration of sexual counselling and sub-fertility and the predominance of these issues in family planning clinics from the 1970s onwards. The production of scientific knowledge of sexual disorders by women doctors remains marginal and has mainly been written about as part of a broad analysis of sexual manuals in general. This chapter therefore analyses a range of hitherto understudied material on sexual counselling and infertility. It examines women doctors' contributions to sex and medical manuals, scientific publications and sexual counselling sessions with their patients from the 1930s to the 1970s, and the extent to which these contributions reflected or challenged the broader conceptions about heterosexuality and gender norms that prevailed at that time. It shows that this new 'positive' dimension of the work of the clinic developed in response to the needs and demands of the patients. Historians, by and large, have presented the patient–doctor relationship before the Second World War as an unbalanced and problematic power relationship where doctors 'knew best' and where patients were pictured as passive agents with little autonomy. It has been shown that this paternalist attitude of the medical profession towards their patients lasted up until the 1960s.[3] I argue that a set of doctors had already planted the seed for a more active role for patients, as they were aware of the significance of the patient's autonomy before the Second World War. Indeed, in contrast to histories that present doctors as all-powerful agents in the patient/client–doctor relationship, the historical practice of sexual counselling in many ways provides a more positive vision of this relationship. By developing an appropriate medical response to the sexual difficulties faced by their patients, women doctors took their patients' demands and needs seriously and used them to shape, to a certain extent, the development and content of sexual counselling.[4]

Integrating sexual disorders into the work of the clinic: 1935–58

Research on the history of sexuality and marital intimacy has underlined the advent of the companionate marriage model that became ideologically dominant in the mid-twentieth century.[5] In this model – mainly put forward by sex reformers and sexologists as well as by members of the medical profession – the sexual pleasure of both spouses was portrayed as the key to a successful marriage. Historical studies have shown the influence of Freud's theory on psychosexual development, which profoundly impacted the medical understanding of sexual disorders, especially that of 'frigidity'. Female sexual disorders became extensively debated around the end of the nineteenth century, at a time when sexology, psychiatry and criminology were developing and mutually influencing each other. Middle-class women were generally constructed and represented as passionless and naturally less sexual than men; they were nonetheless portrayed as having the capacity to be sexually 'heated', and therefore this lack of capacity was referred to as 'coldness'.[6] Freud's theory shifted the emphasis towards women's emotional development. In his view, women who did not experience vaginal orgasm were sexually immature.[7] Indeed, Freud thought that young girls did enjoy sexual pleasure through clitoral stimulation, in the same way that small boys experienced pleasure with their penis. However, during puberty, young women entered a new phase in their sexual development where an erotic transfer took place from the clitoris to the vagina, which became the locus for the mature expression of sexual pleasure. This emphasis on mutual sexual pleasure functioned alongside the idea of the importance of expressing sexual instincts; any attempts to repress them could lead to a neurosis. These ideas influenced the marriage and sexual manuals written in the first half of the twentieth century in that they promoted prescriptive gender roles where wives remained passive sexual agents and husbands, as active agents, had to initiate sexual intercourse while awakening their wives to sexual pleasure.[8] However, many historians have underlined the limited impact of these sex manuals on ordinary individuals; couples struggled to enjoy a happy and mutually satisfying sexual life. Indeed, many studies have shown the prevalence of sexual ignorance among the British that lasted until mid-century. Respectable women were expected to be ignorant of sexual matters, which means that they remained passive.[9]

The history of sexual manuals, marriage guidance and individual behaviours has also attracted growing attention; however, we know little about the practicalities, the nitty-gritty and the content of sexual counselling provided at birth control clinics before the 1970s.[10] The sexual counselling provided by the staff at these clinics has received almost no historical attention.[11] There is some work done on Germany and Australia with regards to psychosexual counselling, but not on interwar and postwar Britain[12]. As there exists no history of sexual counselling in Britain, the first section fills this gap by tracing this history from its early form in the mid-1930s to the first dedicated training seminars in 1958. It offers an overview of the many different actors involved in the subject and the decisive role played by Joan Malleson and Helena Wright in making this new topic a focus of research, expertise and practice.

When the National Birth Control Association changed its name to the Family Planning Association in 1939, its members broadened the scope of the work of the association and extended it to providing advice for women and treatments for 'involuntary sterility, minor gynaecological ailments and difficulties connected with the marriage relationships'.[13] This happened in a context where the mental hygiene movement and social psychiatry were gaining traction in interwar Britain, placing an emphasis on family relations and familial environment as key influences on an individual's behaviour and mental health.[14] Social psychiatry and psychology had great impact on the Eugenics Society, in particular its secretary C. P. Blacker, who was a close friend of Malleson. The latter was a keen supporter of the use of psychological frameworks.[15] In 1935 she had already recognised the necessity to expand the work of the clinics towards the incorporation of advice on sexual disorders, 'suggest[ing] that psychological help might be given at one of the sessions' and offering 'to take this session voluntarily for a little while'.[16] This quotation illustrates the extent of Joan Malleson's commitment to the well-being of her patients, since she agreed to advise them without being paid; it also illustrates the pivotal role she played in developing this new field of work. This work was triggered by her patients' experiences and demands. In 1938, she became head of the clinic for marital difficulties at the North Kensington Women's Welfare Centre. Hence, marriage relationships were elevated to a place of utmost importance in the family planning agenda. In this new arrangement, resolving sexual disorders could lay the foundations for a better marital relationship.

The medical interest in sexual relationships in heterosexual marriage did not appear in a vacuum. The idea that sexuality was central to a successful marriage gained in visibility during the interwar years in a context in which anxieties were aroused around the dissolution of marriages, the relaxation of the divorce law in 1937, the breakdown of family life, the quality of the population, and decreasing birth rates. Many historians have stressed the rise of the ideal of companionate marriage in the interwar years.[17] Marriage reformers were particularly vocal. Historian Marcus Collins defined them as 'a school of thought in favour of measured revision of matrimonial law, enlightened sexual attitudes and a radical restructuring of marital roles in the wake of women's emancipation'.[18] The main leaders of this school were Arthur Herbert Gray, Presbyterian minister and promoter of marriage guidance; Methodist minister David R. Mace; and Dr Edward Griffith, a popular sex-education author and member of the Eugenics Society, the NBCA, and, later, the Family Planning Association. Griffith ran his own birth control clinic in Guildford until the FPA asked him to resign when a recommendation was made to appoint only women doctors at the NBCA.[19] These three male reformers were the founding members of the Marriage Guidance Council (MGC) – a body created in 1938 aimed at promoting marriage and family life, which relied on the help of the clergy and the medical profession.[20] They published sexual manuals hoping to alleviate the suffering caused by unhappy sexual lives, which ultimately led to unhappy marriages. Female sexual pleasure – generally through penetration – became a central component of their idea of the happy marriage.[21] Clitoral pleasure was also discussed and made legitimate, especially if it helped to ease penetration. They also set up advisory sessions on sexual difficulties in married life. Hence, marriage counselling was primarily meant to preserve the stability of the family. As outlined by Claire Langhamer, 'sex and love became tightly bound together within the widely promoted notions of modern marriage'.[22]

Women doctors who provided marital and sexual counselling were in close contact and forged alliances with several members of this new movement aimed at developing harmonious marital relationships. These alliances gave them legitimacy. For instance, Arthur Herbert Gray wrote the introduction to Helena Wright's sex manual, *Sex Factor in Marriage*, published in 1930, as well as Dr Mary Macaulay's *Art of Marriage* in 1952. Mary Macaulay was medical officer to the Liverpool branch of the FPA between 1930 and 1956, and a marriage guidance counsellor. Malleson was a consulting gynaecologist on the advisory board of the Marriage Guidance Council,[23] and she and Wright gave talks on 'sexual difficulties in marriage' and 'how to make a good job of marriage', respectively, for conference days organised by the Marriage Guidance Council in 1938.[24] Wright seemed to have held Griffith in high esteem. According to Lady Houghton, secretary of the

International Committee on Planned Parenthood (ICPP) from 1949, for Wright, 'Edward Griffith could do no wrong'.[25] She shared ideas with Griffith about the organisational aspect of the North Kensington clinic. In 1939 they discussed the opportunity of an 'occasional advisory session on marital difficulties to husbands. [...] It might be possible to run such a session at the same time as Dr Malleson runs hers so that the two could be co-related.'[26] Malleson discussed cases with Griffith and exchanged information on possible treatment and support that could be offered to patients. Many individuals wrote to the Family Planning Association to ask them for advice and guidance on sexual disorders. In 1940, a man wrote to be referred to someone for treatment for impotence. Since the FPA did not yet engage with male patients they wrote to Edward Griffith, asking him to deal with it.[27] Sylvia Dawkins was also active in the MGC, and she was a marriage guidance counsellor. There was, therefore, close collaboration between the members of these different organisations.

In 1948, in London, three centres offered marital sexual difficulties sessions. At the North Kensington clinic, Malleson was the medical officer in charge of the Clinic for Marital Adjustment; in 1950, she was appointed to the contraceptive clinic at University College Hospital, where she later established a dyspaneuria clinic. Meanwhile, Dawkins counselled couples at the Family Planning Centre of Welwyn Garden City.[28] She was trained in contraceptive advice by Wright and in sexual counselling by observing Malleson, with whom she worked: 'In my particular case, Joan Malleson was doing the problems because she was a great pioneer in this and when she was appointed to University College Hospital she said to Will Nixon, half these patients need more time, I need an assistant to do the straight contraception, and that was me. I was very privileged. And so I used to do the contraceptive bit and refer cases to her.'[29]

This interest in psychosexual counselling was not limited to the FPA and MGC. In 1948, the Family Welfare Association created the Family Discussion Bureau, an organisation specialising in marriage problems. Its caseworkers underwent psychotherapy training at the Tavistock Clinic, 'one of Britain's leading flag-ships in psychoanalysis'.[30] Their work focused mainly on marriage difficulties and spousal relationships; the underpinning sexual dimension was not predominant, as was the case in FPA clinics. Illustrating the growing interest in and demand for information on these subjects, the medical conference of the FPA held in 1949 was dedicated to marital difficulties. Here, again, the main organisers and leading figures were women doctors. Wright chaired a morning session on ways to help cases of marital difficulty at FPA clinics, while Macaulay acted as the mediator. Malleson, as an FPA specialist in this work, took the stage to share her experience.[31] She saw this new specialty as inherently connected to the work undertaken in family planning clinics; importantly, she regarded it as a new job opportunity for married women doctors: 'such new lines of work are urgently needed and offer highly suitable opportunities, say to the married women doctors who cannot undertake the full burden of general practice, and to the medical psychologists who would undertake part-time work in the various clinics of the neighbourhood.'[32]

In 1954, the North Kensington Marriage Welfare Centre, following the retirement of Malleson as consultant on sexual disorders, opened a special session on marriage problems under the supervision of Dr Margaret Neal-Edwards, gynaecological surgeon to the New Sussex Hospital and the Lady Chichester Hospital for nervous diseases.[33] In 1955, the conference of clinical medical officers and nurses for the FPA dedicated its meeting to marital difficulties. One of the speakers was Dr A. G. Thompson, a consultant psychiatrist at the Tavistock Clinic, who delivered a speech on 'The Provision of Advice on Marital Difficulties'. He warned the audience that when 'one meets these psychological problems they cannot be dealt with by giving advice to the patients'[34]. He provided a gloomy depiction of what could be done to help the patient by emphasising the limitation of the knowledge and skills available to doctors: 'it has been found at the Tavistock Clinic that every type of worker in this field is dissatisfied with the inadequacy both of their own knowledge and of the recognised technique'.[35] FPA members were then asked to share their own experiences of this topic; many, such as Dr Spicer from North Kensington, underlined that they were not 'educated enough to deal with this problem'[36]. Stemming from the discussion, a resolution was passed at the 1956 general subcommittee meeting stating that the 'FPA nationally and each Branch, within its area and according to its power, should co-operate in programmes for providing education and preparation for marriage and advice on sexual problems, and where existing programmes are not adequate should initiate them when facilities are available'.[37] In 1957, an ad hoc committee on help with sex problems in marriage and related matters was put together. Its aim was to address the growing demand from birth control patients for help with sex difficulties.[38] As a result, the committee agreed on the necessity of offering training for all clinic medical officers prepared to advise on these difficulties.[39] In 1958, the medical committee of the FPA issued a call for enrolling clinic medical officers from London and the Home Counties who dealt with marriage difficulties on a weekend course.[40] The two-day programme included six sessions. The participants' names again highlight the central contribution of women doctors to campaigning for establishing this field as an important part of the FPA's work. Helena Wright and Mary Macaulay discussed the doctor–patient relationship in FPA work. Dr Clifford Allen, consultant psychiatrist in charge of the psychiatric department at the Dreadnought Seamen's Hospital, Greenwich, consultant neuropsychiatrist to the Ministry of Pensions, and the future author of a *Textbook for Psychosexual Disorders* in 1961, approached the question of male problems. Issues linked to dissatisfied couples and failure cases were presented by Margaret Jackson; Dr Margaret Neal-Edwards, consultant gynaecologist and medical officer at the Eastbourne Family Planning Centre and assistant medical officer for maternity and child welfare in Brighton, who had also replaced Malleson at the North Kensington Marriage Welfare Centre, addressed the topic of vaginismus; and Sylvia Dawkins covered relaxation. Here again, women doctors were at the forefront of developing knowledge on the subject. Following these calls for better training on marital problems, training seminars were instituted in August 1958 under the leadership of Michael Balint, directed at family planning doctors.

Before entering into the analysis of Balint's seminar, I turn to the early form of therapy for sexual disorders developed by Wright and Malleson prior to the establishment of Balint's 'unofficial training'. The years 1935–58 were a period of transition in which traditional notions around sexuality were challenged. This time, I argue, should be regarded as a period of experimentation, before the establishment of a more 'conservative' view on sexuality through Balint's seminars, which reaffirmed traditional gender roles in married life. Therefore, the early form of sexual counselling was a radical endeavour, one that laid the foundation for the second-wave feminist criticisms of sexuality as oppressive towards women that were voiced after the sexual revolution.

Centrality of female sexual pleasure: 1935–58

Many significant contributions to the understanding of sexual disorders were made by women doctors, owing to their encounters with patients in birth control, women's welfare and family planning clinics, as well as in their private practices, from 1935 onwards. This section draws on articles and books published by female doctors working in the field of sexual counselling, oral history interviews carried out in the 1980s, and fourteen recordings of sexual counselling sessions carried out by Malleson and held at the Wellcome Library. I use these sources to explore the underpinning motives for addressing female sexual disorders. These sources raise a number of important issues about the relationship between women's sexual pleasure and 'pathology', between natural instinct and education. Moreover, female sexual pleasure served as a forum for a competing vision of female sexuality and a new definition of the realm of doctors' work. Women doctors, therefore, were building a citadel of expertise on birth control, family planning and sexual disorders; in so doing they expanded their professional identities and consolidated a new field of medical intervention. Furthermore, they reinforced their positions among their medical colleagues as forerunners in women's sexual health.

From 1935, Malleson held sexual counselling sessions with patients experiencing different 'sexual disorders', either at birth control and family planning clinics or in her own private practice. Her early form of sexual therapy seemed to have been triggered by her patients' demands. The birth control clinic – a place where birth control was discussed and where women were encouraged to touch their genitals while placing contraceptive devices – at least provided, if not an ideal forum, a safe space for discussing sexual difficulties. Indeed, contraception was only one aspect of the sexual relationship, and patients therefore often hinted at sexual difficulties. Malleson was largely self-taught in her approach to sexual and married counselling. She never underwent any formal training in psychology or psychiatry, and seems to have built her own method out of experience, as she explained in the foreword to her book, *Any Wife or Any Husband: A Book for Couples Who Have Met Sexual*

Difficulties and for Doctors (1950): 'I write as a medical woman whose work deals mainly in women's health and childbearing problems. Although I lack psychiatric qualifications, I am fortunate in sharing cases with colleagues who have this training, and from them and from my patients I have acquired knowledge of sexual disorders. The gynaecologist who takes an interest in such conditions has infinite opportunities to observe and learn.'[41] As a result, psychology and psychiatry informally entered birth control clinics as a new diagnostic tool for understanding sexual disorders. Malleson was well aware that she was a pioneer in the field of sexual counselling and complained that 'psychotherapists apart, doctors have offered relatively little towards the solution of these intimate yet prevalent problems.'[42]

Many colleagues stressed the fact that Malleson's personality was extremely well-suited to this type of work. In a flattering tribute to Malleson after her death, Margaret Jackson, who had known Malleson since they attended University College Hospital together, praised her 'great gifts of sympathy and gentleness'. She 'brought untold comfort to the many couples who came to her with their marital difficulties and problems. Her own experiences of life and particular qualities of temperament gave her a special insight into such matters so that as a medical adviser she possessed a value quite unique and all her own.'[43] In much the same way, Dr Andrew Morland, a Harley Street chest physician, explained that Malleson's 'profound interest in people of all types, her universal sympathy and her failure to pass judgement made her the ideal person to give advice on the problems of marriage, both mental and physical, and it is not surprising that this part of her work soon outstripped the rest.'[44] These quotations reflect the centrality of the human dimension of this new work, which put the patient's well-being and happiness at the centre.

The recordings contain fourteen cases of sexual disorders; one was the case of a menopausal woman and is not considered here. There were eight cases of 'vaginismus', two cases of 'frigidity', and three cases of 'inhibition of orgasm'. Three husbands came along and spoke separately with Malleson. The majority of the patients were referred by other doctors and psychiatrists, showing the increasing esteem in which Malleson's work was held. In one case, a couple who had not consummated their marriage came of their own accord, having read Malleson's book, *Any Husband or Any Wife*. These sessions provide useful and fascinating insights into the way Malleson deployed moral and medical frameworks to treat patients who experienced sexual disorders. These tapes were recorded in the 1950s, before her death in 1956, without her patients' consent. It is worth mentioning that contemporary ethical guidelines did not prohibit the recording of patients' sessions. These sessions seem to have been the only ones that she recorded. To avoid any ethical problems, these tapes have been anonymised and any personal information has been withdrawn. They were recorded plausibly at different locations: at Malleson's private practice, at the Islington clinic, and at the dyspareunia clinic attached to University College Hospital where Malleson worked until her death.[45] Malleson plausibly aimed to use these recordings for teaching, since, as explained by William Nixon, who had convinced Malleson to join the hospital, 'with the realisation of the importance of this subject for general practitioners it was agreed that one student should be present at each session. Many students have expressed their appreciation for the privilege of having learnt from Joan Malleson the way to deal with sexual problems which beset many married women and which if not alleviated lead to the bankruptcy of marriage.'[46] The intentional recording of the session as a teaching tool is also suggested by the fact that, after the sexual counselling sessions, she would make a brief summary of the case, highlighting its main features. In one case, she stressed the patient's difficulty in finding her words and emphasised the benefit of the session as 'good for teaching purposes'. In her view, the session 'shows the sort of expressions the patient would use and perhaps the sort of expressions that she would accept'.[47]

These recordings reveal how she approached the topic of sexual disorders, the type of questions she asked, the dynamic between her and the patient and the emphasis she placed on sexual pleasure. These cases constitute, therefore, a crucial source for illuminating how sexual problems might be understood, not only by practitioners but by the patients themselves. They reveal what was perceived as 'normal sexuality', what was considered pathological, and the type of treatments recommended for curing these conditions. Of course, treating these records as historical evidence is problematic in several ways. First, the doctor–patient relationship is, in itself, a power relationship. Every sexual counselling session was mediated through this relationship. Hence, every answer from the patients might have been an attempt to conform to the expectation of the doctor and to present themselves in a favourable light. However, rather than viewing this as a problem, I argue that this relationship reveals as much about what was perceived as 'normal' or 'pathological' sexual behaviour as the content of sexual counselling itself. These records, therefore, offer a glimpse into the ideas around heterosexuality that circulated at the time, both in lay and medical circles.[48]

Clinics constituted an invaluable place to gain intimate knowledge of difficulties faced by couples. The value of the experience acquired through encounters with patients was made clear in the sex advice manuals and articles that women doctors published. They paid tribute to their patients for providing them with adequate knowledge of sexual disorders: 'the daily work of a gynaecologist brings her into continual touch with married life in all sections of the community. It was not long after I began practice that the dismal act of sexual success which was spoiling the lives of patients showed itself as an unnecessary tragedy compelling attention,'[49] wrote Wright in 1947. Meanwhile, Malleson acknowledged in 1942 that her understanding of some specific types of sexual disorder, and therefore her own devising of therapy, owed much to her patients' explanations:

> Observation of a series of cases has suggested a possible common factor which has not yet received recognition. Cases here studied have been drawn from private practice and from the various departments of the North Kensington Women's Welfare Centre. [...] Many of them have during infancy been conditioned to expect pain in the pelvic region by the insertion of a foreign body, the offending object being usually the enema, the suppository, the old-fashioned soapstick so much employed in Victorian nurseries for the treatment of constipation. The possibility of such an association was first suggested by the chance remark of a woman who had suffered from extreme spasms. At her first examination of the vagina she stated that the examining finger felt exactly like an enema.[50]

This first-hand experience with patients' difficulties convinced Malleson that much of their mental and physical ill health was caused by sexual difficulties due to ignorance. Overcoming sexual ignorance seemed to have been the driving force behind women doctors' writing of sexual manuals. As expressed by Malleson as early as 1935 while writing about women's lack of pleasure:

> It is strange that the parallel syndrome in the male is so widely recognised. The equivalent reaction in the female is incomparably more frequent, but, because it is the custom that women should know little and say less about their sexual reactions, the gynaecological departments are crowded with patients regularly seeking relief from the results of unsatisfactory coitus in the form of a bottle of medicine.[51]

To help women overcome this lack of knowledge, Malleson wrote two books and three leaflets for the Family Planning Association at the end of the 1940s, one on 'Sex Facts in Marriage' and the other two on 'Sex Problems in Marriage'. The targeted audience included female and male patients of FPA clinics who were encountering sexual difficulties and were thought of as being ignorant about sexual intercourse. The first leaflet provided basic information on the functioning of sexual intercourse, since 'the understanding of these facts is the foundation on which a good relationship must be built'.[52] The leaflet depicted the penis, clitoris, and vagina as loci for sexual pleasure, while emphasising that women's pleasure is different from that of men, since women had two places where sexual pleasure could be felt. In the two leaflets addressing sex problems in marriage, Malleson identified five main reasons behind the failure to achieve sexual satisfaction: inability or lack of knowledge 'to give the other the kind of intercourse that she or he needed';[53] the nervousness of one partner, '(usually women)', Malleson added; fear of pregnancy; dissatisfaction with birth control method; and low frequency or absence of intercourse. The second leaflet concentrated on female sexual disorders only. Here, again, Malleson put forward women's ignorance about their own bodies and men's lack of skills in sexual matters as the main reasons behind female sexual dissatisfaction. Building on this idea, she contended that patients could overcome their difficulties if they 'understand a little of how these are caused'.[54]

Malleson was not alone in her belief that sexual ignorance was the main cause of sexual dissatisfaction. Helena Wright clearly laid out the same idea in the foreword of her 1930 book: 'When no trouble is taken to learn how to make sexual intercourse harmonious and happy, a variety of complications arise. Very often wives remain sexually unawakened and therefore inclined to dislike sexual intercourse.'[55] About eighteen years later, she introduced the readers to her new book by referring to her first attempt to arm married people with sexual knowledge:

> The most striking observation is that sexual satisfaction is not obtained by more than 50 per cent of married women, and my study of the effect of this state of things shows that women's lack of sexual satisfaction is an important, though not the only, factor which makes for instability in marital relations. My first impression after a certain amount of work and thought was that this widespread failure was largely caused by general ignorance of the technique of the art of love, and it appeared to me therefore that the remedy would be easy.[56]

In 1982, reflecting on the work she carried out in family planning clinics, she remembered a specific example in which ignorance accounted for sexual dissatisfaction: 'I used to give these patients any chance to talk. I would say now you are perfectly safe you won't have another child. Do you enjoy having intercourse at all? And the patient said these historic words: "But doctor, what is it to enjoy?" Now when you look deeply into that, it was total ignorance.'[57]

Importantly, women doctors actively created a vision and depiction of English women as intrinsically ignorant about sexual behaviours, which had long-lasting and very often dramatic consequences for their married sexual lives.

The work undertaken by women doctors in birth control clinics, while adhering to the vision of preserving the family and the well-being of overburdened mothers, also expanded the notion of sexual pleasure in a more radical way. To these women doctors, sexual pleasure represented a central priority in sexual counselling sessions. Of course, the fact that women doctors were women facilitated conversations about sex and pleasure. Indeed, sex was still a taboo topic, and the fact that the idea of respectability was connected with sexual ignorance might have prevented female patients from broaching the subject freely in the presence of men. As Sylvia Dawkins recalled in an interview for the Television History Workshop in 1988 about work in the clinic: 'it was the situation of women talking to women who accepted that women enjoyed sex, wanted sex. Not only for procreation, that it was a very bonding thing which helped the relationship. Very valuable.'[58] Women's sexual pleasure, or lack of, became a central element of sexual counselling. Women doctors would ask, as related by Dawkins: 'Do you have pleasure, are you enjoying it?' However, ignorance of basic terminology on the part of the patient meant that women doctors did not refer to medical language: 'I didn't use the word orgasm because most of them wouldn't have understood.'[59]

Historian Hera Cook has shown that female sexual pleasure, though through penetration, became a central component of a happy marriage, as described by sexual manuals in the interwar years.[60] What has not been fully acknowledged, however, is the care with which Malleson and Wright emphasised it and the fact that they believed in the educative role of the doctor. This was very much a legacy of the social hygiene movement, where working-class mothers were taught the basics of hygiene in maternal health and antenatal care by medically trained public servants in antenatal clinics.[61]

According to Malleson, the role of the doctor was clearly active, by broaching the subject: 'The practitioner who has knowledge of these important aspects of family life will find what a vast amount of unhappiness is caused by ignorance and sexual maladjustment. It is surprising how frequently help can be given by a little sympathetic and practical advice.'[62] Malleson also explained that 'once the confidence of the patient is gained it is not difficult to ask her whether she is getting her own satisfaction and to explain that if she is capable of getting a climax it is necessary for her health that she should do so.'[63] Similarly, Wright believed in the importance of education for a fulfilled sexual life. There was a constant tension in her writing between the idea that sexuality was a 'natural' thing – 'Sex desire is a natural characteristic of every normal adult woman and man, in itself as beautiful and blameless as moving or breathing'[64] – but that it nevertheless needed to be educated and monitored for individuals to make the most of it and to prevent 'an overwhelming majority of people [from] fling[ing] themselves into marriage, ignorant, unprepared, vaguely hoping for the best'. Wright repeated this argument multiple times in her career:

> As time went on, the sex experience of all adults is universal, the wish to enjoy anything is also universal. Therefore you've got a sympathetic public if you could do two things for them: if you could say 'pregnancy, don't think about it, enjoy your relation with your husband'. It is a natural thing in itself, but it is a thing you must be educated about – it isn't

spontaneous in this country as far as we know. What we were trying to do is to make them realise that education for a good sex partner was as necessary as the one for methods.[65]

However, women doctors' views on sexual pleasure were ambivalent and embodied contradictions. Arguments supporting female sexual pleasure melded traditional and radical visions of sexuality by navigating between established ideas of female sexuality (passive agent that needed to be aroused by the man and the idea of the vagina as the locus of mature sexual pleasure) and the new radical vision of women as active agents in sexual relationships and of the centrality of the clitoris. The coexistence of these arguments not only reflected the transitional period between the 1930s and the 1950s in which social attitudes towards sexuality and female pleasure were shifting, but also the idea that sexuality might be, in itself, multiple, and that there existed different lived experiences. One of the first things Malleson put forward in her 1935 book was the fact that individuals needed different things in their sexual lives; therefore, no clear guideline for behaviours existed: 'It should be remembered that it is always unwise to urge a line of sexual behaviour on another person, for in every case the sexual life of the individual is intricately bound up with his physiological and psychological needs and those of his partner.'[66]

While members of the marriage reform movement underplayed the importance of clitoral orgasm and praised the vaginal one, following the Freudian vision of sexual maturity, Malleson and Wright, informed by the difficulties experienced by their patients in simply reaching climax, rehabilitated clitoral orgasms as a way for the wife to experience sexual pleasure in a marital sexual relationship. For instance, Malleson explained that only one woman out of three could achieve sexual satisfaction through the 'straightforward act of sexual intercourse.'[67] The majority of women seemed to get their 'greatest sexual feelings'[68] from the clitoris, which was its 'sole purpose'. The clitoris was easily aroused if given the right kind of 'caressing movement by the husband's hand', she argued. Following this line of thinking, she explained that vaginal sensations are not easy to feel at the beginning of sexual experience, but that 'time and experience gradually awaken feelings in the vagina.'[69] Two 'conflicting' views coexisted side by side in Malleson's work. She recognised the central significance of the clitoris as the main place for women's sexual pleasure, presenting it as more straightforward than the vagina, while nevertheless acknowledging the vaginal orgasm as a deeper and more rewarding orgasm: 'Although some women cannot distinguish between clitoral and vaginal orgasm, usually the functions are quite distinct. A woman who can get both types of orgasms nearly always values the vaginal one most: normally it evokes deeper emotion and is more satisfying.'[70] At times she challenged the Freudian vision of sexuality by positively emphasising the key role of the clitoris in women's sexuality, though at other times she seemed to agree with the idea that clitoral orgasm was linked with inexperienced sexuality. While emphasising that there were no 'norms' or 'normality' when it came to sexuality, Malleson nevertheless described what she considered to be the 'fairly average standard'. An 'experienced woman' should moisten and penetration should be painless. A vaginal orgasm should 'ideally' take place after a prolonged back and forth movement of the penis inside the vagina. Unless able to attain a vaginal orgasm, she should reach a clitoral climax produced by the husband's fingertips. The clitoral orgasm therefore appears to have been seen as compensation for a failed vaginal orgasm.

This ambivalence was perpetuated in sexual counselling sessions. The following excerpt is taken from the recording of a sexual counselling session with a young unmarried female patient who 'complained she did not get [an] orgasm',[71] as recorded by Malleson when introducing the case. The patient did not seem to mind experiencing no pleasure, but her partner did and wanted her to have an orgasm. This reveals an increasing male interest in female sexual pleasure, plausibly reflecting the stabilisation of the new norm of mutual pleasure; the unmarried female patient said: 'I had intercourse with three men, I didn't really mind, I knew some women didn't. It was sort of pleasant and the chap was enjoying it and I think I didn't really mind. But I have recently met with a man who does mind if I don't. That makes me worry about it.' The patient was anxious to understand what an orgasm was and the difference between a clitoral and vaginal orgasm. Malleson responded by emphasising the significance of sexual experience in the attainment of a vaginal climax. Her answer was testimony to her partial adherence to Freudian principles: 'It's rather the same as an outside one but as you rightly say, it's got different sensations. [pause] I think it's quite early on to expect a vaginal one yet, you know. It takes much more learning. Its err, most little girls can get a clitoral one. Urm, the vaginal one is much more, that of an experienced woman.'[72] However, Malleson nevertheless validated the clitoral orgasm and presented it as a legitimate solution for sexual pleasure:

- Have you not been able to get pleasure from him stroking outside?
- Oh yes I like that.
- Can you get a climax from it?
- Yes
- Oh, but then this isn't so boring for you ...
- (laugh)
- If you get your climax. You speak as though that isn't of any value.
- Oh I ... I suppose it is. I do get pleasure but I always thought the two of you sort of had it together.[73]

Interestingly, the young woman stressed her desire to reach a mutual orgasm, showing how the new norm of mutual sexual pleasure and the centrality of the vagina might have been internalised. Malleson repeatedly emphasised the fact that women who could reach clitoral orgasm were 'not too badly off'.

Another ambivalence found in Malleson's written production and counselling sessions is connected to the role of women in their search for sexual pleasure. She encouraged women to take an active role in guiding their husband towards the provision of adequate caressing of the clitoris in order to trigger their clitoral orgasm. The example of a married woman with inhibition of orgasm illustrates Malleson's commitment to female sexual pleasure. The patient could reach clitoral climax while masturbating, but her husband was unable to sexually satisfy her. Malleson advised the patient to discuss this issue with her husband and to show him how to provide her with pleasure:

- But you see men don't know such a lot about women because, as you say, 'I feel I'm beginning to need an outside climax'.
- Yes. Well I will do that.
- As I grow older I need a little bit more and even if it takes me a long time it would be a help to me. And then of course, show him, take his fingers with yours you see and show him how to rub. Of course, he cannot know by instinct, any woman is different, you see? And I think it would be a mistake to leave your interests aside because however unselfish or cautious you feel, things pile up. Discussion earlier on

which I think could be done without hurting his feelings or your own feelings is important otherwise, things pile up.[74]

While recommending that this patient carefully express her feelings, Malleson nevertheless explicitly warned other female patients against the spoken formulation of their sexual dissatisfaction, which could endanger the husband's confidence in his sexual capacity, thereby threatening his masculinity. Indeed, as the following example shows, Malleson praised one of her patients for her sensitivity in hiding from her partner her lack of sexual pleasure, but paradoxically urged her to take a leading role in the sexual act. The patient was a woman in her mid-thirties who had got married for the second time and was seeking advice about her lack of sexual pleasure and feeling of depression. At the time of the interview, she had been married for a year and was sexually unsatisfied. To a question about her husband's sexual ability, she reckoned that her husband was not 'very competent but he is trying hard'.[75] Afraid of hurting his feelings, she kept her lack of pleasure hidden from him. Contrasting her present experience with that with her ex-husband, she explained that her new husband was quick to come, while with the previous one she had had vaginal orgasms but after longer intercourse of about twenty minutes. Malleson applauded her good reaction and provided advice on the best way to handle the situation:

- Of course, whether we can make him have a longer sexual intercourse is rather difficult to say. He might. After all he is very young ... with judicious teaching, not to make him feel inferior, but encouragement, you might be able [to] get him to do more. A long sexual intercourse is more satisfactory [and] also good for the man – he gets a bigger relief, you see, as well as you. But you might [want] to play your cards carefully. Especially with the second husband. Because they so easily feel inferior. And that is the worst treatment for a nervous man. His sex life becomes less adequate if he feels inferior. The one thing to do is to make him feel confident. And although men aren't to know that consciously, you've done the right thing by not letting him know what you are feeling and so on. But all the same you can judiciously bring in the fact that maybe if you change your position and so on might do better. [...]
- Have you ever tried to take the lead? Does this make him happy?
- No, I haven't.

- Some men love that, especially when they're learners. They like if the responsibility comes from the wife. And it isn't normal for the men to always initiate it. In the happy marriage, the wife will make the first move. That sometimes gives him ... the responsibility is lifted away and he feels release. You should try.[76]

Interestingly, Malleson counselled the patient to initiate sexual intercourse as a means of reassuring the husband that he was desired and loved. Similarly, she encouraged a patient who suffered from vaginismus and 'acute anxiety neurosis' and cried anytime she tried to have intercourse to steady her husband's penis with her hands and guide it towards the vagina. Malleson emphasised the fact that the patient's behaviour, and notably her tears, might have upset the husband who might have lost his confidence:

- Does he ever lose his erection?
- Yes, I think perhaps one of the causes you see – it doesn't seem to be firm.
- But sometimes it is firm?
- Yes.
- But, you see, the more he gets upset about crying the less firm he would be because it takes the confidence away. I think the best you can do is to buy a little textbook I have written for people like yourself, and you find a whole chapter on the difficulties of the young husband ... and that will give him a lot of confidence, and you will also tell him that you were laying in too tightly, that you were not helping him. It is much easier to take the blame yourself cause you see it matters terribly to a man because his self-esteem is involved. Let him learn about the various ways and show him how you lay in the future and he will gain growing confidence – and then you get your feeling in the passage and you will stop crying.[77]

These excerpts show the ambivalence towards male sexuality as well as ongoing constructions of masculinity. Husbands were presented as in need of education on their wife's pleasure, but they nevertheless required a special form of treatment that preserved their feelings of confidence, and therefore their masculinity. The performance of sexuality was intrinsically linked with that of masculinity, and any attempts to criticise the techniques of the husband might lead to feelings of inferiority on his part. Women therefore carried the burden of making sure not only that their husband gave them sexual pleasure, but also that the latter knew how to satisfy them through a careful education on the importance of the clitoris while, at the same time, safeguarding their husband's feelings and masculinity. This inclination of the medical body towards the preservation of the male's virility was not confined to sexual pleasure but extended to treatment for infertility through artificial insemination by donor. Gayle Davis has underlined the fact that the doctors who practised this procedure, such as Mary Barton and Eleanor Mears in London, did not inform the sterile husband of the extent of his sterility, but rather said that he was 'impaired', and consequently mixed his semen with the donor's to preserve the husband's sense of masculinity and virility.[78]

This contradictory injunction led Malleson to recommend that her patients keep trying to have sexual intercourse, despite their lack of pleasure or feelings of pain. She paralleled the learning and development of sexual capacity with the practice of cycling. To a 22 year-old married female patient, who suffered vaginismus and great distress anytime her husband tried to have intercourse, and who, as a result, wanted to 'get a rest' from intercourse, she said: 'But one doesn't learn to do a thing by not trying. Well, if you are afraid to ride your bicycle you shouldn't put it in the shelter. It is not the way to do it.'[79]

Malleson played with prevailing gendered sexual norms, at times challenging them radically and on other occasions counselling the patient to abide by them. However, a fine line was drawn on the necessity for men to have sexual satisfaction. Women should try to reach orgasm, but even if they could not, they were nevertheless urged to satisfy their husband. Malleson's vision of female pleasure during 'problematic' sexual intercourse tended to be more of a psychological and emotional nature rather than of physical one. Giving the husband sexual pleasure, she argued, was in itself a form of satisfaction for the wife. This stance was made clear in the advice she gave to one of her patients; aged thirty-eight, the patient had been married for ten years, but never experienced sexual pleasure. She was sent to Malleson by a psychiatrist who described her as 'an extraordinary crude creature who resents any sign of affection at all from the part of the husband and never had any interest in intercourse.'[80] The patient explained that she told her husband that she didn't get any pleasure at all from intercourse. She further argued that it was not in her nature to show any form of affection; that she had been brought up this way. The husband, hurt by this revelation, no longer wanted to have sexual intercourse. Malleson seems to have been shocked by the detachment of the patient and, as a result, with a gentle, soft voice, nevertheless condemned her behaviour:

- Do you moisten for him or are you dry?
- I moisten.
- So that you're not absolutely unmoved and he gets in all right without hurting you?
- Oh yes!
- How often do you have intercourse?
- I haven't had any for a little while now. It seems to put him off you see? But it used to be once or twice a week.
- Because you told him that you didn't get pleasure.
- Yes – it hurt him I think.
- I expect it has. 'Cause after all you take one thing then another one from him.
- Because he says 'What is wrong?' But I knew I'd hurt him if I tell him, but he says 'Come on, what is wrong?' And I wish I hadn't said it really because it has been really hurting him.
- Now he thinks he can give you nothing, because you don't value his love and you don't value his sex, and you don't want his child. Terrible.[81]

To save their marriage, Malleson suggested to the patient that she should tell her husband that she did enjoy pleasing him:

> I think, if you want to do the proper thing by him, the only thing left to do is for you to tell him that there are other values – for a woman – in having intercourse than just the pleasure she gets out of it. But there is the pleasure of pleasing her husband and being wanted. And you'll have to go along with him a little. It's not in your nature, because you don't really care or think about pleasing him, do you?[82]

Malleson later reflected on this session and reckoned that she 'probably didn't handle it as well as I should. It was hard not to be repelled by her coldness. Perhaps had I approached her differently, a way would have opened.'[83] This disapproval of the wife's behaviour reflects Malleson's view of what a good wife should be – namely a loving and affectionate partner. Her belief that sexual intercourse could be enjoyable for reasons other than sexual pleasure seems to have been widespread at that time. Indeed, similar statements were found by Szreter and Fisher in their oral history study on birth control and sexual behaviour among middle- and working-class people before the sexual revolution. They contended that couples perceived sex as fulfilling when the following conditions were met:

> part of a private relationship in which it was not discussed, when natural, spontaneous and free from cultural interference, when it represented the coming together of pure and clean bodies, and when couples used it to demonstrate the giving, rather than the receiving, of pleasure. Discussions of sexual pleasure were thus intimately connected to a code of respectability, female sexual innocence, caring and sharing, duty and privacy.[84]

Comparatively, Wright's view on female sexual pleasure evolved drastically over time, mainly because of a careful analysis of her patients' difficulties. Wright was more inclined than Malleson, who had a more authoritarian approach to counselling, to reconsider her own views on female pleasure. In her first sexual manual, Wright contended that women needed to be aroused by their husband, a common stance in the sexual manuals at the time, yet their pleasure constituted an essential component of a successful married sexual life:

> At the beginning of the marriage, he [the husband] more often than not has the role of initiator. He is the magic touch that will awaken his wife's physical nature, [and] her future sex happiness will depend to a very large extent on his knowledge, delicacy, imagination and sympathy. To this end, he should study her, discover her latent desires and encourage her to express gradually increasing pleasure in the physical intimacy of sex.[85]

Paradoxically, Wright simultaneously retained an active role for the wife in the enhancement of her own sexual pleasure: 'The wife must decide with all her strength that she wants her body to feel all the sensations of sex with the greatest possible vividness.'[86] Wright strategically valued the clitoral orgasm by comparing the role of the clitoris with that of the penis:

> The clitoris is capable of giving the most acute sensations; the tissue of which it is made is similar to that of the penis and during sex stimulation it has the same power of filling with blood and thereby becoming larger and harder than it is in an inactive state. The only purpose of the clitoris is to provide sensation, a full understanding of its capabilities and place in the sex-act is therefore of supreme importance.[87]

Moreover, the clitoris was the 'gateway' to vaginal sensation. However, after fifteen years of working with patients who found it difficult to reach orgasm, Wright came to a dramatic conclusion – one that prefigured the 1970's discourses about the critics of sexuality as being patriarchal, and the idea that gender identities were socially and culturally constructed. Three reasons, she argued, might explain why 50 per cent of married women did not experience sexual satisfaction during their marital life: failure to identify the difference between 'sexual response in the erogenous zones and an orgasm',[88] underplaying the importance of the clitoris, and adherence to a male definition of sexuality. Indeed, she said that women did not experience pleasure because of their unconscious adherence to a preconceived mental picture of the way they should feel during intercourse, based on the male pattern. This pattern had been established and reaffirmed over time, since the majority of people who wrote about love and sexuality were men:

> In the past, poets, painters, composers and writers have been predominantly men, and in dealing with themes of love and romance have naturally drawn upon their own experiences. Unchallenged by women, men have been able to stamp their kind of sexual pattern on public imagination, and the public has responded with a general and uncritical acceptance of the idea that this pattern is a universal one.[89]

Tradition had defined men as active and women as passive, she argued, and individuals had internalised the fixation on penis–vagina sex. This internalisation of the male pattern, namely the fixation on penis–vagina sex and the active role of men, had prevented women from understanding their own bodies and, as a result, they ignored the function of the clitoris. 'Is the vagina the natural place where a woman should feel an orgasm at the beginning of her sexual life?',[90] asked Wright provocatively. The answer was no, and the clitoris, asserted Wright, was the natural place for female sexual pleasure. To support her claim, she compared the physiology of the penis with that of the vagina: 'Looking at the male and female organs from a sensation point of view, it is immediately obvious that similarity of function exists between the sensitive head of the penis and the clitoris, and not between the penis and the vagina.'[91] The development of the organs during the gestational time was a second indicator of similarity, as was the fact that both organs are covered by 'sensitive mucous membrane and both are protected by a surrounding hood of tissue'.[92]

Wright urged women to identify their clitoris and discover its sensitivity by gently stroking it with an external object such as 'an uncut pencil'. In so doing, they should identify their preferred rhythmic friction and then teach their husband the way they enjoyed being caressed by guiding and moving his hands accordingly. Wright called for a radical reshaping of the way men and women thought about sex. She emphasised the historical gendered construction of sexual identities, in which men were depicted as active agents and women as passive: 'He is the heir to an inheritance of sexual behaviours with a continuous history stretching back to the whole mammalian evolution. For him to take the initiative and to be active in sexual matters is its most natural behaviour.'[93] Women too had inherited a long tradition of sexual behaviours, but theirs went 'in the opposite direction': 'History, society and her own feeling suggest that she should be the one who is sought. To be active and to take initiative in sexual concerns is, for the most majority of women, an unnatural proceeding.'[94] Wright encouraged women to depart from this tradition and to take an active role in their sexual life.

This internalisation of distinctive sexual roles was reflected in Malleson's patients. Indeed, they echoed the 'fixation on the penis–vagina'. Most of them sought help for curing a lack of vaginal sensation, believing that a sexual relationship should be penetrative and enjoyable and lead to a mutual orgasm, due to the prevailing strength of cultural and social constructions of female and male pleasure. Malleson, in particular, negatively denounced the new pressure to conform to the new sexual norm of reaching orgasm that women were encountering: 'I think it is a difficulty of your generation because twenty to thirty years ago hardly any women got orgasms, and it was not talked about. Now it is talked about everybody feels that it should be a standard measurement and wonders if there is something wrong with them if they are not exactly like someone else they've heard about. It's miserable. Everybody is different. You cannot compare with somebody else.'[95]

Sexual disorders in women: identification and therapeutics

Just as sexual pleasure was becoming central to the work of Wright and Malleson, the latter, triggered by an accumulation of cases that underlined the difficulties for many women in experiencing sexual pleasure, published several articles in medical journals that offered a scientific classification and description of female sexual disorders and suggested therapy for them. Replicating the strategy of asserting their legitimacy through the medicalisation of the issue, a strategy that had successfully been used for birth control (see Chapter 1), these pioneer women published articles in respected medical journals and spread scientific knowledge of sexual disorders. This medicalisation of sexual disorders, which paradoxically relied on informal psychology, was a strategic move to make this new field of inquiry respectable.

Distinguishing between frigidity, lack of sexual capacity, vaginismus, vaginal anaesthesia and inhibition of orgasm, Malleson first endeavoured to provide an accurate description of each term in an attempt to position sexual disorders as a new scientific field of research. Frigidity referred to the absence of emotional and physical response to '*the sexual relationship under discussion*'.[96] This condition should be differentiated from that of women who could experience erotic feelings, but lacked the intensity to bring about orgasm. She suggested referring to these women as 'lacking orgasmic capacity'. This condition did not necessarily imply difficulties in health or in their married life; 'the fact remains that many women with no such capacity are perfectly healthy and stable'.[97] She also pursued the description of 'vaginismus'; the term denoted a condition of 'vaginal spasm varying from a constriction at the beginning of coitus (so slight that it may merely discomfort the woman herself) up to the extreme case in which the spasm causes acute pain to the woman and entirely prohibits any penetration by the husband'. Another condition was that of vaginal anaesthesia, which varied in degree and persistence from women capable of a little sensation to women suffering complete and permanent anaesthesia. This condition appeared to be common in newly married women. While reaching vaginal orgasm might be difficult for these women, some of them would experience a clitoral orgasm and have a happy and enjoyable sexual life. Inhibition of orgasm – a condition in which sexual feeling and erotic sensation were present but no orgasm could be reached – represented another sexual disorder. Women affected by this condition experienced sleeplessness, depression, frustration, aching back and pelvis the day after intercourse, and eventually symptoms of anxiety neurosis. A potential result of this condition might be secondary frigidity, which went hand in hand with distaste for sexual intercourse.

Malleson developed a sophisticated therapy over the course of her career, from the early 1930s to her death. Her therapeutic framework was psychological. As early as 1935, in a manual published for fellow practitioners, she resorted to specialist psychological vocabulary, which clearly indicates her knowledge of the field: 'The recent understanding of anxiety-neurosis has thrown a floodlight onto types of functional ill health which make up of the work of a general practitioner. Among the factors which cause this condition must be considered the sexual (and therefore contraceptive) adjustment of the patient.'[98] The relationship between anxiety and 'interferences with the satisfactory completion of the sexual act' therefore became a central aspect of her work. This relationship had profound implications for the way Malleson understood her patients' sexual difficulties and the type of treatment and therapy that she would prescribe. She drew on Freud's ideas on the psychosexual development of men and women, though she did not adhere entirely to his vision of female sexuality. She was recognised as a Freudian by her colleagues, as shown by her response to a letter from Griffith in which he asked whether the Freudian school approved or disapproved of the practice of stretching the hymen: 'I have certainly never heard of any condemnation of the practice by a Freudian.'[99] In a tribute to Malleson published in the *New Statesman and Nation* after her death, the journalist Kingsley Martin, who knew Malleson during the last years of her life, wrote that she 'early discovered that it was impossible to divide gynaecology from psychology [...] She could argue about Freud and Jung with psycho-analysts, and no doubt she found the key to many neuroses in their works. But a prolonged course of psychoanalysis is not a useful remedy to recommend to a woman with a family and a husband earning 10 pounds a week.'[100] Furthermore, publishing in different medical journals, she referred to the Freudian idea of psychosexual development of the child: 'In fact, psychologists assert that the earlier in infancy the trauma is experienced the more indelible will be its impression.'[101] In her sex manual for couples, she stated: 'What writers have largely failed to recognise, perhaps because they cannot tolerate the acceptance – is that many people's sexual handicaps are, since childhood, deeply engrained [...] I shall hope to show that most sexual disorders have a nervous origin.'[102]

For Malleson, what was at stake in trying to help couples face and overcome – if possible – their sexual difficulties was informing them about the unconscious barrier that prevented them from fully achieving climax. This approach was applied for inhibition of orgasm and vaginismus. She believed that most sexual disorders derived from emotions and from an inhibition of erotic impulses, restricted since early childhood. As a result, she asked her patients to talk and sought to find causes for 'inhibition' and 'vaginismus' in childhood traumatic experiences or unconscious conflicts. For instance, Malleson treated four cases of vaginismus and two cases of inhibition of orgasm at her clinic at University College Hospital. In the first case of vaginismus, the patient, attending for the second time said she had made some progress: 'I feel more relaxed and I feel much better and I feel less pain. I still feel in my mind that I need to relax. It is not physical, it is in my mind, and I cannot find a way to do that.' Malleson encouraged her to dig into her childhood memories to find any cause of possible trauma, as shown by the following excerpt:

- I have the impression that this wasn't only just the fear of being touched, but it was more likely to be a fear of some sort of memory from childhood that had frightened you. Your body might have a 'feeling memory'. You might not have a memory in words, but your body might have a feeling memory, and that any sort of sexual activity triggered early fears, very early fear also, and it was my impression that this feeling triggered early childhood fear, that you could quite forget. Did you not think of that yourself when we talked?
- I couldn't think of anything.
- But well, you know, it's even before remembering time. I think I did ask you if you slept with your parents and what sort of experiences you'd had? [...]
- I had a happy childhood. I was clean baby.
- You are an only child?
- No, I have two brothers.
- Well you probably slept with your parents quite a while. You might have seen things of which you were frightened. Babies are quite aware of sexual intercourse at eight, ten, twelve months – we know that. And when you have your own you must remember that you see. That can scare a child very deeply. But they won't be able to put it into words [...] You are afraid of an early experience happening to you again. Something that is good now and proper, but the fear still remains. I'd like you to think along those lines.[103]

Sexual disorders and infertility

She followed the same type of procedure with each patient, pushing them to explain what was going on in their sexual life and why they were seeking advice. By encouraging the patient to speak and reflect on their own sexual life, she challenged the sexual culture that told women to be ignorant and passive. She mediated between the prescriptive and the subjective, leading the patient to reflect on their own history; but also very often she put words into the patient's mouth, imposing, to some extent, her own views about their sexual life. Sexual counselling was an intense negotiation between patients' individual experience and needs and an expert's prescriptive advice. Indeed, while encouraging the patient to self-diagnose, Malleson nevertheless discouraged self-diagnosis when it came directly from the patient herself without having been first mediated by her, as shown by the following example with a 37 year-old divorced and remarried woman who lacked sexual pleasure in her current married life:

- Would you say your mental health has been better or worse since this last marriage?
- Much worse. Well, I think it's a reaction from the years before, opposition from my husband's parents. They like me but my circumstances, having been married once and having a daughter and, hum, I accepted that. There wasn't opposition to our marriage so much as an intense disapproval. His mother is very kind and very good, but she is a rather weepy type.
- So, don't let's wonder what caused it, but tell me the symptoms. Are you sleeping less well?[104]

In one case she also used the concept of transference, without naming it, which showed her deep knowledge of psychological concepts. To the frigid patient who did not express her love to her husband, she suggested that her cold behaviour reflected the hate she felt for her father instead of her husband:

- I believe your parents were really cruel to you. You're not being very nice back to your husband, are you? [...]
- My father had a terrible temper. After the last war, he came home like that. He was a changed man. My mother had a terrible life with him.
- You chose a husband of a very different sort from your own father, didn't you?
- Oh yes.
- But you're still treating him as if he were your father, aren't you?

- It's born in me really.
- No, it isn't born in you, it's made in you. And anything that is made in you, like a bad habit, is open to get over a little bit. You see, when your husband says: 'Do you love me?', what you ought to be saying is 'I hate my father and so you're getting it', instead of saying 'What is love?', which is a horrible answer.[105]

Besides developing a therapy based on discussion and in-depth reflection on the sexual experience of her patients, Malleson also elaborated practical means to improve female sexual life. For instance, she encouraged 'tight' women to dilate their hymen themselves: 'it is my own habit to show a woman how to do it for herself, and I imagine this reduces any psychological trauma to a minimum. I find only a very few cases which need a whiff of gas, or any real procedure.' She lent them different sizes of dilators to take home and ensured they came back for checking. Second, for women with secondary frigidity or vaginismus, she taught them the lying position they must adopt to relax the entrance of the vagina, which should ease the penetration of the penis. Through simple exercises that they practised within the office, Malleson educated and corrected her patient: 'It's all a matter of learning various sorts of tricks with your muscles to relax because you see it is not that a person is too small, it is about being too tight; they hold themselves too tight because they're frightened. If I show you some way to relax, it's easy to cure this disorder. It doesn't go on for ever, but you do need rather a special help.'[106] Vaginal lubrication was routinely prescribed by Malleson as a means to improve sexual relationships. She was convinced that a great deal of sexual disorders could be resolved by adequate lubrication, vaginal lubrication being of 'inestimable value'.[107] For women who lacked moisture and found penetration difficult, she would explain:

> You know the use of artificial lubricant is everything. The clue to the situation. No woman likes to be touched when it is dry and irritating instead of pleasant and even though he is not experienced he will sense if you are not moist and that you are not wanting him. It is like trying to eat a meal when you have a dry mouth it wouldn't work you see.[108]

Meanwhile, the therapy developed by Wright was based on her own experience with sexuality. Being married to a man five years younger, who was a virgin, meant that her sexual experiences had not been enjoyable from the beginning. In a private conversation with her biographer Barbara Evans, Wright explained:

> Peter being the kind, kind man he was, and having been brought up so far away from this idea, never thought in the least about it. I had to tell him. 'Peter', I said, 'I find this a bore'. It wasn't boring to him. He had his orgasm all right. 'Oh dear' he said, 'I am so sorry'. As if he'd broken a teacup.[109]

Already before marriage, Wright, anxious to have pleasant intercourse, looked for information in textbooks about her hymen and the way to stretch it herself. As a result, she recalled that the 'first intercourse wasn't painful, but everything felt dead. I didn't want to wound Peter, but I thought to myself, "there must be some way of doing this".'[110] She sought inspiration in books: she read the Kama Sutra and the six volumes of Havelock Ellis's *Studies in the Psychology of Sex* (1896). She then encouraged Peter to experiment with their sexual life, and 'they did'. During their married life, Wright had several lovers. Drawing on her readings and personal experience, Wright devised a method for the patient who consulted her about sexual difficulties. She would first begin the appointment with a physiology lesson with the help of a drawing of a nude male to give the patient a basic understanding of the sex organs. She would then go on with a lesson in the female and male anatomy and the sensitive part of their bodies. Using a mirror, she showed the patient the precise location of the clitoris and let her discover the joy of caressing it.[111] She then urged the patient to teach her partner her preferred rhythmic friction and emphasised that the man should also play his part and adapt to his partner rhythm for the patient to have an enjoyable sex life.

The seminars, set up after Malleson's death, derived from women doctors' will to meet their clients' needs. For instance, Dawkins remembered that when Malleson died in 1956, she 'had to take on her clinic' at University College Hospital. Having the feeling that she did not know enough, she attended Michael Balint's seminar on psychosexual counselling. Over a period of two years, the scheme provided weekly case seminars conducted by Balint, modelled on those provided by him at the Tavistock Clinic for General Practitioners. Balint was a Hungarian psychoanalyst who lived in London and worked as a consultant at the Tavistock Clinic in London. He developed a method to 'train' as opposed to 'teach' the general practitioner in psychotherapy based on the relationship between patient and doctor and group seminars. In Balint's view, more than one quarter of the work of the general practitioner consisted of providing psychotherapy. However, the general practitioner responded inadequately to these cases as, most of the time, his or her role was limited to prescribing a bottle of medicine or reassuring the patient that 'nothing organically wrong has been found'.[112] To remedy this problem, the general practitioner should acquire new skills: 'the doctor has to discover in himself an ability to listen to things in his patient that are barely said, and, in consequence, he will start listening to the same kind of language in himself'.

Formalising psychosexual training: the setting up of Balint's seminar 1958–74

To sum up Balint's main idea, the consultation between a doctor and patient is a moment of human negotiation in which the patient 'offers' his or her illness, which might not be the main reason for the consultation, and the doctor offers a response to it through listening, reassuring and suggesting a treatment. In so doing, the doctor 'helps the patient to organise an illness around certain symptoms'.[113] However, the way the doctor answers the demands of his or her patient in turn influences what a patient expects and says. Moreover, the doctor's answer is shaped by what Balint called the 'apostolic function of the doctor', which is the meaning and perception that the doctor gives to his or her work. The doctor's training, the mores within the medical profession, and the doctor's personality are all factors influencing this apostolic function, creating an 'automatic pattern of response'. Therefore, in addition to the patient, the doctor should also be considered an object of study so as to free himself or herself from this automatic pattern. The training provided by Balint consisted of a group of eight to ten doctors led by a 'supervisor' or 'leader'. Each doctor was instructed to share his or her own experience with ongoing cases and to describe, as frankly as possible, his or her difficulties. The cohesion of the group would enable the doctor to identify mistakes, blind spots and limitations, allowing a better understanding of his or her problems. Sharing their experiences encouraged the doctors to experiment, thereby breaking the automatic behaviour.

From 1958 onwards, a group of ten women doctors followed this training scheme and met under the guidance of Balint to discuss individual cases of 'sexual and marital disharmony'. The group included Sylvia Dawkins, who had worked with the FPA for over twenty years when she started the training; Rosalie Taylor, who had twenty-five years of experience in medical gynaecology; Jean Pasmore, a general practitioner; Mary Pollock, a gynaecologist; Alison Giles, a general practitioner who had worked for the FPA for ten years; Eleanor Mears, who had seventeen years of experience in medical gynaecology; Margaret Blair, a general practitioner with an interest in medical gynaecology; Rosamond Bischoff, a specialist in medical gynaecology and obstetrics; Ruth Lloyd-Thomas, a general practitioner; and Eileen Mallinson, a maternity and child welfare medical officer.

As explained by Balint, the aim of these meetings was to 'develop therapeutic techniques by combining the routine gynaecological and the psychotherapeutic examination into one integrated approach to the patient's problems'. Since most of the patients coming to family planning centres were women, members of the training scheme primarily discussed female sexual difficulties, the more common ones being non-consummation and dyspareunia. The group shed light on the main reason behind these sexual difficulties, which they attributed to the female patient's inability to accept her own body as a site of pleasure for both her and her partner. In addition, the group identified various 'nightmarish phantasies' about what a sexual relationship should be. The therapy developed by the group to resolve these difficulties consisted of trying to find the reason for the patient's rejection of her own body.[114] Three main publications resulted from these meetings: in 1961, Alison Giles published 'Learning to deal with sexual difficulties' in the *Family Planning Journal*, while Sylvia Dawkins and Rosalie Taylor wrote 'Non-consummation of marriage' for the *Lancet* and, in 1962, Leonard Friedman released *Virgin Wives: A Study of Unconsummated Marriages*. The book offered an analysis of non-consummation in marriage based on the classifications of patients into three categories. The first category was the 'sleeping beauty' – namely patients who 'restrict conscious awareness of sexual feelings. They use the defence mechanism of "not knowing" about their sexual organs to ward off anxiety.'[115] The second category was 'aggressive women', who made their husbands impotent. In these cases, the doctor had to be able to decode the behaviour of the patient while simultaneously being aware of his or her own feelings towards the latter. The last category was women who were still virgin, but nevertheless became virgin mothers through the injection of their husband's semen into their vagina with a syringe. In all cases, the therapeutic method developed is one of interpreting the patient's conflicts rather than reassuring her. One recurrent element, emphasised by numerous doctors who undertook this psychosexual training, was the fact that patients revealed their deepest anxieties, fears and fantasies during the vaginal examination. Consequently, several doctors referred to it as 'the moment of truth'. Doctors encouraged their patients to describe what they thought their vagina and uterus looked like and, to dissipate any misconceptions, urged them to explore it and feel it for themselves.[116]

Aside from Balint's training, two other leaders oversaw psychosexual training: Dr Tom Main, director of the Cassel Marital Clinic, and Dr Thompson, a senior member of the staff of the Tavistock Clinic. There was resistance from the FPA headquarters to the formal implementation of sexual counselling and its connected training, in part due to financial constraints and in part to do with the nature of the service provided. Prudence Tunnadine recalled the way people working in sexual counselling were deemed a 'lunatic' fringe:

> It was very interesting that in the beginning of our work in psychosexual medicine, which arose because in those years, in the '50s, there were no, not all this wide and wild variety of sex therapy that [there is] today, and we recognised quite early that one thing people hoped for, without even necessarily being able to dare to say so, was help with the quality of their sex lives. And those of us who tried to find ways to help them, quite seriously studying the emotional aspects, um, found quite a lot in the hierarchy of the FPA and of their lay workers who thought this was very lunatic fringe stuff indeed, um, and it's been an awful struggle.[117]

Thus, seminar training arose from a grassroots base; it emerged from the pressure of many doctors requesting help to deal with their patients' sexual problems. First established informally, they grew in numbers, and formal, official training was put together in 1974.[118] These seminars appeared to be more conventional than subversive in terms of the gender roles they conveyed, since they relied heavily on Freud's vision of sexuality and urged male and female patients to comply with and perform the traditional gender roles of the feminine and loving wife and the masculine, active and virile husband.

Under the training of Balint and Main, women doctors developed a more gendered, differentiated perception of sexual behaviours, linked with notions of femininity and masculinity. Indeed, in the 1966 *Handbook on Family Planning*, Jean Pasmore, who was trained by Balint, presented frigidity as the expression of a woman's 'fear or dislike of physical relationship with the man, her difficulty in accepting the social role of being a woman and her resentment against the man'.[119] In her 1970 book, based on her individual practice as a sexual counsellor in a family planning clinic and her training under Thomas Main, Prudence Tunnedine presented a case of secondary frigidity: a mother who could no longer experience orgasm. Resorting to gendered expressions of femininity, Tunnedine argued that her patient's childhood explained this lack of sexual pleasure:

> The patient had been tomboyish in childhood, intolerant of silly girly things and her mother has said that she could be feminine but not in an obvious way. She could accept the doctor's interpretation that perhaps she could be motherly but not sexy, and was able to discuss her difficulty with tenderness [...] She presented as jolly and hearty, and the doctor was able to show her that this tomboyish heartiness was a defence system against her fears of foolish girlish tenderness. She returned looking more feminine with a new fluffy hairstyle and pretty clothes, her sexual life already improved.[120]

Tunnadine also narrowed the notion of frigidity as described by Malleson from an absence of feelings to the inability to achieve vaginal orgasm within the act of intercourse; therefore, she adopted the penis–vagina fixation denounced by Wright. When she acknowledged the role of the clitoris in sexual pleasure, she asserted that, departing from Masters and Johnson's analysis of vaginal orgasm as the result of the penis petting the clitoris, this type of orgasm conveyed a different emotional signification: 'the togetherness, mutual abandonment of control systems, the emotional acceptance of the penis and all it implies in terms of the man, and of the vagina and all it implies in terms of the woman, make this a unique experience that is not mimicked emotionally by mutual masturbation, however loving'.[121] Her approach to frigidity was deeply rooted in Freud's theory of child development. Indeed, she further invoked the concept of 'penis envy' to explain why some women could not achieve vaginal orgasm: they unconsciously envied 'man, the organ and all it represents and reacted against them with resentment, anger and the need to control and destroy'.[122] This depiction of female sexuality would be strongly criticised by second-wave feminists. As this example illustrates, although the 1960s are often perceived as a period of sexual radicalism, this does not hold true for sexual counselling. In terms of sexual counselling, the period featured a return to traditional values around gendered responsibilities within marriage.

Sterility session

The second orientation of the work done under the label 'sub-fertility' was the handling of sterility cases and difficulties conceiving. Again, this service was grounded in patients' demand for advice on the issue. From the 1920s, scientific developments took place within the field of infertility; tubal insufflation and the salpingogram became used as tests for tubal patency. Despite these new techniques, surgeries were still rare and women's chances of conceiving remained low. Semen analysis was increasingly practised, but there was no consensus on the number of sperm needed for successful conception.[123] Until the setting up of specialised sessions in family planning clinics, medical 'treatments' for infertility were still only available on a private basis. For instance, Margaret Moore White was the first assistant at the gynaecology department of the Royal Free Hospital, where she treated infertile patients from the mid-1930s onwards. Mary Barton counselled infertile patients in her private practice. The latter was famous for practicing artificial insemination by donors – the sperm came from anonymous donors, among them her second husband, Dr Berthold Wiesner, who was said to have fathered more than a hundred babies – and many patients who wrote to the FPA in the late 1940s asking for advice on this practice were referred to her. Other famous male professionals, such as Wiesner and Kenneth Walker, also specialised in infertility.

However, it was only after 1930, when Margaret Jackson started to advise and treat couples for infertility in the Exeter and District Women's Welfare Centre, that the possibility of seeking medical treatment opened up for working-class and middle-class patients. Out of the total number of patients attending the clinic in 1933, only 1 per cent sought advice on infertility. In 1943, this had increased to 33 per cent, totalling 161 patients.[124] Initially, Jackson wished to refer the patients in need of full investigation and treatment 'elsewhere', but she rapidly realised that there were no facilities to deal with them and if this type of work 'was to be done at all', members of the clinic 'had better do it themselves.'[125] Consequently, she actively looked for financial and material help with developing this new area of work through three essential steps: acquiring new skills and instruments, access to an X-ray department, and access to a laboratory that could run semen analysis and examine biological materials. These requirements were met through the support of the Royal Devon and Exeter Hospital and their radiology department, and the University College of the South West of England, which allowed the free use of their facilities; this was where the medical secretary of the clinic, Mrs Clare Harvey – who had previously been trained as a biologist – could examine vaginal and seminal fluid and cervical mucus. Based on this specialised work, Exeter grew in reputation and patients were sent to the clinic from general practitioners and hospitals.

Exeter was not the only place that endeavoured to answer patients' cries for help in sub-fertility matters. In 1942, Helena Wright suggested to the medical committee of the North Kensington Women's Welfare Centre that a new session be started, dedicated to the investigation of sterility cases.[126] Similarly, Joan Malleson encouraged the FPA to address the needs of patients through the opening of 'motherhood clinics' where patients could be advised on sexual disorders and sub-fertility. In 1943, at the height of wartime mobilisation, the president of the FPA, Lord Horder, published an article in the *Lancet* that informed his colleagues of the relevance of the work done in FPA clinics at a time of declining birth rate: 'In view of the fact that at least 10 per cent of married couples suffer from involuntary sterility, it is obvious that the problem of such sterility is one of great national importance, not only because of the personal unhappiness it may cause, but because [of] the urgent need to increase our present birth-rate if a falling population is to be averted.'[127] This anxiety about the state of the British population should be understood in view of the fact that, in 1943, Britain was looking ahead of the war, as the Beveridge Report testifies, and was increasingly thinking about rebuilding the country. In this context, the state of the population was put on the political agenda, as exemplified by the setting up of the

Royal Commission on Population in 1944. Horder announced the creation of an ad hoc committee 'which intended to organise clinics to deal with cases of sterility either by referring them where necessary to the appropriate hospital centres or where these do not exist by providing such expert attention as facilities permit'. The committee was made up of leading experts in infertility: Margaret Jackson, Joan Malleson, Margaret Moore White, Annis Gillie, Alex Bourne, William Nixon, Cedric Lane Robert, Kenneth Walker and Albert Sharman. To assess practitioners' willingness to offer sterility sessions, the subcommittee sent out a questionnaire to all clinic medical officers. While some of them saw no necessity to develop this work, since local hospitals took care of this aspect, a great number of medical officers had seen enough interest and demand from patients to want to integrate this aspect, as shown by the answer from Dr Gwendoline Smith: 'This question of sterility is a problem in our Carlisle Clinic. I get quite a lot of it, and so far have been able to do very little for the women and I am very glad this subject is considered and hope something really helpful will be the results.'[128] These answers led the subcommittee to prioritise the opening of a laboratory in London for semen analysis. In 1944, following several months of debate and tension between members of the subcommittee on the best strategy to adopt – i.e. whether to open a sub-fertility clinic or use the resources of St Mary's Hospital, London to carry out seminal tests – a seminological centre opened in London under the supervision of Dr Hans Davidson, expert in seminology. The clinic saw an average of 2,000 patients per annum.[129] In September, an infertility conference was held in Exeter, where Margaret Jackson and Claire Harvey taught medical officers the basics of semen analysis. From then onwards, the FPA organised an annual sub-fertility conference where participants covered male infertility in depth, and basic procedures for testing husbands and wives were presented.[130]

Following this new emphasis on sub-fertility, the North Kensington Women's Welfare Centre appointed a consultant gynaecologist, Dr Kathleen Harding, to their sub-fertility clinic in 1945. The work was slow to develop, since many clinics maintained their close relationship with local hospitals and referred their patients to them. In 1950, Kathleen Harding pleaded for more sub-fertility clinics in the work of the FPA at the general meeting. Based on her own experience, both in North Kensington and in hospital, she urged FPA clinics to develop this aspect of the work, since it required 'more patience, understanding and perseverance than most aspect[s] of obstetrics and gynaecology'. Such work was better suited to FPA clinics than to hospitals, where time was a central issue. Supporting her claim, she put the patient's emotions at the centre of her argument, emphasising that well-being was central in FPA clinics and that it 'means a great deal to a patient who is so sensitive about her failure to reproduce (as it was still the woman who sought treatment first)'.[131] While the work was slow to grow, mainly due to lack of funding, it nevertheless expanded. In 1957, twelve clinics held special sub-fertility sessions, and out of the 220 family planning clinics 170 gave preliminary advice and referred their patients to local hospitals.[132] The work continued to develop in the 1960s.

The topic of infertility was, however, not confined to the world of the clinic; it broke out in the wider medical circle in the mid-1940s. A great number of articles were published in medical journals to inform doctors about the issue of infertility, trying to offer lines of inquiry and suggestions for treating sub-fertility and infertility from the interwar years onwards. Again, a great number of these articles were authored by women doctors who encountered this problem in their private practice and at family planning clinics. Chief among them were Margaret Jackson, Margaret Moore White, Mary Barton, Katherine Harding and Joan Malleson. Their main contribution was the articulation of a guideline of extremely detailed medical procedures that doctors should follow in order to identify, diagnose and handle sub-fertility cases. They covered the array of laboratory techniques to diagnose and identify the causes of infertility, published their latest results, and helped advance the state of research in the field.[133]

They published together, as shown by the joint paper from Margaret Moore White and Mary Barton published in 1951 in the *British Medical Journal*.[134] Beyond the focus on medical procedure, women doctors actively challenged the gender dynamic underpinning fertility diagnosis. In fact, infertility was commonly perceived as a female pathology, since 'diseases affecting reproductive health were principally addressed under the auspices of gynaecology during the nineteenth and early twentieth centuries, thereby establishing infertility as a female problem'.[135] It was against this background that women doctors tried to dismiss the assumption that the causes of infertility must be related to the woman. For instance, in 1935, Frances Huxley, member of the

Medical Women's Federation and birth control activist, published *The Clinical Study of Sterility Cases with Notes and Treatment* in the bulletin of the federation. Drawing on the knowledge gained after a visit to fertility clinics in the US, she familiarised her female colleagues with this topic. She introduced her readers to different methods of determining sterility: insufflation of CO_2 into the uterus and tubes, and the battery of tests made by a clinic that not only tested the wife but also the husband. She then presented a step-by-step description of the way she handled sterility cases. She first showed how to diagnose sterility and reviewed all the possible causes. She dealt with the wife *and* the husband, insisted on obtaining a 'report of the doctor who made the examination',[136] and used the Huhner test, which detects active spermatozoa. Similarly, in an article presenting the work she carried out at the Exeter and District Women's Welfare Centre in 1944, Margaret Jackson insisted on investigating the husband: 'too often women are subjected to examination and operation without their husbands having been asked to submit a seminal specimen for examination'.[137] This emphasis yielded positive results; during the 1947 FPA conference on infertility, a speaker underlined that both spouses should be examined:

> it was perhaps natural that in the earlier years, the study of infertility should be largely concerned with the part played by the woman; she is usually the first to become impatient at her failure to conceive, and the grosser conditions that may impair fertility are readily detected. It may even be suggested that one of the reasons for initially one-sided investigation was that the majority of investigators could not allow their scientific impartiality to overcome their human vanity and admit that their own sex could in this sense be the weaker one.[138]

Similarly, Margaret Moore White, in a 1947 article published in *The Practitioner*, reminded the reader:

> two persons are concerned in a fertile mating and an average of four to five [factors] militate against conception in every unfertile couple. In most cases, some measure of responsibility rests on both sides, and from the methods of investigation at present available, it would appear that male is equally as responsible as female ... Care should be taken to ensure that one party does not embark on some expensive treatment until it is known whether any absolute contraindication is present in the other.[139]

The acknowledgement of the possibility that men could be responsible for sterility seemed to have won acceptance in 1960, to the extent that Kathleen Harding affirmed: 'the fact that the man is responsible in quite one-third of the couples is now accepted'.[140] This shift plausibly reflected a change in attitude towards gender roles in heterosexual relationships, as the rise of companionate marriage meant that a more egalitarian relationship was encouraged.

Aside from these technical publications, more accessible work was published by the FPA, such as the leaflet *Childless Wife*, which offered detailed but simple explanations of possible causes for infertility and a step-by-step guide to seeking medical help. The leaflet started by asserting that infertility was not a given and couples should seek advice:

> A delay of even a few years does not necessarily mean that the marriage is going to be barren. A couple who have had two years of regular married life together without conceiving a child are wise to get help. It is probable that in England about one couple out of ten is unable to have children; and of these probably at least one third could be set right with proper medical attention.[141]

The leaflet offered basic information on the biology of reproduction and provided advice on the best bodily position to adopt for increasing the chance of conception and the optimal time for conception. It described the possible causes and means to diagnose infertility in the husband and the wife, such as post-coital tests, semen analysis, tubal insufflation, support of the womb in the vagina, electric heat and glandular injections. In cases where total infertility was diagnosed, adoption was to be recommended. Women were urged to seek treatment, and those who failed to get pregnant without trying all the other alternatives were said not to deserve sympathy: 'The woman who is disappointed should not really ask for sympathy until she has consulted a doctor and undertaken every possible measure he suggests.' This excerpt shows the pressure women were under and the gender expectations underpinning fertility treatment. This pathologisation of the sterile wife that accepted her situation without looking for medical advice indicated a faith in medicine and the new role taken by doctors in the handling of sexual lives.

Connected to infertility was the hotly contested topic of artificial insemination by donor (AID), or what were commonly called 'test-tube babies'. Margaret Jackson, Mary Barton, Margaret Moore White, Joan Malleson and Helena Wright defended and/or practised this procedure in their private practices as early as the late 1930s. The FPA, which still had difficulties establishing its legitimacy, was reluctant to engage with this controversial topic. As a result, the association provided advice on treatment for infertility and then referred patients who wanted AID to Mary Barton and Margaret Jackson. Malleson also designed a syringe for artificial insemination that was manufactured by Allen & Hanburys.[142]

A debate on AID took place in the House of Lords in July 1943, followed by an answer from Mary Barton in the *BMJ*, which triggered dozens of letters in the column of the journal. This debate has been analysed in detail by historians Angus McLaren, Naomi Pfeffer and Andrew Hanley.[143] What needs to be remembered is the crucial role played by women doctors in the advocacy for artificial insemination. Also, these debates focused mainly on the ethical and moral aspects of AID, to the great despair of Margaret Jackson, who complained in the *BMJ*:

> there can be few subjects which call forth more emotional (as opposed to intellectual) [response] than AID [...] It is of prime importance that doctors should think about and weigh these things in the light of their special knowledge and experience, setting aside in so far as they can, or at any rate recognising, their own emotional particular bias in the matter.[144]

Nevertheless, the debates eased public concern about the subject and gave rise to numerous letters to the FPA from childless individuals who wanted to try this method. These letters revealed the agency of patients, who were proactive in searching for advice and treatment on the issue of sub-fertility; patient agency was an important element in the development of sub-fertility services.[145]

The issue of AID remained a contentious one throughout the 1950s, as shown by the setting up of the Feversham Committee in 1958. Its aim was 'to enquire into the existing practice of human artificial insemination and its legal consequences; and to consider whether, taking account of the interests of individuals involved and of society as a whole, any change in the law is necessary or desirable'.[146] Several doctors who practised the method were appointed as experts, more than half of them being female doctors: Margaret Jackson, Eleanor Mears, Mary

Barton and Helena Wright. Their role was therefore recognised as an important one in the issue of infertility. The debate took place between opponents of AID, who viewed this procedure as sinful and considered it beyond the scope of the medical profession, and partisans of it, who regarded it as a valuable means to help childless people. The outcome of this fierce debate was that AID between consenting adults should not be prohibited. In her report for the *Journal of the Family Planning Association*, Margaret Jackson commented on the selection of experts for the Feversham Committee:

> There would seem, however to be one glaring omission from this formidable list of individual and corporate witnesses – nobody from the select band of barren couples was called … without whom the notion of A.I. would not have arisen and whose views and experiences are surely of some importance.[147]

Her remark has two key interests. First, it shows Jackson's awareness of the need to listen to and integrate the individual experiences of sterile couples, which had been absent from the public debate on infertility until then. It reflects her own medical ethic, which placed individual experiences and needs at the core of her practice. Second, it shows that infertility, while known by everyone, was not publicly recognised. Despite the repeated attacks on the practice, women doctors persisted in helping the patients who asked for AID. The procedure therefore continued to be practised alongside new assisted reproductive technologies, such as in vitro fertilisation.

Conclusion

During the interwar years, in a context of fears about marriage – thought of as the cornerstone of British society – and population at the fore of political concerns, women doctors developed sexual counselling and infertility advice as a way of preserving the stability of marriage as an institution. They framed this side of their work as the positive side of family planning and medicalised sexual disorders. However, while their aim could be called 'traditional' from our post-feminist perspective, the methods and ideas they developed were radical and challenged common assumptions around gender roles. Indeed, with the issues of sexual disorders and infertility, they called into question the lack of acknowledgement of women's sexual pleasure for the former and the strong bias towards women's responsibility for infertility for the latter. They also spread information, through medical articles and sexual manuals, on the sexual relationship and its associated difficulties. Hence, women doctors were pivotal in developing sexual counselling in interwar Britain. They did so as a result of the sexual disorders their patients faced. By listening to their patients' needs, difficulties and emotions, they forged therapeutics that emphasised the role of the clitoris as the place for sexual pleasure. In so doing, they challenged the central role of the vagina. While their views might have been at some points contradictory, they nevertheless opened the way for more female agency in the realm of sexuality. Wright was ahead of her time in her gendered analysis of sexual roles, while Malleson anticipated the second-wave feminist criticism of the increasing pressure to achieve orgasm, or what she called the 'fallacy of orgasm'. The period in which they actively pressed the extension of the work of the clinic (1930–56) should be considered as a peak of radicalism that would die down when formal training in sexual counselling was established in the 1960s.

Regarding the issue of sub-fertility, here, again, women doctors met their patients' needs by creating sub-fertility sessions and practising AID in their private practice. They also advocated for testing the husband, therefore breaking with the tradition of performing long and, too often, useless invasive treatments and surgical procedures on the female body only. But invasive investigations on women continued once the husband had been tested and found to have adequate sperm. Family planning clinics therefore offered a privileged space for developing new skills and fields of expertise, as well as cutting-edge therapy in sexual health. Women doctors working in these spaces created a new professional identity that revolved around a holistic approach to family planning where their patients' needs were taken seriously. All in all, looking at the historical development of sexual and infertility counselling helps to correct the myth of all-powerful doctors counselling passive patients.

Notes

1 Wellcome Collection, London, PP/MAL/4, 'J. Malleson, 2 clinical studies of women who failed to get orgasm'.

2 The purpose of this chapter is not to reify the nomenclature used by these women doctors, since recent works have shown how problematic it was. See in particular: P. Cryle and A. Moore, *Frigidity: An Intellectual History* (Basingstoke: Palgrave Macmillan, 2011); C. Beccalossi, 'Nineteenth-century European psychiatry on same-sex desires: pathology, abnormality, normality and the blurring of boundaries', *Psychology & Sexuality*, 1:3 (2010), pp. 226–38; I. D. Crozier, 'The medical construction of homosexuality and its relation to the law in nineteenth-century England', *Medical History*, 45:1 (2001), pp. 61–82; R. Beachy, 'The German invention of homosexuality', *The Journal of Modern History*, 82:4 (2010), pp. 801–38.

3 A. Mold, 'Repositioning the patient: patient organisations, consumerism, and autonomy in Britain during the 1960s and 1970s', *Bulletin of the History of Medicine*, 87:2 (2013), p. 226.

4 This was not only the case with sexual counselling. Anne Digby argued that patients appreciated female practitioners' commitment. Women doctors 'appear to have achieved an empathy, a personal closeness that was more rarely found (or at least acknowledged) amongst their male colleagues'. See Digby, *The Evolution of British General Practice*, p. 185. A similar conclusion was reached for the US: see R. Morantz-Sanchez, *Sympathy and Science: Women Physicians in American Medicine* (Oxford: Oxford University Press, 1985).

5 L. Davidoff et al., *The Family Story: Blood, Contract and Intimacy* (London: Longman, 1998); J. Finch and P. Summerfield, 'Social reconstruction and the emergence of companionate marriage, 1945–59' in D. Clarke (ed.), *Marriage, Domestic Life and Social Change: Writings for Jacqueline Burgoyne (1944–88)* (London: Routledge, 1991), pp. 7–32; Rebreyend, *Intimités amoureuses*. For the US see also Simmons, *Making Marriage Modern*.

6 A. Moore, 'Relocating Marie Bonaparte's clitoris', *Australian Feminist Studies*, 24:60 (2009), pp. 149–65.

7 S. Freud, *Three Essays on the Theory of Sexuality: The 1905 Edition* (New York: Verso, 2017).

8 H. Cook, 'Sex and the doctors: the medicalisation of sexuality as a two-way process in early to mid-twentieth-century Britain', in W. de Blécourt and C. Usborne (eds), *Cultural Approaches to the History of Medicine* (Basingstoke: Palgrave Macmillan, 2004), pp. 192–211; M. Jackson, *The Real Facts of Life: Feminism and the Politics of Sexuality, c.1850–1940* (London: Taylor & Francis, 1994); R. Porter and L. Hall, *The Facts of Life: The Creation of Sexual Knowledge in Britain, 1650–1950* (New Haven: Yale University Press, 1995); J. Neuhaus, 'The importance of being orgasmic: sexuality, gender, and marital sex manuals in the United States, 1920–63', *Journal of the History of Sexuality*, 9:4 (2000), pp. 447–73.

9 Szreter and Fisher have however nuanced this depressing depiction of marital sexuality. Szreter and Fisher, *Sex Before the Sexual Revolution*.
10 Irwin has analysed the 1970s and 1980s. See R. Irwin, 'To try and find out what is being done to whom, by whom and with what results': the creation of psychosexual counselling policy in England, 1972–79' *Twentieth Century British History*, 20:2 (2009), pp. 173–97; R. Irwin 'Recalling the early years of psychosexual nursing.' *Oral History*, 39:1 (2011), pp. 43–52.
11 Cook, 'Sex and the doctors'.
12 L. Featherstone, 'The science of pleasure: medicine and sex therapy in mid-twentieth-century Australia', *Social History of Medicine*, 31:3 (2018), pp. 445–61; A. Grossman, *Reforming Sex: The German Movement for Birth Control and Abortion Reform, 1920–50* (Oxford: Oxford University Press, 1995), pp. 66–70.
13 Wellcome Collection, London, SA/FPA/A16/1, 'Ninth Annual Report of the Family Planning Association'.
14 On the history of the mental hygiene movement see J. Toms, 'MIND, anti-psychiatry, and the case of the mental hygiene movement's 'discursive transformation', *Social History of Medicine* [online], hky096, available at: https://doi.org/10.1093/shm/hky096 (accessed 25 June 2020). See also J. Toms, *Mental Hygiene and Psychiatry in Modern Britain* (Basingstoke: Palgrave Macmillan, 2013). For an overview of developments in mental health service see J. Busfield, 'Restructuring mental health services in twentieth century Britain' in M. Gijswijt-Hofstra and R. Porter (eds), *Cultures of Psychiatry*, Clio Medica 49 (Amsterdam: Rodopi, 1998), pp. 9–28.
15 On Malleson's training in psychology see C. Rusterholz, '"You can't dismiss that as being less happy, you see it is different". Sexual therapy in 1950s England', *Twentieth Century British History*, 30:3 (2019), pp. 375–98.
16 Wellcome Collection, London, SA/FPA/ NK225, 'Psychological advice: Minutes of the 23 medical committee meetings, 22 march 1935'. See also the article by Irwin, '"To try and find out"'.
17 For a history of this concept see: Szreter and Fisher, *Sex Before the Sexual Revolution*; Davidoff et al., *The Family Story*; Finch and Summerfield, 'Social reconstruction'; Fisher, *Birth Control*.
18 Collins, *Modern Love*, p. 90.
19 Wellcome Collection, London, SA/FPA/A14/32, 'Letter from the secretary of the N.B.C.A to Edward Griffith, April 14th 1939'.
20 On the history of the Marriage Guidance Council see J. Lewis, D. Clark and D. Morgan, *Whom God Hath Joined Together: Work of Marriage Guidance* (London: Routledge, 1992).

21 See in particular Collins, *Modern Love*, chapter 4; Brooke, *Sexual Politics*, pp. 117–23.
22 Langhamer, *The English in Love*, p. 6.
23 Wellcome Collection, London, PP/EFG/A.2, 'Marriage Guidance advisory board, 1938–9'.
24 Wellcome Collection, London, SA/FPA/A13/69/1, 'Marriage Guidance Council leaflets'.
25 Wellcome Collection, London, PP/PRE/J.1/22/19, 'Interview carried [out] by Barbara Evans with Lady Houghton, 1982'.
26 Wellcome Collection, London, SA/FPA/A14/32, 'Letter from Edward Griffith to Acting Secretary of the FPA, undated 1939'.
27 Wellcome Collection, London, SA/FPA/A14/32, 'Letter from Acting Secretary of the FPA to Edward Griffith 16th January 1940'.
28 Wellcome Collection, London, SA/FPA/A3/5, 'Letter from Mrs Bowmer, secretary of the Women's married centre at Welwyn Garden City to Mrs Robins, 4 June 1948'.
29 Wellcome Collection, London, GC/105/26, 'Interview with Sylvia Dawkins, In the Club'.
30 While in Britain psychoanalysis and psychology were at first met with reluctance among the elite in medicine, education and caring professions, after the Second World War psychology was embraced by the majority and came to be used on a daily basis. The incorporation of psychology into marriage guidance counselling, as funded by the welfare state in postwar Britain, has been a subject of recent interest. See T. Chettiar, 'The Psychiatric Family: Citizenship, Private Life, and Emotional Health in Welfare-State Britain, 1945–79'. PhD dissertation, University of Evanston, 2013; Lewis, Clark and Morgan, *Whom God Hath Joined Together*; Langhamer, *The English in Love*, in particular chapters 7 and 8; Collins, *Modern Love*.
31 Wellcome Collection, London, SA/FPA/A5/88, 'Minutes of the medical sub-committee, 24th January 1949'.
32 J. Malleson, *Any Wife or Any Husband: A Book for Couples Who Have Met Sexual Difficulties and for Doctors* (London: Penguin Handbook, 1950), p. 153.
33 Wellcome Collection, London, SA/FPA/NK26, 'Letter from Joan Malleson to Dr Irwin, 12 July 1954'.
34 Wellcome Collection, London, SA/FPA/A6/10, 'Report of a Conference of Clinic Medical Officers and nurses held at the Queen Mary Hall, London, Saturday 26th November 1955', p. 5.
35 *Ibid.*
36 *Ibid.*, p. 6.
37 Wellcome Collection, London, SA/FPA/A5/109, 'Training and reorientation of doctors'.

38 Formed of Dr Balint, Dr Rosamond Bischoff, Mrs Burrell, Dr Dawkins, Dr Edwards and Neal Edwards, Dr Hinds, Mrs Raphael, Dr Smelt, Dr Swyer and Dr Rosalie Taylor.
39 Wellcome Collection, London, SA/FPA/A5/98, 'Minutes of the meeting held in London, 7th November 1957, Ad hoc committee on help in sex problems in marriage and related matters within the scope of the Association's objects'.
40 Wellcome Collection, London, SA/FPA/NK70, 'Letter from Margaret Blair to Clinic Medical Officers, 28th March 1958'.
41 Malleson, *Any Wife*, p. 11.
42 *Ibid.*, p. 143.
43 'Obituary', *Lancet*, 267:6926 (1956), p. 810.
44 'Obituary', *British Medical Journal*, 1:4977 (1956), p. 1242.
45 J. Borge, 'The Psychosexual Counselling Tapes of Dr Joan Malleson: New Theories'. Unpublished MA thesis, Institute of Historical Research, School of Advanced Study, University of London, 2012.
46 W. C. W. Nixon, 'Joan Malleson', *British Medical Journal*, 1:4978 (1956), p. 1304.
47 Wellcome Collection, London, J. Malleson, PP/MAL/3, '4 short cases of vaginismus'.
48 I analysed these tapes in detail through an emotional history lens. See Rusterholz, '"You can't dismiss that as being less happy"'.
49 H. Wright, *More about the Sex Factor in Marriage* (London: Williams and Norgate, 1947), p. 9.
50 J. Malleson, 'Vaginismus: its management and psychogenesis', *British Medical Journal*, 2:4259 (1942), pp. 213–16.
51 Malleson, *The Principles of Contraception*, p. 63.
52 Wellcome Collection, London, SA/FPA/A16/24/19, 'Sex Facts, Married Life, 1949'.
53 Wellcome Collection, London, SA/FPA/A16/24/19, 'Sex problems in Marriage I, A doctor advises, 1949'.
54 *Ibid.*
55 H. Wright, *The Sex Factor in Marriage: A Book for Those who Are, or are About to Be, Married* (London: Noel Douglas, 1930), p. 6.
56 Wright, *More about the Sex Factor in Marriage*, p. 7.
57 Women's Library, London School of Economics, London, 8SUF/B/149, 'Interview with Helena Wright'.
58 Wellcome Collection, London, GC/105/26, 'In the club, interview with Sylvia Dawkins'.
59 *Ibid.*
60 See in particular Collins, *Modern Love*, chapter 4; A. McLaren, *Reproduction by Design: Sex, Robots, Trees, and Test-Tube Babies in Interwar Britain*

(Chicago: University of Chicago Press, 2012), chapter 3; Brooke, *Sexual Politics*, pp. 117–23.
61 J. Lewis, *The Politics of Motherhood: Child and Maternal Welfare in England, 1900–1939* (London: Croom Helm, 1980); J. Lewis, 'The working-class wife and mother and state intervention, 1870–1918' in J. Lewis (ed.), *Women's Experience of Home and Family, 1850–1940* (Oxford: Blackwell, 1986). On medically trained public servants see J. Welshman, *Municipal Medicine: Public Health in Twentieth-Century Britain* (Oxford: Peter Lang, 2000); S. Szreter, *Health and Wealth: Studies in History and Policy* (Rochester, NY: University of Rochester Press, 2005), pp. 281–341. On antenatal clinics see S. Al-Gailani, '"The mothers of England object": public health, privacy and professional ethics in the early twentieth-century debate over the notification of pregnancy', *Social History of Medicine*, 33:1 (2020), pp. 18–40.
62 Malleson, *The Principles of Contraception*, p. 25.
63 Ibid.
64 Wright, *The Sex Factor in Marriage*, p. 12.
65 Women's Library, London School of Economics, London, 8SUF/B/149, 'Interview with Helena Wright'.
66 Malleson, *The Principles of Contraception*, p. 83.
67 Wellcome Collection, London, SA/FPA/A16/24/19, 'Sex problems in Marriage I, A doctor advises'.
68 Ibid.
69 Wellcome Collection, London, SA/FPA/A16/24/19, J. Malleson, 'Sex Facts, Married Life'.
70 J. Malleson, 'Sexual disorders in women, their medical significance', *British Medical Journal*, 2:4746 (1951), p. 1480.
71 Wellcome Collection, London, PP/MAL/4, J. Malleson, '2 clinical studies of women who failed to get orgasm'.
72 Ibid.
73 Ibid.
74 Wellcome Collection, London, PP/MAL/4', 'Inhibition of orgasm'.
75 Wellcome Collection, London, PP/MAL/2, 'Scottish woman having acute anxiety neurosis 1950s?'.
76 Ibid.
77 Wellcome Collection, London, PP/MAL/10, 'Record of a most severe vaginismus'.
78 G. Davis, 'A tragedy as old as history, medical response to infertility in Britain' in Davis and Loughran, *The Palgrave Handbook of Infertility in History*, p. 371.
79 Wellcome Collection, London, PP/MAL/3, '4 short cases of vaginismus'.

80 Wellcome Collection, London, PP/MAL/5, 'This couple were referred by a psychiatrist for marriage guidance'.
81 *Ibid.*
82 *Ibid.*
83 *Ibid.*
84 Szreter and Fisher, *Sex Before the Sexual Revolution*, p. 319.
85 Wright, *The Sex Factor in Marriage*, p. 31.
86 *Ibid.*
87 *Ibid.*
88 Wright, *More about the Sex Factor in Marriage*, p. 46.
89 *Ibid.*, p. 47.
90 *Ibid.*, p. 49.
91 *Ibid.*, p. 57.
92 *Ibid.*, p. 58.
93 *Ibid.*, p. 65.
94 *Ibid.*
95 Wellcome Collection, London, PP/MAL/4, 'Inhibition of orgasm'.
96 Malleson, 'Sexual disorders in women', p. 1480.
97 Malleson, *Any Wife*, p. 42.
98 Malleson, *The Principles of Contraception*, p. 15.
99 Wellcome Collection, London, PP/EFG/A.3/1, 'Letter from Joan Malleson to Edward Griffith, 7 November 1944'.
100 Wellcome Collection, London, SA/FPA/A14/58.2, K. Martin, 'A beloved physician', *New Statesman & Nation* (26 May 1956).
101 J. Malleson, 'Vaginismus: its management and psychogenesis', p. 215.
102 Malleson, *Any Wife*, p. 15.
103 Wellcome Collection, London, PP/MAL/3, '4 short cases of vaginismus'.
104 Wellcome Collection, London, PP/MAL/2, 'Scottish woman having acute anxiety neurosis'.
105 Wellcome Collection, London, PP/MAL/5, 'This couple were referred by a psychiatrist for marriage guidance'.
106 Wellcome Collection, London, PP/MAL/3, '4 short cases of vaginismus'.
107 Malleson, *Any Wife*, p. 57.
108 Wellcome Collection, London, PP/MAL/2, 'Scottish woman having acute anxiety neurosis'.
109 Evans, *Freedom to Choose*, pp. 151–2.
110 *Ibid.*
111 *Ibid.*, p. 150.
112 M. Balint, 'Training general practitioners in psychotherapy', *British Medical Journal*, 1:4854 (1954), pp. 115–20.
113 M. Balint, 'Psychotherapy and the general practitioner: I', *British Medical Journal*, 1:5011 (1957), p. 157.

114 M. Balint, 'The marital problem clinic – a problem child of the FPA', *Family Planning*, 9:1 (1960), pp. 18–20.
115 L. J. Friedman, *Virgin Wives: A Study of Unconsummated Marriages* (London: Tavistock Publications, 1962), p. 39.
116 On the vaginal examination as an element of truth see: P. Tunnadine, *Contraception and Sexual Life: A Therapeutic Approach* (London: Tavistock Publications, 1970).
117 Wellcome Collection, London, GC/105/4, 'In the club, interview with Prudence Tunnadine'.
118 On this formal training see Irwin, '"To try and find out what is being done to whom"'.
119 P. Tunnadine and J. Pasmore, 'Sexual problems in marriage in women' in Pollock, *Family Planning*, p. 123.
120 Tunnadine, *Contraception and Sexual Life*, p. 51.
121 Ibid., p. 54.
122 Ibid., p. 55.
123 Davis and Loughran, *The Palgrave Handbook of Infertility in History*.
124 M. Jackson, 'The organisation of a sterility service within a Family Planning Association clinic', *Post-Graduate Medical Journal*, 20:225 (1944), p. 237.
125 Jackson, 'A medical service for the treatment of involuntary infertility', p. 117.
126 Wellcome Collection, London, SA/FPA/NK22, 'Minutes of the medical committee of the North Kensington Centre, 30 September 1942'.
127 L. Horder, 'Sterility', *Lancet*, 241:6247 (1943), p. 664.
128 Wellcome Collection, London, SA/FPA/A5/103, 'Letters and papers relating to the sub-fertility committee'.
129 Ibid.
130 Wellcome Collection, London, SA/FPA/A16/8/22, 'Programme of a sub-fertility conference'.
131 Wellcome Collection, London, SA/FPA/A3/21, 'Kathleen Harding'.
132 Wellcome Collection, London, SA/FPA/A3/26, 'Sub-fertility'.
133 See, for instance, Jackson, 'The organisation of a sterility service'; Jackson, 'A medical service for the treatment of involuntary sterility'; M. Moore White, 'The endocrine treatment of sterility', *Post-Graduate Medical Journal*, 20:225 (1944), pp. 215–22; M. Moore White, 'The problem of sterility, its investigation and treatment', *The Practitioner*, 158:946 (1947), p. 279; K. Harding, 'Sterility in the female', *The Medical Press* (29 April 1953); M. Barton and B. P. Wiesner, 'The receptivity of cervical mucus to spermatozoea', *British Medical Journal*, 2:4477 (1946), pp. 606–10.
134 M. Moore White and M. Barton, 'Conception in spite of extreme oligozoospermia', *British Medical Journal*, 1:4709 (1951), p. 741.

135 H. Andrew, '"The Reluctant Stork": Science, Fertility and the Family in Britain, 1943–60'. PhD dissertation, York University Toronto, 2016.
136 F. Huxley, 'The clinical study of fertility cases with notes and treatments', *Medical Women's Federation Journal* (1 July 1935), pp. 28–37.
137 Jackson, 'A medical service for the treatment of involuntary sterility', p. 118.
138 Wellcome Collection, London, SA/FPA/SR 22/9, 'FPA Conference on Infertility, 1947'.
139 Moore White, 'The problem of sterility'.
140 K. Harding, 'Management of infertility', *The Medical Press* (November 1960), p. 436.
141 Wellcome Collection, London, SA/FPA/A16/24/3a, 'Childless Wife'.
142 A. Malleson, *Discovering the Family of Miles Malleson 1888–1969* (2012) [online], available at: https://books.google.co.uk/books?id=WBVhkj_JAJ8C&printsec=frontcover&dq=discovering+the+family+of+miles+malleson&hl=en&sa=X&ved=0ahUKEwib0bDQ6MPlAhX4RBUIHebwB1gQuwUILTAA#v=onepage&q=discovering%20the%20family%20of%20miles%20malleson&f=false (accessed 30 October 2019).
143 Andrew, '"The Reluctant Stork"'; N. Pfeffer, *The Stork and the Syringe: A Political History of Reproductive Medicine* (Cambridge: Polity Press, 1993); McLaren, *Reproduction by Design*, chapter 5.
144 M. Jackson, 'Artificial insemination', *British Medical Journal*, 1:4512 (1947), p. 945.
145 For a detailed analysis of these letters see chapter 2 in Andrew, '"The Reluctant Stork"'.
146 Quoted in Davis, 'A tragedy as old as history', pp. 359–81. Gayle Davis offers an insightful analysis of these debates.
147 M. Jackson, 'Human artificial insemination', *Family Planning*, 9:3 (1960), p. 6.

3

Medicalising birth control at the international conferences (1920–37): a British–French comparison

During the interwar years, women doctors medicalised birth control in Britain by developing a number of strategies to position themselves as experts in contraception and sexual disorders.[1] Among these strategies were publication of medical articles on birth control and participation in medical conferences. Yet these forms of dissemination of medical knowledge were not restricted to the national sphere; British women doctors also took part in international conferences on birth control. In fact, in a context where the quality and quantity of the world's population was an object of intense scientific debate, birth control was receiving increasing attention. These meetings were determinant spaces for doctors working in birth control, not only for gaining knowledge on new contraceptive methods and updates about clinical trials but also for asserting their expertise and debating the social and medical benefits of contraception. The international role of women doctors' work reveals how birth control and its medicalisation needs to be understood as a history of internationalism.

This chapter compares the roles of British and French women doctors in advancing knowledge of birth control at international conferences. By focusing on women doctors from two countries with strikingly divergent legal access to contraception, relationships with population issues, and women's political rights, this chapter explores the way national experiences shaped international debates.

In France, the sale and publicity of contraceptive devices was made illegal by the 1920 law, which was the culmination of years of pronatalist campaigning fuelled by anxieties around depopulation. After 1920, a radical minority mostly comprised of anarchists and neo-Malthusians continued to promote birth control; some of these activists, such as

Eugène and Jeanne Humbert and Madeleine Pelletier, were arrested as a result. While the French context, compared to the British one, was repressive in terms of access to information and contraception, women's place within society also differed drastically. British women aged over 30 who met specific qualifications obtained suffrage in 1918, and this right to vote was extended in 1928 to all women on the same terms as men, while French women only gained political rights in 1945. However, French women benefited from more state protection and support under the Third Republic than women in Britain.

Notwithstanding this difference in political power, when it came to women's position within the medical community, both British and French women occupied only a peripheral place within the male-dominated field of medicine. In France, although women had been able to practise medicine since 1870, it remained a profession for the masculine elites until after the Second World War, owing to the fear of overcrowding. Male doctors tried to restrain women from entering 'their' field, but the state 'allowed for moderate, steady progress toward equality'.[2] Between 1900 and the Second World War, the number of women medical students multiplied by six, though they still represented only 2 per cent of all potential doctors in 1928. Women doctors were assigned to 'feminine' fields and to more precarious hierarchical positions in both countries, such as public and community health, gynaecology and general practice in Britain, and medical gynaecology in France. In 1931, a survey of the 275 members of the French Association of Women Doctors revealed that the largest concentration of women doctors worked in the field of gynaecology and obstetrics.[3] Whereas obstetrics and gynaecology were unified in Britain after the First World War, this was not the case in France, where these two fields remained distinct from each other. The process of medical specialisation – including reproduction-related specialties – in France has a complicated history.[4] In 1949, four different specialties were recognised in France: obstetrics and gynaecology; surgical gynaecology, which was the most prestigious field and predominantly male; obstetrics; and medical gynaecology, which was almost entirely populated by women.[5] One important difference between the British and French situations was that British women doctors were strongly involved in the birth control movement, whereas French women doctors were not, as a consequence of the 1920 law.

This chapter assesses the relationship between national politics and birth control stances by comparing the norms of contraceptive practices articulated by British and French female doctors as transcribed in proceedings of international conferences on birth control. In addition, the chapter looks at the gender dynamics around positions on birth control expressed at international conferences. I try to determine whether women doctors held different stances on the subject as compared to male doctors, and how their position within the national medical landscape impacted their stances at the international level.

Internationalising birth control

The first decade of the century witnessed the advent of an international birth control movement led by the Malthusian League and later by Margaret Sanger, the well-known US birth control activist. Neo-Malthusians considered that excessive population resulted in poverty, and consequently they believed that limiting the size of the population would favour prosperity.[6] Founded in 1877 by the famous Annie Besant and Charles Bradlaugh, convicted and sentenced for having republished an 'obscene pamphlet' written by Charles Knowlton, the Malthusian League promoted the education of individuals in sexual matters and contraceptive use so as to reduce poverty. The League published its first leaflet, entitled *Hygienic Methods of Family Limitation*, in 1913, the first medical birth control publication of the twentieth century. The League began its international path in 1900. At the turn of the century, a wide range of international activities and associations flourished in relation to a diversity of topics: overpopulation, health, tropical medicine and labour, to name a few.[7] These international connections were also reinforced by the expansion of colonial empires. The issue of population, in particular, became an international concern. A first international meeting was held in Paris (1900), then further meetings in Liège (1905), The Hague (1910) and Dresden (1911). This movement brought together scientific experts and doctors from Britain, the United States, the Netherlands, France, India, Sweden, Belgium and Spain to discuss and share knowledge on the 'population problem'. The period between 1900 and 1911 was referred to as 'the high era of international meetings' by Alison Bashford.[8] Close cooperation was therefore sought between activists from different countries. The scope of these conferences, argued Bashford, was broader than birth control alone and encompassed many aspects of the population question: the issue of space, world resources, food, population growth, eugenics, political economy and natural history, among others.

These international meetings paved the way for the increasing importance of conferences as spaces for knowledge acquisition and transfer across national borders. In the following decade, three international neo-Malthusian and birth control conferences took place: London (1922), New York (1925) and Zurich (1930). For the first time, birth control was included in the title, suggesting that the idea had become accepted. Representatives from Britain, the United States, Germany, Austria, Holland, Denmark, France, India, China, Japan and Sweden were present. In addition, Margaret Sanger, with the help of the British feminist and birth control activist Edith How-Martyn, set up the World Population Congress (WPC) in Geneva in 1927 to promote scientific interest in contraceptive research. At this congress, however, birth control was left off the agenda in favour of more demographic and economic concerns linked to the population question.[9] These conferences again gathered experts from different fields: demography, medicine, sociology, agriculture, economics, biology, etc. The majority of the male experts were strong supporters of birth control methods, but not because of concerns over women's health. Here lies the main difference between the stances taken by women doctors and many of the male attendees. As Bashford convincingly demonstrated, for these male experts birth control represented a 'means by which food scarcity might be ameliorated, war averted, and global security achieved. As a rule, geopolitics not gender politics energised these prominent men.'[10] The quality and quantity of the population was also a key motive for British male speakers, whereas women doctors, in contrast, understood birth control as a way of improving women's health and giving them reproductive autonomy. The strategist Margaret Sanger understood that a mixture of arguments between population, food resources, issues of war and peace, and women's health was necessary to attract international support for the cause of birth control.

Following the Geneva conference, an International Birth Control Information Centre, which functioned as an advice and teaching hub for members' countries, was set up in London under the direction of the British suffragist Edith How-Martyn and the leadership of Margaret

Sanger. At the same time, international associations were created, such as the Medical Women's International Association (MWIA) in 1919. Set up in New York by unifying national branches of women's medical associations, this association aimed at 'providing means of communication between all medical women, promoting their general interests and furthering friendship and understanding between the medical women of the world. At the same time [affording] opportunities to confer upon questions relating to the health and well-being of humanity.'[11] The MWIA, based on its membership, organised a conference on birth control in 1934 in Stockholm and another on maternal mortality and abortion in 1937 in Edinburgh, showing how women's reproduction had become an international health concern. Meanwhile, other international meetings were also organised by the World League for Sexual Reform, an organisation officially created in 1928 by Magnus Hirschfeld and aimed at reforming social attitudes about sex. Among the aims of the association was support for the dissemination of information on birth control and the self-determination of couples in terms of conception or non-conception.[12]

Thus, the period between 1920 and 1937 saw the institutionalisation of international conferences and the positioning of birth control as a matter of international significance that attracted a broad range of experts including doctors, biologists, economists, statisticians, demographers and so on. In this new international network, British women doctors were to play an increasing role in the medicalisation of birth control, contributing to framing it as an international health concern and aligning with American, German and Austrian female doctors in their call for medical and reliable forms of contraception to safeguard women's health.

1922–30: towards medical arguments

Organised in 1922 in London by the New Generation League – the rebranded name for the British Malthusian League – the Fifth International Neo-Malthusian and Birth Control Conference was divided into seven sections: individual and family aspects of birth control, economics and statistics, morality and religion, eugenics, national and international perspectives, medical perspectives, and contraceptives.[13] While British doctors were present and actively involved in these debates, there was only one French birth control advocate among the speakers. Plausibly due to the 1920 law, Gabriel Giroud, a neo-Malthusian activist who had attended prewar international conferences, participated in the conference under the pseudonym G. Hardy, and described the legal situation in France and the risks incurred in publicly supporting birth control. Out of thirteen British delegates who presented papers during the 1922 conference, four were doctors. They were Dr Norman Haire, former medical director of the Walworth Women's Welfare Centre in London; Dr Killick Millard, medical officer for health in Leicester and a convinced eugenicist; Dr Binnie Dunlop, Scottish doctor and leading member of the Malthusian League and of the Eugenics Society who proffered birth control advice to working-class mothers in East London in 1914;[14] and the only woman doctor, Dr Frances Mabel Huxley,[15] gynaecological surgeon to the Marie Curie Hospital and founding member and then in 1928 president of the Medical Women's Federation. In 1929, Huxley was elected as a Foundation Fellow of the Royal College of Obstetricians and Gynaecologists.[16]

In all contributions to the 1922 conference, British male doctors advocated for birth control with the aim of improving national and sometimes even global welfare. Even though they invoked the medical dimension of birth control, these doctors softened its significance by drawing on eugenic or neo-Malthusian rationales. Their close affiliation and previous engagement with the Eugenics Society and the Malthusian League might explain this ideological orientation.[17] While he was not a medical doctor, it is worth developing the view of the president of the 1922 conference, Charles Vickery Drysdale, son of the famous birth control activists Dr Alice Vickery and physician Charles Robert Drysdale, since he set the tone of the debates.[18] Eugenics arguments permeated his opening. He appreciated that birth control would 'remove untold suffering from millions of hapless men, women and children[,] make early marriage and social purity possible, [and] improve the quality of the race'.[19] He urged public health authorities to provide birth control instruction 'to all whose circumstances or bodily or mental characteristics render them unfit for satisfactory parenthood'.[20] Drysdale linked women's agency with the eugenics argument, since birth control empowered women and this would eventually benefit the whole of society: 'By being able to have her children only when she feels able to do justice to herself and them, she becomes mistress of her fate, and from the point of view of the race the eugenic effect of birth control would be enormous.'[21] But Charles Drysdale did not aim at empowering women per se from an individual welfare perspective, but rather at achieving a eugenics society, for 'global welfare'. The contributions of male doctors presented the audience with the same strategy of legitimising birth control with eugenic or neo-Malthusian rhetoric. In his keynote address during the first evening's public event, Killick Millard resorted to eugenic arguments when he called for the spread of birth control to tackle the issue of 'the reckless lack of caution of the C3 class'.[22] He asserted that the fertility of the C3 class (the expression derived from the classification of substandard military recruits) represented a 'world-wide danger' for 'the individual, the nation and the race'. Binnie Dunlop gave a paper entitled 'Contraception is necessary for the elimination of poverty and is therefore moral' in the morality and religion session; in this paper, he underlined the threat that a high birth rate represented for the world's inhabitants: 'if God disapproves of contraception, He must approve of poverty'.[23]

Killick Millard chaired the medical session. Nine papers were presented; eight were by male doctors and scientists and one by a female doctor. Millard opened the session with a paper on 'Birth control and the medical profession' and called for medical men and women to study 'the various medical problems connected with Birth Control which are [awaiting] solution'. He provided the audience with a brief overview of the work of the founder of the Malthusian League and went on to present the results of two inquiries he had made into the views on birth control held among the medical profession in Britain. The first inquiry was made in 1918, when questionnaires were sent to medical men and women; seventy-four were returned. Fifty-two respondents stated that they did not think birth control methods were 'injurious to health under ordinary circumstances'. The answers that considered birth control as detrimental to health were not backed up with 'any actual experience'. But Millard quoted the answer of a woman doctor who supported birth control by referring to her clinical experience: 'In nearly thirty years' practice among women, of which nearly twenty years have included experience on the staff of a women's hospital, I have not met a single case in which I could trace ill-health to this cause.'[24] The second inquiry was made by Millard with the help of Dunlop in 1921. They addressed 160 questionnaires to 'eminent gynaecologists', and 'some women doctors of standing were also included'; sixty-five had been returned. The questionnaires revealed that medical men and women who approved of birth control were three times more numerous than those who disapproved, and condoms came out as the 'favourite' method of birth control. By providing an overview of his inquiry and sharing the results at the international conference, Millard sought to make the point that 'it cannot be claimed in the future that the medical profession condemns contraception'.[25]

The other contributions by British males referred to doctrinal elements. A resort to the eugenics argument was central to the speech of the famous sexologist and medical practitioner Norman Haire, chief honorary medical officer of the Walworth Women's Welfare Centre, a birth control clinic in central London. He spoke about the 'sterilisation of the "unfits"', a negative eugenic measure to prevent their 'multiplication'.[26] Similarly, Dunlop's paper in the medical session explicitly referred to doctrinal aspects and was entitled 'A Malthusian view of death rates and on the average duration of life'.

In comparison, the only British medical woman to address the 1922 conference limited her contribution to her personal medical experience of birth control. This attested to a different vision and construction of expertise, foregrounded on facts and applied knowledge rather than on moral considerations. British female doctors were strikingly underrepresented in these conferences. Having only one paper from a British woman does not allow me to make any conclusive or general arguments. However, her contribution, based on medical grounds, appears to be unusual in comparison to the general trend towards moral considerations in the medical session. She limited herself to describing her medical experience, in an attempt to underline the scientific legitimacy of birth control. Frances Huxley delivered a talk on 'Birth control from the point of view of a woman gynaecologist'. As the title made explicit, her practical experience in Britain formed the core of her paper. She clearly explained that she came to support birth control due to what she found in 'the course of her work' and the observation of 'facts and conditions'.[27] Her use of a neutral scientific vocabulary, such as 'facts' and 'conditions', helped objectify birth control, reducing the moral components in favour of a scientific, objective and medical approach to the subject. Birth control, after all, explained Huxley 'is here with us now',[28] and she called for a 'rational' answer from the medical profession. Based on her clinical experience, she advanced three arguments in favour of birth control. First, the self-determination of married couples to decide upon their family size: 'it is they who are responsible for the wellbeing of their children, and it is they alone who can judge their sexual needs'.[29] She presented the knowledge of birth control as a 'right': 'it is the right of every married couple to know, if they wish to know, how best to regulate the size of their family'. Secondly, she urged her listeners not to label birth control as an antinatalist measure, as she asserted that married women from all classes wanted more than one child, and that 'birth control will not alter this'.[30] Third, she turned to medical considerations on the advantage of spacing births for the health of the mother, irrespective of her social class, thus mirroring a shift in the understanding of birth control away from eugenic and moral considerations towards individual welfare: 'a woman has the right to expect to be as well after the birth of her family, as before it'.[31] Huxley specifically stressed the benefit of birth control for working-class women, who were generally ignorant of birth control, which resulted in the bad health of both the mother and the child. In support of her claim she presented the example of a 'woman of thirty-six, looking forty-six, who has had twelve confinements and three miscarriages, seven children now living. She has never time to recover from one confinement before the next is upon her.'[32]

She then turned to the methods available. Discouraging coitus interruptus, she advocated four requirements for the choice of birth control methods: 'to be ideal the methods used should be aesthetic, safe, harmless and inexpensive [...] and precautions should be taken by the wife'.[33] (The word 'aesthetic' refers to the notion that contraception should not disturb intercourse due to any odour or the mode of application.[34]) These recommendations would later form the basis for birth control clinics, reflecting the medical expertise of Frances Huxley which anticipated the main leitmotiv of scientific recommendation of birth control. By giving responsibility to the wife, Frances Huxley nonetheless recognised women as sexually active agents. She ended her speech by calling for further 'scientific investigation' into birth control methods.

What is compelling in Huxley's speech is her reference to her medical experience. She was able to use experience gained at the national level and to turn it into an asset for legitimising birth control on medical grounds at the international level, to a male-dominated audience. Thus, the 'feminine' domain of expertise made women doctors not only particularly aware of their patients' concerns about additional pregnancies, but also well equipped and qualified to deal with this problem in a scientific manner at international conferences. Moreover, while the title of her talk did refer to her gender, she only presented 'objective' and medical facts to support birth control, and clearly put forward the health of the mother as the main reason for birth control. However, her position was marginal in the 1922 medical session since a resolution was taken that underlined the eugenic character of birth control despite acknowledging the medical responsibility for birth control issues: 'Birth control instruction should become part of the recognised duty of [the] medical profession, and such instruction should especially be given at all hospital and public health centres to which the poorest class and those suffering hereditary disease or defectiveness applies for relief ....'[35] Only in 1930, when British women doctors were becoming the leading figures in the birth control movement at the national level, were they also able to influence the debates at the international level.

Finally, the last session on contraception was chaired by Haire. This session was private and reserved for members of the medical profession, showing that information on techniques of contraception was thought to be within the realm of doctors alone. This session was attended by 164 members of the medical profession.[36] Haire read a paper on contraceptive techniques. He first denounced the medical profession's neglect of the issue, which, he argued, resulted in failure to help women avoid pregnancy as the appropriate means to do so were not being described and explained; this failure, he maintained, 'opened the way for the quacks and charlatans'.[37] Haire was assuredly reacting to the commercialisation of contraceptive powders and devices by laypeople.[38] He concentrated on the advantages and disadvantages of different methods of birth control, stating that 'all methods but one are faulty',[39] praising the Dutch Mensinga pessary, which he claimed he had introduced into England. He underscored the necessity of the device being fitted by a medical professional for correct choice of size, which ensured protection, therefore placing birth control under medical responsibility. He also recommended permanent sterilisation for people considered unfit for parenthood, who might 'contaminate the race', testifying to his eugenic ideology. He urged the medical profession to undertake 'research and experiment' in the field of contraception and called for the opening of birth control clinics. Frances Huxley participated in the debate that followed Haire's presentation, showing the expert position she held on the subject. She put forward the necessity of recommending methods that were efficient both for the wife and the husband. She explained that she prescribed condoms, but so far had not had the opportunity to try the female pessary. However, she held the view that women who wanted to use birth control should have personal help, 'because the anatomical structure is so different in different women'. She questioned the accuracy of Haire's affirmation of the reliability of the Dutch pessary, arguing, 'I should have thought there was sufficient gap there (between the rim and symphysis) to be a danger to the patient, although Dr Haire says it is not.' She put efficiency, reliability and harmlessness at the centre of her argument, testifying to her concern about providing couples with efficient ways to avoid pregnancies. This concern was undoubtedly dictated by her patients' needs.

The Sixth International Neo-Malthusian and Birth Control Conference was organised by Margaret Sanger and held in New York in 1925. Again, birth control was directly associated with eugenics. The French jurist, anthropologist and racial eugenic theorist Georges Vacher de Lapouge gave a paper entitled 'Eugenic birthrate for France'. The British physician, sexologist and social reformer Havelock Ellis delivered a talk on 'The evolutionary meaning of birth control', while Norman Haire spoke on 'Health aspects of birth control'. In his talk, Haire referred to the necessity of preventing unhealthy parents from reproducing, via birth control advice. While his views were embedded in eugenic ideology, he nevertheless placed birth control under the sole responsibility of the medical profession and called for the provision of birth control advice in 'every hospital, every dispensary, every asylum and every welfare centre'.[40] There were no British or French female doctors in this session.

1930: birth control as a (female) medical responsibility

By 1930, a change in argumentation was noticeable at the international level; there was a detachment from the doctrinal perspective of eugenic and neo-Malthusian considerations of global welfare in favour of scientific objectivity, where facts and evidence were central. Thus, a process of medicalisation of birth control was under way. Women doctors played an influential role in this shift. Apart from British ones, prominent voices among female doctors came from the American doctor Hannah Stone, close friend of Margaret Sanger and in charge of the New York Birth Control Clinic, Dr Rachel Yarros, a gynaecologist, social hygienist and director of the Illinois Birth Control League who opened the second birth control clinic at Hull House, and German doctors such as the physician, abortion activist and founding member of the German Birth Control Committee Martha Ruben-Wolf, and the member of the Frankfurt Advice Bureau Dr Lotte Fink.

This process was made visible at the seventh International Birth Control Conference held in Zurich in 1930, organised by Margaret Sanger. In preparation for the event, Sanger asked every national birth control movement to fill in a questionnaire 'relating to the methods and organisation of birth control clinics'.[41] The questionnaire covered the history of the clinics, the number of patients admitted, the marital situation of the patients and the practical running of the clinic (who prescribed and then instructed birth control methods, the types of methods prescribed and the number of failures for each method, as well as the follow-up policy). This conference was one of the first to categorise birth control as an international health measure which was part of preventive medicine. Sanger triumphantly underscored the radicalism and the international dimension of this gathering, as shown by the following quote from her introduction of the proceedings of the edited collection:

> On September 1, 1930, an earnest group of experts – men and women – from various parts of the civilised world gathered quietly together in Zurich, Switzerland. These men and women were delegates to the Seventh International Birth Control Conference. They came together in the interest of the scientific quest for contraceptive knowledge. For 5 days, more than one hundred scientists, physicians and clinicians discussed the technical problems of contraception. They compared notes, reported progress made in research laboratories and birth control clinics, and proved beyond doubt that the much troubled subject now universally known as Birth Control had entered a new phase of development.[42]

She drew attention to the unprecedented aspect of the meeting by saying that the 'Zurich conference represents a milestone in the history of modern civilization'. Moreover, she flagged up the new direction taken by the science of medicine from the 'art of curing to the art of prevention'.[43] In this new paradigm, birth control had to play a vital role in improving the conditions of life.

Experts framed birth control as a medical responsibility through the use of scientific vocabulary and by focusing on its practical aspects. The 1930 conference covered four themes, among which three were indicative of this new 'medical' and scientific orientation: reports from birth control leagues and clinics; contraceptive devices and techniques; and birth control in relation to the health and economic conditions of men, women and children.[44] The titles of the papers also reflected this process of medicalisation. Among the 130 physicians, clinicians and researchers who attended the 1930 sessions, the eugenicist C. P. Blacker spoke on the 'Need for research on contraception'; the British specialist in spermicide, Dr Cecil Voge, talked about 'Future research upon sterilisation and contraception'; and Dr John Baker, another British specialist in spermicide, delivered a paper on 'Chemical contraceptive'. These three male experts were all members of the BCIC and spoke on the research aspect of birth control. Women doctors, as we shall see, focused on their practical experience in working in birth control clinics, and, as I have shown in Chapter 1, acted as liaisons between research carried out in the laboratory and patients' experiences with contraceptive methods.

The conference clearly defined birth control as a medical subject by stating that it was the first birth control symposium to focus on 'practical, medical, and scientific considerations of birth control'. Even though one can still find traces of eugenic rhetoric, especially from the male doctors' contributions,[45] this conference aspired to remove such doctrine by emphasising 'the impersonal and scientific abstraction'[46] of the issue. It is worth remembering that contraception was not part of any medical training in either country until long after the Second World War (see Chapter 1 for Britain). Thus, it is not surprising that the only way to inform medical considerations on birth control was to rely on the practical experience of doctors dealing with the issue in their individual exercise of medicine; these were predominantly women doctors.

The fact that the practical aspects of birth control as reported 'by those actively engaged in the movement'[47] were the focus of the Zurich conference meant that numerous women were present and taking an active part in the medical debate on birth control. Until then, male scientists dominated the conferences in terms of both number and the orientations of the debates. Thus, this medicalisation process opened the door for women doctors' involvement at international conferences, as they were the experts in the practical aspects of birth control. Indeed, as shown in the previous chapters, the majority of British birth control clinic workers who dealt with the day-to-day aspects of birth control were female. This was also the case in Germany, and German women doctors were also present in great numbers. The experience acquired at the national level constituted a valuable source of knowledge of contraception that women doctors used to position themselves as experts at the international level. In addition, male experts increasingly described contraception as a female medical responsibility. The American obstetrician and birth control advocate Robert L. Dickinson urged women to be involved in birth control activism since the issue was a feminine one, relying upon gendered expertise: 'In the past, a few physicians and a number of prominent masculine thinkers have been advocates for birth control. But in a movement for mercy for mothers, and particularly in urgency for widespread practical application, the vigorous leaders have to be women: mothers, nurses, scientists, social workers, women doctors.'[48] The majority of the women doctors that attended the 1930 conference were working in birth control clinics and were also members of the MWF, such as Dr Helena Wright and Dr Joan Malleson.[49] Whereas the individual members of the MWF increasingly supported birth control, especially from the mid-1920s onwards, the organisation as a whole 'maintained a somewhat cautious attitude towards this increased dissemination of contraceptive knowledge'.[50] The following examples illustrate this new role of women doctors as legitimate experts and agents of knowledge transfer on birth control. British women doctors and laywomen speaking on behalf of the birth control clinic staff medicalised contraception in different ways.

First, they placed contraception under the medical flag by affirming that a medical consultation and supervision were necessary and essential steps for choosing an appropriate method. For instance, the lay birth control activist Flora Blumberg, who introduced the audience to the work carried out in the Salford clinic in Manchester, insisted that a female doctor was in charge of seeing the patient and performed a thorough vaginal examination with the help of the speculum. The use of the speculum had been advocated by Wright (see Chapter 1) to spot any abnormalities or diseases that could affect the choice of method. Similarly, Evelyn Fuller, the secretary of the Society for the Provision of Birth Control Clinics, explained that in each of the association's centres, every patient 'was given a gynaecological examination by a woman doctor'.[51] This requirement was aimed at boosting women doctors' professional standing and framing contraception as a technical medical specialty.

Female speakers also discussed in great detail the advantages and disadvantages of various methods of birth control. For instance, one of the most prominent birth control activists in Britain, Wright, discussed the presentation given by Dr Ernest Gräfenberg, a German scientist, on the intrauterine device.[52] Her speech at the international conference revealed her engagement with the production and assessment of scientific knowledge about birth control and her willingness to learn new methods. As I will show in Chapter 5, she met Ernest Gräfenberg in Berlin. She then started to study the use of the Gräfenberg ring in her own private practice in England, fitting patients with this contraceptive device, and thus translating the knowledge she gained from him into practical research. She presented her first results based on a case study of fifteen patients she had fitted with the Gräfenberg ring. She then asked Gräfenberg questions about the difficulties she had encountered when placing the ring into the vagina, showing her interest in improving the method. Taking into account the different knowledge she acquired, Wright continued her research and published her results in 1931.[53] She also presented two papers, 'Notes on the North Kensington Women's Welfare Centre' and 'Indication for the use of the Dumas and Prorace cervical caps'. Based on her own practical medical experience, she elaborated on the advantages and inconveniences of these methods, their effectiveness and the possible problems one could encounter when placing Dumas and Prorace cervical caps. Here again, she articulated her description in scientific and medical terms:

> The cap lies in the roof of the vagina with its concavity upwards. The circular ring fits closely to the vaginal mucous membrane just outside the circle of the upper limit of the intravaginal part of the cervix, and therefore occupies all four fornices. The mucous membrane surrounding the external os uteri should not be in contact with the dome of the cap.[54]

Several other women doctors also conveyed observations they gained from their practical work and shared advice on the best way to insert a cap, using diagrams to illustrate their explanations. Chief among them was the American Dr Hannah Stone, who worked closely with Margaret Sanger.

In addition to describing methods of birth control, women doctors provided statistics based on clinic records and case cards. The latter served the purpose of challenging the assumption that use of contraceptives led to sterility, but it was also a means of showing the extent of their accumulative experience and asserting their authority and expertise on the matter. For instance, Evelyn Fuller reminded the audience that methods prescribed at the centre did not cause permanent sterility. To support her statement she referred to the 'many cases in which the patients have deliberately conceived after a long period of using the appliances'.[55] A member of the MWF, Dr Lily Butler, gave a talk on her work at the Walworth and East London clinics, focusing on the failure of contraceptive methods, based on the 7,000 cases of patients attending the clinics between 1921 and 1927. She said that 3,596 patients failed to report and 2,893 had 'been successful with the appliance recommended', and then provided insights into the reasons why the other women failed to apply the methods.[56]

These statistics reveal that there existed no methods of birth control that were truly reliable. Consequently, while acknowledging the significance of gathering statistics for the basis of research, Fuller nevertheless warned against too much effort wasted on their collection and too much reliance on their accuracy. There were different definitions of the term 'failure' across the centres, and therefore the lack of a common denominator did not allow for definitive results. She suggested instead that there was an urgent need for 'further research work'. She used the international platform to call for an effort to be made towards discovering the ideal contraceptive: 'The results we hope for from this world wide conference is that an impetus be given to the search for the ideal contraceptive.' Such a contraceptive should be 'aesthetically suitable', reliable, simple and inexpensive. She painted this search as a feminist imperative to 'place within every woman's reach the power to control her own destiny'.[57] This use of language suffused with medical terminology, combined with a scientific precision in describing the diverse methods of birth control, contributed to positioning women doctors as active and legitimate agents in the handling of birth control issues and the shaping of production of sexual scientific knowledge at the national and international levels.

In addition, British female doctors paid great attention to the experience of their patients with birth control, showing the amount of practical experience they gained from being in direct contact with this subject in their own offices or at birth control clinics. Furthermore, this reveals their commitment to putting individual welfare at the centre of the birth control issue. For example, during the 1930 conference, Helena Wright commented on Baker's paper on 'chemical contraceptives' with regard to applied experience with her patients of a laboratory-based study carried out on guinea pigs. During her comment, she referred to patients' concerns and experiences. Adopting the 'point of view of poor patients'[58] who did not have running water, she recommended the use of a specific spermicide that did not require women 'to douche when using it [...] the pellet costs the patient just about one penny each.'[59] Meanwhile, Lily Butler justified the follow-up appointment with patients after their first visit by referencing their vulnerable psychological situation during their examination, since they were 'nervous and frightened.'[60] Thus, a second visit appeared to be the best way to ascertain that the patients understood the instructions given to them. Similarly, Evelyn Fuller pointed out the centrality of the patient in the way the work is carried out: 'the desire to meet the patients' point of view is one of our guiding principles. The main thing is to get the confidence of the women – to treat them not as so "many cases" but as individual human beings to whom a knowledge on birth control is a matter of vital and urgent importance.'[61] Interestingly, Fuller also called for patients not to be used 'experimentally as test cases' for new contraceptives, putting the emphasis on the fact that the factor of paramount importance for the patient who attended the clinic was that they should not conceive, and therefore only the most reliable contraceptive should be prescribed to them. Flora Blumberg also drew attention to the relationship between patients and doctors. She explained that women doctors dealt with patients with 'great patience and care.'[62]

Thus, this conference provided the ideal platform for sharing the latest updates on birth control methods and practical experiences among practitioners, and especially among women doctors. Here women doctors functioned as agents of the transfer of knowledge about birth control between the national and international spheres. As such, they helped to develop a system of legitimate knowledge of the effects of contraception on the female body. The method on which they seemed to reach a consensus was the combined use of mechanical devices preventing contact between sperm and egg, such as a diaphragm or a cervical cap, and chemical spermicide substances. These methods were to be the responsibility of the female patients, as these female doctors wanted to give women control over their reproductive functions.

The knowledge that British women doctors gained at the international level was brought back to Britain, where it nurtured their own work. They enabled the circulation of contraceptive knowledge by drawing on international scientific research in the medical manuals they published. For instance, Dr Gladys Cox referred to the presentations of other doctors made at the Zurich international conferences, such as Dr Hans Hehfeldt from Berlin, on the advantage of the cap in her handbook on contraception.[63] She also displayed four diagrams on the adjustment of the diaphragm pessary that she had borrowed from Dr Hannah Stone. She was not the only one to make use of Stone's work. Dr Joan Malleson extensively quoted data collected in birth control clinics in Britain, but also drew on the work of other scientists, Stone in particular, to support her demonstration of the harmlessness of birth control to fertility. With these references to other works, she showed her awareness and knowledge of contemporaneous international debates on this topic.

French versus British women doctors: 1934–7

The close analysis of British and French women doctors' positions on birth control at the 1934 international conference offers a valuable lens through which to assess the impact of the national context. One prior assumption is that French and British women doctors would have shared similar views on birth control due to their shared understanding of the female body. But national reproductive politics and women's previous engagement played a determinant role in shaping French women doctors' views on birth control. Whereas British women doctors were involved in the running of the clinics – and many of them held feminist stances, given that they sought to advance knowledge on contraception to give women power and control over their reproduction – this was not the case in France. In a context of lacking political representation, the French feminist movement, mainly reformist and familial, tended to fight for causes in line with the mainstream political agenda (motherhood as a social duty) to rally male politicians to support women's enfranchisement.[64] In addition, campaigning for birth control, an action prohibited at home though not at international conferences, was at odds with the mainstream political involvement of many women doctors in familial feminism, as I show.

The 1934 conference brought together the national branches of the MWF, and delegates from member countries took part in the event. Anna Louise McIlroy, Professor of Obstetrics and Gynaecology at the Royal Free Hospital, University of London, presented a report on birth control based on the answers to the questionnaire sent by the MWIA to members for Britain, the US, New Zealand and India.[65] Out of the thirteen British contributors to the report, eight were already involved with the birth control issue. Of these, those previously discussed in this book include Dr Lily Butler, Dr Helena Wright and Dr Frances Huxley; other contributors were the general practitioner Dr Annis Gillie, member of the Royal College of Physicians and later member of the executive committee of the Family Planning Association; Dr Olive Gimson, appointed doctor at the Manchester, Salford and District Mothers' Clinic in 1926 and at the birth control clinic at Withington Hospital in 1931;[66] Dr Mary Macaulay, medical officer for the Liverpool branch of the National Birth Control Association; Dr Lilias Jeffries, general practitioner and gynaecologist at the New Sussex Hospital in Brighton; and Dr Louisa Martindale, British physician and surgeon and Fellow of the Royal College of Obstetricians. McIlroy and Martindale had a more traditional attitude towards birth control than their colleagues, due to their adherence to social purity feminism. A late nineteenth-century construct, the social purity movement aimed at eradicating prostitution and the sexual double standard. It was a movement that sought to elevate morality from a Christian perspective and improve the sexual treatment of women by advocating for sexual restraint. In 1921, Martindale delivered a talk on birth control to the London Association of the Medical Women's Federation, where she expressed her anxiety that birth control risked 'encouraging sexual excess and the possibility of eventual sterility'. Her talk was in line with social purity feminists that considered women to be less sexual and consequently morally superior to men. Similarly, McIlroy, who testified in favour of the Catholic doctor Halliday Sutherland during his trial for libel against Marie Stopes in 1923, also belonged to the social purity feminists. In the special issue on birth control published in *The Practitioner* in 1923, she wrote that contraceptives 'will not bring to women freedom but worse slavery in sexual matters, for they will remain the instruments of men's uncontrolled desires'.[67]

For the French report, Dr Denise Blanchier explained that only 15 of 300 members of the French Association (5 per cent) answered the questionnaire about birth control from the MWIA. She completed the report using answers from thirty-one male doctors, gynaecologists and psychiatrists. The national difference here is noticeable. French women doctors did not refer to their position as women doctors only, and indeed sought the opinion of their male colleagues, suggesting that birth control was not perceived as a female medical responsibility in France. This situation reflected both the absence of training on the subject for these women and the power relationship within the French medical profession and more broadly in French society, where women were not enfranchised.

What is clear from the French report is that the French branch would not have approached this subject if it were not for this international conference. Indeed, due to the 1920 law, French women doctors could not have addressed the subject of birth control publicly. Thus, it was 'under constraint' that the national French branch was 'forced' to address this issue. As Blanchier explained, she struggled to obtain answers from physicians, possibly because they were afraid of getting into trouble with the law, and was able to do so only when she presented the subject as a foreign one, imposed by foreign branches from countries where the movement for birth control was already widespread.[68] Moreover, she added that the term 'birth control' was difficult to translate into the French language due to its foreign etymology and foreign meaning, which were unknown to the French way of thinking. She used the British word 'birth control' alongside 'prophylaxis anticonceptionnelle' in the French report.[69] Notwithstanding this attempt to distance the term 'birth control' from the French experience, the conference did give the French branch the opportunity to understand the birth control movement. Dr Germaine Montreuil-Strauss, president of the French association, wrote a historical report on the evolution of birth control.[70] In a neutral style, she presented the arguments for and against birth control. Since more than half of the article was devoted to introducing French members to the work of the birth control movement in Britain and the wide range of support it received, one could argue that the tone of the report was positive; this long historical introduction might be perceived as an attempt to overcome the 1920 law. Though her historical presentation was politically and morally neutral and scientific, she nonetheless familiarised women doctors with the issue of birth control, providing them with arguments to support the movement.

Secondly, the French report did not follow the recommendation to leave moral and political aspects out of the debates. The questionnaire recommended focusing only on the physiological and medical point of view in order to avoid any 'political and religious controversy'.[71] In its introduction, for instance, the French report underlined the 'tendentious character'[72] of the questionnaire, perceived as being in favour either of a feminism 'that allowed women to live a free sexual life without any dangers as do men'[73] or of licentious propaganda that led to 'ethnic national suicide and moral depravation'.[74] Both qualifications were negatively depicted and reflected the fears of depopulation that pervaded the French elite. In addition, sexual relations, in the Catholic context, were meant for procreation and not for pleasure. Separating sexuality and reproduction was condemned by the Catholic Church. Furthermore, the report clearly stated that hygiene and morals could not be distinguished: 'one can only advise a woman, in the name of hygiene, of the two alternatives to sexual life that are not anti-biological: motherhood or chastity'.[75] These positions were again in line with those of the Catholic Church, reflecting the possible influence of the latter, and more broadly with those of the conservative position of the French association.[76] Indeed, historian Anne Cova has shown the involvement of women, and among them women doctors, in the natalist movement, and she has shown how Catholic women were at the forefront of the interwar development of family policy.[77] However, this position was not shared by all women doctors; Blanchier reported having noticed a slight difference between the answers from female and male doctors, with women tending to be more tolerant of birth control when it came to protecting the individual well-being of a child. She attributed their answer to 'maternal nature'.[78] Thus, an essentialist vision of motherhood permeated this report. This is not surprising given the fact that many French women doctors were part of the 'familial' feminist movement.

Historian Karen Offen defined familial feminism as a type of feminism that 'predicated a biologically differentiated, family-centred vision of male–female complementarity'.[79] Thus, familial feminists tended to emphasise motherhood as a social duty. In addition, French women doctors were active in advancing social and familial reforms in the interwar years, and played an important role in the fight against venereal disease. For instance, many French women doctors were members of familial associations – associations that fought for the defence of the family and familial Christian values. Denise Blanchier and Germaine Montreuil-Strauss were members of the Committee for Female Education of the French Society for Sanitary and Moral Prophylaxis, a group that promoted sex education as a way to fight venereal diseases through 'biological education for maternity';[80] Denise Blanchier and Dr Madeleine Thuillier-Landry belonged to the National Committee for Childhood, a committee promoting child hygiene; and from 1936 Denise Blanchier was a member of Medicine and Family, an association bringing together parents of numerous children.[81] Although many female doctors were involved in providing sex education to young women after the First World War through the Committee of Female Education, the topic of contraception was never approached.[82] Women doctors were absent from the debate on birth control during the interwar years, with the notable exception of the radical feminist Dr Madeleine Pelletier, who advocated abortion and birth control.[83] This familialist feminist orientation of the association was clearly stated in the French report. In fact Blanchier negatively referred to the feminist 'emancipatory rhetoric' supporting birth control, while emphasising that 'we do not accept this definition of feminism'.[84] Apart from being part of the familialist feminist movement that supported natalist policy, French women doctors, as suggested by historian Yvonne Knibiehler, might have tried to secure their respectability in the battle for access to medical positions by holding natalist stances.[85] In this context, campaigning for an immoral subject such as birth control might have been perceived as an obstacle to achieving this.[86] Thus, this essentialist vision of motherhood has to be understood as part of their position within the French medical scale and society.

Only one remark on the 'maternal nature' was found in the British report and unsurprisingly came from Martindale. She maintained that 'maternity is the normal and natural state for women and if well taken care of there is physiological benefit'.[87] Despite this essentialist vision, the conclusion of the British report advised 'the use of contraceptives in the case of married women, who because of social and economic stress are unable to rear their children in a condition of health and happiness'.[88] In addition, chastity, while strongly recommended before marriage, was described as non-natural after marriage as it could lead to neuroses. Furthermore, British medical women kept to the practical aspects of the subject of birth control and based their observations on their own professional experience.

Thirdly, judgements about the medical effects of birth control practices on the female body differed between the French and British reports. In the former, birth control practices were in general depicted as both inefficient and dangerous. Going against biological laws or the 'law of nature' (maternity) was 'anti-medical', since maternity was beneficial for 'the normal female organism'.[89] For Blanchier, this argument should have convinced doctors to refrain from considering contraception as part of 'hygiene' to be taught to healthy individuals. She drew on the pronatalist argument to reject the idea of creating birth control clinics, arguing for encouraging births in a context of declining fertility.[90] British doctors, meanwhile, recommended the combination of either the male condom or the Dutch rubber vaginal cap with a spermicidal jelly – with a slight preference for the latter. This recommendation was in line with the conclusions of the Zurich conference but also reflected the strong preference for female-controlled devices in birth control clinics in England. British women doctors put forward the autonomy of women as the main advantage of the Dutch rubber vaginal cap: 'Easy to insert and remove by the woman herself when taught properly [...] Can be used by woman without cooperation of the husband'.[91] Thus, through these advantages, women doctors placed responsibility for birth control in women's hands. This autonomous rhetoric was not surprising in a context of enfranchised working women doctors who were used to working in birth control clinics created to give every woman control over her own fertility.[92] These feminist British women doctors drew upon psychology and patients' individual experiences to support their stance, stressing the psychological benefits of birth control for individuals. For instance, a specialist in psychological medicine, Dr Doris Odlum, 'very rarely found the use of contraceptives harmful as the relief from the fear of pregnancy is so beneficial'.[93] In her feminist opinion, women had a right to pleasure, and relieving them from the anxiety of pregnancy encouraged sexual satisfaction: 'In women, orgasm is slower than in men and intercourse is, therefore, distasteful if no satisfaction is obtained. It is of the greatest importance physiologically that all conscious or unconscious anxiety should be removed during coitus.'[94]

Fourthly, the conclusions of the reports differed between the two countries. In the French report, women doctors agreed not to present a conclusion officially because of the divergent opinions among the medical body, but most probably because of the 1920 law. This testifies to two things, namely the lack of agency of French women doctors, who were unable to speak openly on the subject, even though some of them were clearly in favour of spreading information on birth control, and the adherence of French doctors to familial feminism. In the British report, a majority of women doctors were in favour of birth control and called for the integration of this subject into medical curricula and the development of scientific research to find a cheap and reliable method of contraception that was accessible to women of all social classes. The only female doctor who expressed some form of hesitation was Martindale, and this was not surprising given her previous stance on birth control and her adherence to social purity feminism.

Two similarities in the reports deserve to be mentioned. The first is that female doctors from both countries disapproved of public propaganda, feeling that birth control should remain within the scope of the medical body. The other similarity was that sterilisation and abortion received little attention in either report. Although birth control was thought to reduce the number of abortions according to both reports, women doctors tried to distinguish birth control from abortion. French women doctors were, nonetheless, reluctant to recommend the prescription of birth control methods, presumably for fear of legal consequences linked with the 1920 law. They appeared over-determined by the legal context but also by lack of suffrage and civil power.

Contrastingly, the issue of abortion was debated at length in 1937 at the Edinburgh conference. The theme was suggested by the British branch; abortion was topical in Britain at the time, notably due to the inquiries on maternal mortality commissioned by the Minister of Health in 1932 and 1937. The latter had led to the establishment of an interdepartmental committee on abortion by the Home Office and the Ministry of Health.[95] Here again, the French position remained highly traditional and familial compared to the British one. The questionnaire devised for the conference addressed the legal situation in each country and public opinion on this contentious issue. The French report, written by Dr Anchel-Bach, the former chief of the obstetrics clinic in Paris, underlined that while therapeutic abortion was legally forbidden, exceptions were made when the mother's life was endangered by an additional pregnancy. In that case, doctors were held morally responsible for making the decision and undertaking the procedure. Anchel-Bach contended that public opinion supported abortive procedures when the mother's health was in danger. However, she added that 'the medical pretext served as a screen for the desire to have an abortion',[96] betraying the conservative views shared by the majority of the pronatalist medical profession, who depicted abortion as an abominable practice and denied women the agency of making their own informed decisions. The report nevertheless suggested that the law should be changed, if only for medical reasons, to grant immunity to women who undertook illegal abortions so that women in need of medical help would no longer be afraid of seeking it, and to prosecute only the abortionists. The British report, written by Janet Campbell, senior medical officer at the Ministry of Health, in contrast, showed how much more tolerant British female doctors and British public opinion were towards the practice. The report explained that while abortion was unlawful, therapeutic abortion could be obtained with 'no difficulty'[97] when it was 'genuinely needed on medical grounds'. Public opinion could be divided between two 'extremes of opinion': Catholics, who regarded abortion as a sin, and people who considered that a woman 'has a right to decide for herself whether or not she will bear a child or terminate her pregnancy'.

The French and British means for reducing the number of illegal abortions and their related casualties diverged from one another, reflecting again the legal, religious and political conditions of each country and, moreover, the familial inclination of French doctors who suggested pronatalist solutions to illegal abortion. French women doctors advocated three means. First and foremost, they foregrounded the necessity to address the main causes of abortion, namely poverty, the social conditions in which women found themselves, and the selfishness shown by rich and well-off families, by developing appropriate policies to support single, unmarried and poor women and their families. The second way they proposed to limit illegal abortions was to spread information among the public on their dreadful consequences and dangers, and the third was to apply the law on the matter with rigour and severity. No mention was made of any form of information on birth control, not even natural methods. In stark contrast, British women doctors asserted the necessity of educating wife and husband on birth control, since 'successful contraception is a positive means of reducing the incidence of illegal abortions'.[98] Educating the public on the danger of abortion was also credited, as well as the need to encourage women in difficult situations to seek postnatal advice. These considerations indicated that British women doctors did not consider abortion as a means of birth control, but as a last resort procedure that could be avoided by adequate teaching of birth control to married people. Although British women doctors appeared more liberal than their French counterparts, they remained nevertheless limited by the traditional framework of the married couple, ignoring the significant number of abortion-seekers that were unmarried young girls.

Conclusion

In the interwar years, British women doctors, although not numerous in the medical field, were transnational agents for the legitimacy of birth control. In the national medical field, as shown in Chapter 1, they tried to make birth control a new specialty of medicine by opening clinics, fitting individuals with contraceptive devices and writing scientific articles. Empowered by this experience grounded in their daily practice of medicine, they were vocal on the international scene and tried to medicalise birth control. While birth control tended to be framed in eugenic or neo-Malthusian terms by male doctors before 1930, it gradually became a medical subject in which scientific vocabulary and individual welfare predominated. Women doctors played a major role in bringing about this shift. The international conferences on birth control and population issues positioned women as experts in this medical field, but also revealed national differences. While British women doctors acquired recognition for their work at an international level and shaped the debate in favour of the more practical and medical aspects of birth control from the 1930s onwards, French women doctors, by contrast, were either absent from those debates or publicly aligned themselves with the politically sanctioned and legally safe pronatalist stances of their male colleagues. This difference could be explained by the lack of practical experience of the latter about contraception due to the 1920 law. In France, it would have been extremely difficult for French women doctors to publicly support the birth control movement without risking legal consequences, including imprisonment. Another significant element is their engagement with familialist associations that fought social scourges such as venereal disease. As members of familialist feminist associations, French women doctors adopted natalist stances. Thus, the two different conceptions of feminism and population policy and reproductive health greatly contributed to positioning British women as comparative leaders in reproductive knowledge.

Notes

1 An earlier version of this chapter appeared in *Social History of Medicine*: see C. Rusterholz, 'English and French women doctors in international debates on contraception (1920–1935)', *Social History of Medicine*, 31:2 (2018), pp. 328–47.
2 J. Fette, 'Pride and prejudice in the professions', p. 61.
3 *Ibid.*, pp. 69–70.
4 P. Pinell, 'Champ médical et processus de spécialisation', *Actes de la Recherche en Sciences Sociales*, 1 (2005), pp. 4–36.
5 I. Löwy and G. Weisz, 'French hormones: progestins and therapeutic variation in France', *Social Science & Medicine*, 60:11 (2005), pp. 2609–22.
6 R. A. Soloway, 'Neo-Malthusians, eugenists, and the declining birth-rate in England, 1900–1918', *Albion*, 10:3 (1978), pp. 264–86.
7 M. Roemer, 'Internationalism in medicine and public health' in D. Porter (ed.), *The History of Public Health and the Modern State* (Amsterdam: Rodopi, 1994), pp. 403–22; D. Neill, *Networks in Tropical Medicine: Internationalism, Colonialism, and the Rise of a Medical Specialty, 1890–1930* (Stanford: Stanford University Press, 2012); C. Sylvest, 'Continuity and change in British liberal internationalism, c.1900–1930', *Review of International Studies*, 31:2 (2005), pp. 263–83; J. Hodder, S. Legg and M. Heffernan, 'Introduction: historical geographies of internationalism, 1900–1950', *Political Geography*, 49 (2015), pp. 1–6.

8 Bashford, *Global Population*, p. 44.
9 On the organisation of this conference see Bashford, 'Nation, empire, globe'.
10 Bashford, *Global Population*, p. 212.
11 Wellcome Collection, London, SA/MWF/B/3/6, Journal 1967, Jubilee file 2 of 2.
12 See I. Crozier, '"All the world's a stage": Dora Russell, Norman Haire, and the 1929 London World League for Sexual Reform Congress', *Journal of the History of Sexuality*, 12:1 (2003), pp. 16–37; F. Tamagne, *La Ligue Mondiale Pour La Réforme Sexuelle: La science au service de l'émancipation sexuelle?* (Paris: Editions Belin, 2005); R. Dose, 'The World League for Sexual Reform: some possible approaches', *Journal of the History of Sexuality*, 12:1 (2003), pp. 1–15.
13 R. Pierpoint, *Report of the Fifth International Neo-Malthusian and Birth Control Conference: Kingsway Hall, London, July 11th to 14th, 1922* (London: William Heinemann Medical Books, 1922).
14 On this subject see Debenham, *Birth Control*, p. 114.
15 She was not a relative of the famous eugenicist Julian Huxley who attended the 1922 conference without presenting a paper.
16 Manchester Medical Collection, Manchester, Biographical files, GB133 MMC/2/Huxley, 'Frances Mabel Huxley'. See also 'Obituary notice', *British Medical Journal*, 2:5657 (1969), p. 638.
17 For the influence of eugenics on Killick Millard as a medical officer for health in Leicester see J. Welshman, 'Eugenics and public health in Britain, 1900–40: scenes from provincial life', *Urban History*, 24:1 (1997), pp. 56–75. For the involvement of Binnie Dunlop in the Malthusian League see R. Ledbetter, *History of the Malthusian League, 1877–1927* (Columbia: Ohio State University Press, 1986), pp. 206–9. For the many connections of Norman Haire with the Eugenics Society and the Malthusian League see Wyndham, *Norman Haire*.
18 On Charles Vickery Drysdale and the way eugenic and neo-Malthusian ideas influenced him see Klausen and Bashford, 'Fertility control'.
19 Pierpoint, *Report of the Fifth International Neo-Malthusian and Birth Control Conference*, p. 7.
20 *Ibid.*, p. 5.
21 *Ibid.*, p. 58.
22 *Ibid.*, p. 219.
23 *Ibid.*, p. 115.
24 *Ibid.*, p. 230.
25 *Ibid.*

26 *Ibid.*, p. 234.
27 *Ibid.*, p. 246.
28 *Ibid.*
29 *Ibid.*
30 *Ibid.*, p. 246.
31 *Ibid.*
32 *Ibid.*
33 *Ibid.*, p. 247.
34 Fisher and Szreter have shown the different meanings attached to this word. See Szreter and Fisher, *Sex before the Sexual Revolution*.
35 Pierpoint, *Report of the Fifth International Neo-Malthusian and Birth Control Conference*, p. 267.
36 *Ibid.*, p. vii.
37 *Ibid.*, p. 269.
38 On the market of contraceptives see C. L. Jones, 'Under the covers? Commerce, contraceptives and consumers in England and Wales, 1880–1960', *Social History of Medicine*, 29:4 (2016), pp. 734–56.
39 *Ibid.*
40 N. Haire, 'Health aspects of birth control' in M. Sanger (ed.), *Medical and Eugenic Aspects of Birth Control: The Sixth International Neo-Malthusian and Birth Control Conference, Volume III* (New York: American Birth Control League, 1926), p. 95.
41 Wellcome Collection, London, SA/FPA/NK73, 'Letter from Marjorie Martin on behalf of Margaret Sanger to Mrs Marjorie Farrer, 14 June 1930'.
42 M. Sanger, 'Introduction' in M. Sanger and H. Stone (eds), *The Practice of Contraception: An International Symposium and Survey* (Baltimore: Williams & Wilkins, 1931), p. viii.
43 *Ibid.*, p. xviii.
44 Sanger and Stone, *The Practice of Contraception*.
45 For instance C. P. Blacker used eugenic rhetoric such as 'the effect upon the race of present day contraception is probably on balance dysgenic', in Sanger and Stone, *The Practice of Contraception*, p. 163.
46 Wellcome Collection, London, PP/CPB/B.4, 'Seventh International Birth Control Conference to be held in the Konzertsaal zur Kaufleuten Pelikanplatz Zurich, Switzerland'.
47 Sanger and Stone, *The Practice of Contraception*.
48 *Ibid.*, p. 12.
49 Debenham has also shown the influence of feminist movements on women doctors working in birth control clinics who were also members of feminist associations. See Debenham, *Birth Control*.

50 Hall, 'A suitable job for a woman', p. 142.
51 Sanger and Stone, *The Practice of Contraception*, p. 211.
52 With the support of pictures, Ernest Gräfenberg explained how to insert the Gräfenberg ring into the vagina. Based on his case studies with his female patients, he also presented the contraindications for such a method and the precautions doctors needed to take to avoid any harmful procedure against the female body.
53 Wellcome Collection, London, PP/CPB/C.2, 'Report of the Birth Control Investigation Committee, 1931'.
54 Sanger and Stone, *The Practice of Contraception*, p. 15.
55 *Ibid.*, p. 211.
56 *Ibid.*, pp. 216–8.
57 *Ibid.*, p. 215
58 *Ibid.*, p. 93.
59 *Ibid.*
60 *Ibid.*, p. 216.
61 *Ibid.*, p. 210.
62 *Ibid.*, p. 222.
63 G. M. Cox, *Clinical Contraception*, 2nd edition (London: Butterworth-Heinemann, 1937), p. 59.
64 Allen, *Feminism and Motherhood in Western Europe*.
65 Wellcome Collection, London, SA/MWF/K8/3, 'Report on Birth Control by Dame Louise McIlroy, MWIA 3rd congress Stockholm'.
66 Debenham, *Birth Control*.
67 A. L. McIlroy, 'The harmful effects of artificial contraceptive methods', *The Practitioner*, (July 1923), pp. 25–35.
68 D. Blanchier, 'Compte-rendu de l'enquête faite à propos du "Birth control"!', *Bulletin de l'Association française des femmes médecins*, 15 (1933), p. 6.
69 *Ibid.*
70 G. Montreuil-Strauss, 'Le Birth control: Exposé historique par Montreuil-Strauss', *Bulletin de l'Association française des femmes médecins*, 12 (1933), pp. 3–22.
71 Bibliothèque interuniversitaire de Santé, Paris, *Bulletin de l'Association Internationale des femmes médecins*, 7 (1932), p. 15.
72 Blanchier, 'Compte-rendu', p. 7.
73 *Ibid.*
74 *Ibid.*
75 *Ibid.*, p. 25.
76 C. Carribon and A. Duetto, 'Le Bulletin de l'Association française des femmes médecins (1929–40). Un discours médical spécifique aux femmes ?', *Le Temps des medias*, 23:2 (2014), pp. 46–8.

77 A. Cova, *Au service de l'Eglise, de la patrie et de la famille: femmes catholiques et maternité sous la III République* (Paris: L'Harmattan, 2000).
78 Blanchier, 'Compte-rendu', p. 30.
79 Offen, 'Depopulation', p. 654; K. Offen, *Les féminismes en Europe (1700–1950): une histoire politique* (Rennes: Presses Universitaires de Rennes, 2012).
80 M. J. Maynes, B. Søland and C. Benninghaus, *Secret Gardens, Satanic Mills: Placing Girls in European History, 1750–1960* (Bloomington: Indiana University Press, 2005).
81 This information came from the database created by Fabrice Cahen and Adrien Minard on the organisations and affiliated members involved in combating 'social scourges' and aiming at protecting 'life'. See F. Cahen and A. Minard, 'Les mobilisations pour "la vie" et contre les "fléaux sociaux" dans l'entre-deux-guerres: essai de cartographie sociale', *Histoire et Mesure*, 31:2 (2016), pp. 141–70.
82 Y. Knibiehler, 'L'éducation sexuelle des filles au XXe siècle', *Clio. Femmes, Genre, Histoire*, 4 (1996), pp. 419–82. Gelly has shown how medical training on birth control was scarce and biased even after 1990. See M. Gelly, *Avortement et contraception dans les études médicales: une formation inadaptée* (Paris: Editions l'Harmattan, 2006).
83 C. Bard, *Les filles de Marianne: Histoire des féminismes; 1914–40* (Paris: Fayard, 1995); C. Mitchell, 'Madeleine Pelletier (1874–1939): the politics of sexual oppression', *Feminist Review*, 33 (1989), pp. 72–92.
84 Blanchier, 'Compte-rendu', p. 10.
85 Knibiehler, 'L'éducation sexuelle des filles au XXe siècle'.
86 Allen, *Feminism and Motherhood in Western Europe*, p. 140.
87 Wellcome Collection, London, SA/MWF/K/8, 'Martindale quoted in L. McIlroy, "Report on birth control"', p. 18.
88 *Ibid.*
89 Blanchier, 'Compte-rendu', p. 24.
90 Bibliothèque interuniversitaire de Santé, Paris, Fonds Dalsace, Dalsace birth control, 11.1 'Rapport sur le "birth control" par le Dr Ludmilla Dewetterova, 3e Congrès quinquennal de l'Association internationale des Femmes-Médecins, Stockholm du 7 au 12 août 1934'.
91 Wellcome Collection, London, SA/MWF/K/8, 'McIlroy, Report on birth control'.
92 On the relationships between feminism and birth control in England see Debenham, *Birth Control*.
93 Wellcome Collection, London, SA/MWF/K/8, 'McIlroy, Report on birth control'.
94 *Ibid.*

95 On the issue of abortion in Britain see S. Brooke, '"A new world for women?" Abortion law reform in Britain during the 1930s', *The American Historical Review*, 106:2 (2001), pp. 431–59.
96 M. Anchel-Bach, 'La mortalité maternelle et l'avortement', *Bulletin de l'Association français des femmes médecins*, 18 (1937), p. 29.
97 J. Campbell, 'Abortion in relation to maternal mortality', *Journal of the Medical Women's Federation* (May 1936), p. 27.
98 *Ibid.*

4

Building a transnational movement for family planning: 1928–70

This chapter delves into the many ways in which British women doctors pressed for the development of an international movement for birth control and family planning, from the first attempt in 1928 to create an international organisation to the establishment of the International Planned Parenthood Federation in 1952.[1] In addition, this chapter pushes the transnational approach even further by showing how the circulation of actors and knowledge from Britain to France eased the creation of a French family planning movement and family planning centres. As shown in Chapter 3, from the mid-1920s, British female doctors were decisive agents of the medicalisation of birth control at international conferences. These conferences gathered scientists, doctors and activists – the majority of whom were male – and advocated the use of birth control, but on different grounds. Alison Bashford has argued that population, food security and world resources were central motives behind famous scientists' participation in this movement.[2] Women were also present, and chief among them was the American birth control activist Margaret Sanger. The British women who took part in these international conferences were strongly feminist and envisaged birth control as a means of improving women's health. At the 1930 Zurich International Conference on Birth Control, female British doctors, alongside female German, Swedish and American doctors, shaped the debate in favour of the medicalisation of the issue. They drew on their practical experience acquired at national levels to move away from moral considerations of birth control, and instead concentrated on applied scientific knowledge of contraceptive methods. This experience made them skilled in debating the issue at international levels, reinforcing their expertise and positioning them as experts on these issues.

British women doctors were also instrumental in the creation of the first international movement specifically dedicated to spreading the 'gospel of birth control' in the interwar years, namely the Birth Control International Information Centre (BCIIC). After the Second World War, this international campaign for birth control spawned the International Planned Parenthood Federation, in which contraception was formally established as a medical issue. In the reactivation of this movement, British women doctors assumed prominence, along with their Swedish, American and Dutch colleagues. Drawing on the proceedings of international conferences on contraception and family planning; the archives of the Medical Women's Federation, the Family Planning Association, and the Mouvement Français pour le Planning Familial; and female doctors' publications, this chapter demonstrates the agency of British female doctors from 1930 onwards at the transnational level. In doing so, this chapter first looks at their contribution and their role in the first attempt to create a Birth Control International Information Centre, before analysing their contribution to setting up the International Planned Parenthood Federation (IPPF). Finally, a discussion of the influence of British women doctors on French doctors and the French movement for family planning closes this chapter.

Going international: the Birth Control International Information Centre

As briefly explained in Chapter 3, following the 1927 Geneva conference, and under the leadership of Margaret Sanger and Edith How-Martyn, in 1928 a first attempt was made to create an official organisation for people working on birth control. It resulted in a London-based centre, the Birth Control International Information Centre, aimed at 'disseminating applied knowledge on contraception'[3] through a network of *women physicians*, social workers and birth control activists. The centre provided information, literature, and updates on the 'latest and most hygienic measure known'[4] for avoiding pregnancy. Besides spreading information, the centre collaborated with birth control clinics in London to offer training in contraception to foreign doctors; this teaching was under the leadership of Helena Wright. Her expertise and experience in pushing for training facilities in Britain (see Chapter 1) made her the ideal person to take up this new work, and it illustrates how Wright easily navigated between the national and international spheres, using the skills and knowledge she acquired at both levels to advance the cause of birth control.

Numerous leaflets presenting the work of the centre called attention to the fact that 'urgent appeals from doctors and social workers in all parts of the world' had reached the centre. This shows how calls for birth control advice originated from the grassroots activism of people in touch with the needs of mothers, as well as mothers themselves, who 'begged' the centre 'to help them with knowledge and advice for limiting and spacing their family'.[5] The centre had correspondents in many countries, such as Poland, Spain, South Africa, Japan, Norway, Sweden, Finland, Soviet Russia, Canada, India, Japan, China and France. These correspondents testify to the onset of an international movement. Interestingly, the French correspondents who were invited to present the situation in France to members of the centre were not native French, but migrants who lived in France; these included Susanna Green (1855–1937), a British-born educator who lived in France, and the Dutch writer, traveller and mistress of H. G. Wells, Odette Zoé Keun, who lived with Wells in Grasse. Both visited the Birth Control International Information Centre and spoke about the French situation. They also received training in birth control.[6] In addition, Green distributed leaflets provided by the BCIIC to French public health officials. The fact that it was non-French individuals who advocated birth control is revealing of the repressive context in which many French individuals found themselves.

Finally, the centre organised international conferences on birth control. As explained by Lord Horder when opening the 1933 London conference, organised by the BCIIC on the subject of birth control in Asia, the main goal of the centre was 'missionary, that is to say, it aims at making known as widely as possible, and … in as many countries and languages as possible, the gospel of birth control'.[7] The term 'missionary' evidences the legacy of colonialism and the view held by BCIIC on the leading roles of its members in educating other countries. This form of knowledge transfer implies an assumption of superiority on the part of BCIIC members. Representatives of Japan, India,[8] China and Ceylon were present. Helena Wright opened the session on the practical problems of contraception in the East. Lord Horder, introducing her to the audience, emphasised her expertise in birth control in Britain but also stressed the fact that she had lived in China and had 'studied the problem there',[9] thereby portraying her as both a national and international expert. Wright started by presenting what she considered to be the essential element for setting up an international movement for birth control, namely the fact that the input should come from within each country. She adopted a stance that she would keep while reactivating the international movement of planned parenthood after the Second World War: while acknowledging that financial and advisory help could prove fruitful, she emphasised that 'control of the movement ought to be in the country in which the work is taking place'.[10] This position would later clash with that of Margaret Sanger, as I will show in the following section. To foster the development of national birth control movements and centres, Wright explained that she had already trained a female Chinese doctor in contraception: Dr Ling, who was willing to open a training centre in Peking. Wright's strong case in favour of national self-determination to develop birth control infrastructures in foreign countries was picked up again and made central by Edith How-Martyn while closing the conference, showing how influential Helena Wright's ideas were. The movement was very much a Western movement, however, attempting to spread its own views to other countries by educating members about Western values and methods.

Between 1930 and 1940, in a context of fear of declining fertility, supporters and militants for birth control foregrounded the positive aspects of their work. Besides relying on arguments connected to the health of the mother – where eugenic, neo-Malthusian and feminist arguments were invoked at international conferences – they increasingly referred to 'planned parenthood' alongside 'birth control', a way to stress the right of parents to decide the size of their family as well as the individual welfare of the child. For instance, the 1936 leaflet advertising the BCIIC distinguished between birth control in the Western world and 'uncontrolled fertility elsewhere',[11] and epitomised birth control in modernity. Accepted by most 'progressive people',[12] birth control was 'one of the greatest achievements of modern science'.[13] While parental health, especially that of mothers, had been an essential argument for the legitimation of the use of birth control in the previous decade, individual responsibility for the well-being of the child was central in the leaflet:

> By making the birth of a child dependent on foresight and deliberate choice, birth control has enabled parents to exercise a civilised regard for the rights of the children whom they voluntarily bring into the world. The knowledge of this power to control conception has heightened the self-respect of men and women, and immensely increased their sense of personal responsibility for the good management of their own lives, and for the welfare of their children.[14]

Framed in the rhetoric of rationalisation typical of the post-Depression era, when the UK and US encouraged economic planning, this quotation encompasses all the propositions that would constitute the motto of the IPPF: the parents' responsibility to decide on the size of their family, the emphasis on voluntary and rational child-rearing, and, most importantly, the right of children to be wanted and to have a good life.[15] The concept of planned parenthood aimed to improve the environment in which children were born and raised so as to make every child a wanted child. This idea opened up the path to a new medical research field focusing on infertility and harmonious matrimonial relationships as instrumental to good child-rearing. Female doctors invested in these new fields in great numbers, as we saw in the previous chapter.

This international movement was halted for a decade by war, before resurfacing afterwards in 1946. The prevailing context was no longer one of declining fertility, but of the growth of the global population and of an intensive population explosion in Asia, Latin America and Africa, raising fears of shortages of food and resources.[16] As the following section shows, women doctors again played a pivotal role in rebuilding and expanding this international movement.

Women doctors as creators of the international movement for planned parenthood

Women doctors were instrumental to the creation of the international movement for planned parenthood after the Second World War. Sweden hosted the first postwar international Conference on Sex Education, Family Planning, and Marriage Counselling in Stockholm in 1946, organised by Elise Ottesen-Jensen from the National League for Sex

Education, who was also present at the 1930 international conference.[17] Ottesen-Jensen invited Joan Malleson to attend the conference as a representative of the FPA.[18] During the conference, a resolution was passed on the need to recreate an international association of family planning and population professionals. This call quickly came to fruition. With the financial support of Margaret Sanger, and under the auspices of the FPA, an international congress on Population and World Resources in Relation to the Family was held in Cheltenham, Britain. It brought together scientists from more than twenty-two different countries. Elise Ottesen-Jensen and Margaret Sanger were both present. Several British women doctors participated in the conference and played a pivotal role in its organisation; Wright was the chairwoman of the organisation committee. She described this role as 'a key position that has to be handled very technically and carefully since you mustn't frighten the people around you whose ideas are smaller'.[19] In other words, the position required the negotiating skills that Wright acquired in her fight for birth control in Britain. She first contacted the leaders of the birth control movement in China, the US, Sweden and Holland, and she later remembered: 'Quite early here was the chance of making the beginning of an international link but nothing had to be said yet'.[20] At the opening of the conference she described the aim of this international meeting: the conference would result in no less than 'well-considered, powerful action which will eventually change the conditions of the world. We cannot have a bigger aim than that, and we have to prove ourselves worthy of it.'[21]

Among the chairwomen of the sessions were Lady Denman, chairwoman of the FPA; Wright; Margaret Jackson, medical officer of the Exeter and District Women's Welfare Centre, which she had also contributed to setting up; and Malleson. These women had all been present at the international conference on contraception held in Zurich in 1930. Thus, they were central to the continuity of the movement for birth control and its reconfiguration into the planned parenthood movement.[22] Wright would later explain that she was very well suited to being in charge of the organisational aspect of the conference, since she was 'a curious personality because [she was] essentially international and [she] got to know these people in Zurich.'[23] They were not exceptions in Britain; several male scientists, such as London's eugenics leader, Carlos Paton Blacker, who intervened in the 1930 Zurich conference, were also present. Male scientists still held highly visible positions in the conference and were in the majority as speakers; they included Abraham Stone, vice-president of the Planned Parenthood Federation of America; Professor Whelpton from the Scripps Foundation for Research in Population Problems at the University of Miami; and Sir John Boyd Orr, Director-General of the United Nations Food and Agriculture Organization. This situation reflected the need to gain recognition from the international community.

While Wright was supposed to chair the last session of the conference, she ceded her chair to one of her famous American male colleagues, Frank Lorimer, Professor of Sociology at the American University in Washington. Her retreat is symptomatic of the work carried out by female doctors: practical work that occurred behind the scenes, though it was essential to organising such an international network. Although women doctors' roles were less visible, they were highly influential since they were the ones who organised the conference and decided who to invite.

Only one French scientist was present, Jean Sutter from the National Institute of Demographic Studies. He presented the pronatalist policy in France, explaining that 'all French Governments are opposed to contraceptive propaganda, because of the state of our population, and for fear of accelerating the present trend and having a population which will decline, with incalculable speed, until it totally disappears'.[24] This position clashed with the increasing recognition of the importance of family planning underlying the conference. Consistently, the session's chair was quick to remind him that 'it was not merely a matter of family limitation; to many people, the object of providing contraceptive information was to give women freedom to decide for themselves the number of children that they wished to have'.[25] He drew attention to the idea of planned parenthood as disconnected from the natalist vision and encompassing the well-being of the family: 'the problem is not one of the large families but of happy families, and happy families could be attained only through freedom of choice and desire on the part of the parents themselves'.[26] Helena Wright recalled that, for France, they had chosen 'the wrong leader but we had to deal with it'.[27]

The resolution taken during the conference underlined the fact that 'wanted children who can be given a reasonable standard of living are the first essential for the building of a happy and stable family life'.[28] This led to the creation of a provisional international committee, made up of British (Wright), Dutch (Dr Conrad van Emde Boas), Swedish (Ottesen-Jensen) and American (Margaret Sanger and Abraham Stone) delegates; it was set up in London, due to the efforts of Wright and Margaret Pyke, secretary of the FPA, in an office provided by the Eugenics Society. The purpose of the committee was to exchange information and foster research on family planning – i.e. contraception, fertility and sub-fertility – by providing contraceptive information to clinics and doctors. To this end, it established contact with family planning organisations in over twenty countries. Finding a name proved difficult as soon as the idea of formalising the movement arose. Helena Wright remembered the complexity of finding a common ground between these personalities as they met for several hours each evening of the Cheltenham conference:

> We began to have long evening meetings. The personalities were so different. Conrad had to disagree with everything. Three and four evenings, three to four hours, we, four countries' leaders, beckoned, unable to find words. We had the idea, in our minds it was quite clear, but to find a word in English that would be acceptable to all personalities was our first experience of how difficult that was, but we succeeded.[29]

The correspondence between Helen Donington, secretary of the provisional centre, Margaret Sanger and Helena Wright attests to the conflicting views on the direction that the organisation should take. The common aim rested on the need to appoint an advisory board in each country, made up of distinguished and high-level individuals, to give status to the organisation as well as giving 'access to valuable data'[30] on the individuals in need of this service. In the British case, the names put forward were those of Lord Horder, physician and president of the Eugenics Society; Julian Huxley, the evolutionary biologist; and Sir John Boyd Orr, doctor, biologist and Director-General of the United Nations' new Food and Agriculture Organization (FAO) and a future Nobel Prize winner (1949). Margaret Sanger encouraged the British branch to have 'several population men' on its committee, reflecting her desire to orient the work of the organisation towards this subject.

Sanger was convinced that in order to gain support from American fundraisers the organisation needed to distance itself from the resolution taken at Cheltenham, since 'there is nothing in the resolution relative to world resources and a very great deal is said about family planning, marriage counselling and other aspects of the movement, which in the opinion of many people here, is not as important a need in the educational field as the subject of population and world resources'.[31] But while agreeing that close collaboration with eminent individuals working in the field of food resources was to be encouraged, British members were of the opinion that fundamental research on this topic, as suggested by Sanger, remained beyond the scope of the organisation and they would prefer to see this type of research undertaken by other bodies specialising in the area, such as the UN or UNESCO.[32] Indeed, as underlined by the British members, as a voluntary body, the organisation was free from 'political and religious pressure', and they were reluctant to 'burden themselves with this area of work'. In addition, the British members, Helena Wright and Margaret Pyke in particular, acted as mediators in the controversial issue of naming the international committee. Tensions arose between Margaret Sanger, a strong proponent of population control who suggested the name 'International Population Planning Committee', and the Swedish, Dutch and British members, who were in favour of addressing the sexual needs of individuals and were sensitive to the diverse attitudes towards sexuality among the peoples of the world. Eventually, they settled on the International Committee on Planned Parenthood (ICPP).[33] The ICPP helped to organise an International Congress on Population and Family Planning in India 'to begin definite preparations for a permanent world organisation'.[34] This conference resulted in the creation of the IPPF, to which Sanger was appointed honorary co-president.

The headquarters of the ICPP and later IPPF was in London and functioned as a central hub for help and advice on family planning for all member countries. At Wright's instigation, a medical subcommittee was formed in 1954 with the mission of collecting and circulating information on family planning services and setting standards of organisation for clinics.[35] Headed by Jackson, it aimed at 'reaching international agreement on tests and standards for contraceptive products'.[36] The headquarters also hosted training courses on contraceptive techniques and received the visit of a French delegation, as made clear in the first report of the IPPF.[37] To sum up, the federation again relied on women doctors to organise and provide the training of foreign members. Wright also travelled around India after the Bombay conference to give lectures and training in contraceptive techniques. In 1960, she undertook a teaching tour in Poland, as did Cecily Mure, of the Walworth Branch of the FPA, in Pakistan.[38] From 1963 onwards, Jackson, Wright, Eleanor Mears (1917–92, a gynaecologist, member of the MWF and medical secretary of the FPA) and Mary Pollock (clinical assistant at the Gynaecological and Fertility Department of the Royal Free Hospital) were members of the medical committee of the IPPF region for Europe, the Near East and Africa, testifying to the key roles they held in the IPPF.[39] Women doctors also circulated international work and contributed to the publication of handbooks. Mears edited a British issue of *Babies by Choice or by Chance* by Alan Guttmacher, the president of the IPPF. Wright, Jackson and Mears all wrote chapters in the *Medical Handbook on Contraception*, published by the IPPF in 1964. This handbook reviewed the latest advances in contraceptive methods and included contributions from international doctors.

Framing planned parenthood as a human right

This section analyses how planned parenthood became increasingly promoted as a basic human right, thanks, in part, to women doctors. This happened in the postwar context of the growth in discourse around 'human rights' (e.g. the Universal Declaration of Human Rights, 1948) and at a time when this concept became part of the language of everyday life and a marker of 'modern civilisation'. At the 1948 Cheltenham conference, four sessions were dedicated specifically to family planning. Study groups were also organised around the medical aspects of family planning, such as sub-fertility, sex education and marriage guidance, revealing the new stance of the family planning movement. In one of the family planning sessions, Jackson underscored the need for a different approach to family planning according to particular national priorities – for instance, encouraging birth regulation in Britain but birth limitation in parts of the world facing overpopulation.[40] This call would form the basis of the policy of the IPPF. The IPPF's country-specific approach would increasingly be recognised as the 'proper' family planning policy by policymakers all over the world.

A constitution for the new federation was finalised at the Fourth International Conference in Stockholm in 1953. It stressed knowledge of contraception as a 'fundamental human right'.[41] By referring to contraception as a 'human right', this constitution pinpointed the international dimension of this right, beyond the individual rights of Western citizens. It reflected the view that birth control had to become an international priority and that every human should consider birth control and plan their family accordingly. In addition, this rhetoric diluted the feminist perspective usually linked with birth control, in favour of a more 'gender-neutral' approach to family planning, where gender specificities were less visible. Framing birth control as a human right was also a means to ally politicians and governments, who might plausibly have been reluctant to support a feminist narrative. Another aim was to stimulate appropriate research in the following subjects: 'the biological, demographic, social, economic and eugenic implications of human fertility and its control; methods of contraception; fertility, sub-fertility and sterility; sex education and marriage counselling',[42] thus broadening the concept of 'planned parenthood'.

This cultural script of human rights became predominant, and it was found at the international conference in Vienna in 1968, organised by the International Women's Federation and entitled The Hungry Millions, a clear sign that family planning was again being seen through the lens of the 'population bomb'. Contemporary fears of population explosion and food shortages permeated all dimensions of the proceedings of this conference. Female medical doctors presented family planning as 'a basic human right' and underlined the need for medical responsibility in 'participating in a variety of methods of family planning which need to be carefully selected for their applicability to the people for whom they are advised'.[43] Education, rather than imposition, was presented as the best way of spreading family planning. These positions greatly reflected those of the IPPF, strengthening the cultural script spread by the federation. As pointed out by Nikolas Rose and Alison Bashford, individual freedom was the cornerstone of reproductive rights, and planned parenthood was to be achieved 'through the self-government of individual women: the exercise of a "universal" right to reproductive choice'.[44] Female doctors, among them Wright and Jackson, were thus instrumental in creating an international movement of planned parenthood after the Second World War and providing training to members from different countries in order to make 'this universal right' of contraception widely available. Their role was not only general, working in the larger international sphere; they exercised a great influence on French doctors in particular.

British women doctors' influence on French family planning centres (1950–70)

In 1956, more than thirty years after the 1920 law was enacted forbidding the dissemination of contraceptives and information on contraception, the French female gynaecologist Marie-Andrée Lagroua Weill-Hallé and the housewife Evelyne Sullerot, along with women from the middle and upper classes, created the Association of Happy Motherhood (Maternité Heureuse). This association was set up following the widely publicised 'Bac affair', where a young married couple was accused of accidental manslaughter following the death of their fifth child. The trial revealed that the mother was completely exhausted after five consecutive pregnancies. During the trial, witnesses were called to defend the couple, Lagroua Weill-Hallé being one of them. Ignorance about contraception was therefore perceived to be the reason behind this dramatic case. The fact that its founding members were all mothers gave the association respectability at a time when promotion of birth control was still illegal. Its aim was to fight ignorance, considered to be the main cause of backstreet abortions and unhappiness within marriage, through the spreading of information on contraception to its members thanks to the collection of scientific research on this topic carried out in France and abroad. The association was renamed the French Family Planning Movement (le Mouvement Français pour le Planning Familial) and became a national branch of the IPPF in 1959.

In 1967, after more than fifteen years of lobbying and intense activism from members of the movement, the Neuwirth Law legalised contraception in France. The history of the liberalisation of contraception and abortion has received much attention from historians.[45] However, what remains overlooked is the influence of the international network on the establishment of family planning centres in France. Recent research from Bibia Pavard has shown the importance of transnational exchange in the creation of the French Family Planning Movement. She has underlined how foreign experience of birth control, especially that in the US, helped to 'legitimate the cause of birth control in France'.[46]

A transnational movement for family planning 181

This last section extends Pavard's work by showing how the British case constituted a resource and model for family planning in France. In the French pronatalist and familialist context, where contraception and public propaganda on birth control were banned, approaching the subject of birth control through the lens of the debate in Britain and the US facilitated the advent of a similar but adapted debate in France. Similarly, recent research has shown the influence of British doctors in the contraceptive training of doctors in Spain and Poland.[47]

British women doctors represented a channel of birth control information for French doctors from 1935 onwards. The first French birth control clinic, a clandestine experiment that lasted no more than two years, opened in the city of Suresnes in 1935 due to the common efforts of Dr Jean Dalsace, an activist in the Association d'Etudes Sexologiques, who became a loyal supporter of birth control and contraception in France and one of the major figures of the movement, and Henri Sellier, the Popular Front's minister for public health. Henri Sellier built a garden city based on social hygiene in Suresnes, where they established a prenuptial clinic and distributed information on sex education and diaphragms as a way to prevent illegal abortions. As early as 1931, Edith How-Martyn from the Birth Control International Information Centre replied to a letter from Dalsace asking her for information on birth control, and she forwarded him literature on the subject. In 1934, one year before opening his birth control clinic in Suresnes, Dalsace wrote to Gladys Cox and Margaret Jackson, asking them to describe their work in the clinic and on infertility, as he was keen to learn more about this issue. Jackson replied, explaining that she referred patients with possible sterility to hospitals and private medical centres. The aim of birth control clinics 'is providing advice on birth control, [as] such information could not be found in other medical organisations'.[48] Dalsace seems to have used this material not only as a resource for opening 'his' centre in 1935 – little is known about the history of this clinic[49] – but also for documenting his 1934 conference paper, entitled 'Birth Control', for the Groupe d'Etudes Philosophiques et Scientifiques pour l'Examen des Tendances Nouvelles. He started his talk by expressing his reluctance to use the word 'birth control', a reluctance he felt not only towards the English expression but also due to its diverse translations in French. He argued that using 'control' meant the 'incursion of the State or the doctor or a third party into the couple's private intimacy'.[50] The various tentative translations into the French language were no better, in his view, which is why he would use 'birth control' in its English meaning and translation for lack of a better phrase. He emphasised the fact that due to the 1920 law he would not be able to present and explain birth control methods as such. He then offered a history of birth control and emphasised the leading role of Marie Stopes in Britain. He characterised Britain, a country generally depicted by the French as a 'hypocritical country', as honest with regard to sexual matters and praised its efficiency and simplicity in taking care of the issue through setting up birth control clinics. Britain was therefore presented as an example to follow, a country in which 'birth control is officially recognised and where it is perceived as a humanitarian charity',[51] whereas France was portrayed as a fickle country where birth control was widely practised but health authorities refused to take the issue under their care.

After the Second World War, and while creating the Mouvement Français pour le Planning Familial, French leaders of the movement such as Lagroua Weill-Hallé and Jean Dalsace made numerous references to Britain, presenting it as an example of the standard towards which modern medicine should strive. In 1953, in her article published in *La Semaine Médicale*, Lagroua Weill-Hallé presented the work carried out by US and UK family planning centres. She also tried to translate 'planned parenthood' into French, settling on *'maternité dirigée'* (directed motherhood), a clear refocus from parenthood to motherhood. She immediately refined her argument, emphasising that it meant giving parents the opportunity to have a wanted child. This labelling attests to Lagroua Weill-Hallé's desire to adapt the American and British experience to the particular circumstances of the French familialist and pronatalist climate. Indeed, to gain public support, especially from the medical profession, Lagroua Weill-Hallé had to distance herself from neo-Malthusianism and instead align her rhetoric with mainstream familialist language, which was dominant not only within the Ordre des Médecins – the medical association of doctors created during the Vichy Regime – but also among population experts such as the demographer Alfred Sauvy, director of the National Institute for Demographic Studies, who was against any change to the 1920 law. Lagroua Weill-Hallé called for a revision of the 1920 law and explained that such a stance was 'not incompatible with a pronatalist policy'.[52] She presented the US and the IPPF as sources of inspiration for her movement, explaining that she had first discovered birth control clinics while travelling in the US with her husband in 1947 and was introduced to the subject by Abraham Stone. She equally referred to the Cheltenham conference as a founding moment where different countries gathered to acknowledge the advance of '*maternité dirigée*'.

This was not Lagroua Weill-Hallé's only reference to the foreign context. In her speech at the Académie des Sciences Morales et Politiques on 'considerations about voluntary motherhood', advocating the dissemination of birth control information as a tool to prevent abortions, she underlined that 'opposition to birth control is unjustifiable in a country which flatters itself on permitting the individual the free exercise of his conscience. In other countries such as the US, Britain, Holland and Sweden, birth control has been accepted as a social measure.'[53] By comparing the French situation with that of other countries, she implicitly highlighted the French backwardness in terms of reproductive politics, and she called for a change in the law. This speech was reported in the bulletin of the IPPF, revealing that the French situation was closely followed by the IPPF's members who therefore considered France as a probable future member of the movement. Lagroua Weill-Hallé published a book in 1958 entitled *La liberté de la conception à l'étranger* (*The Freedom of Conception in Foreign Countries*), which described all the contraceptive methods available in family planning centres in the US and Britain, the Netherlands and Sweden based on the documentation provided by the FPA and that she acquired on a study trip she made to Britain and Netherlands. Moreover, Lagroua Weill-Hallé recognised the key role played by the British FPA in the creation of the French movement in a letter addressed to Margaret Pyke in 1961 about the inauguration of the first centre of the Mouvement Français pour le Planning Familial in Paris: 'We never forget to tell the numerous members of the movement that if British members did not contribute through their concern, help and generosity towards our work, we wouldn't have been able to develop the movement in France. In particular, our doctors know the pivotal role you played in helping them satisfy their medical prescriptions.'[54]

Following the Bac affair, birth control loomed large in the French press, and here again supporters of its use took Britain as a model. In 1961, the journalist Madeleine Franck published a series of articles in *France Soir*, relating a trip she undertook in Britain. Entitled 'Birth

Control: Yes or No', this series was aimed at providing the reader with accurate information to answer a set of specific questions:

> A husband and wife, can they and ought they to choose the most propitious moment for the birth of a child? Would it be desirable in everybody's interest, that scientific means be legally supplied to French women – as they are to English, American, Dutch and Scandinavian women – to control and plan their birth rate? Ethically, by making birth control easier, shall we take a step forward in civilisation, or on the contrary, a step backwards? If the sale of contraceptive pills were authorised in France, as has just been done in England, would you approve?[55]

To answer this question Madeleine Franck met Jean Medawar from the Family Planning Association in London. Jean Medawar was the joint editor of *Family Planning* from 1959 and had joined the FPA executive in 1960. In addition, she was a receptionist at the Islington Family Planning Clinic. Married to the Nobel Prize winner for medicine, Peter Medawar, the couple were the parents of four wanted children, born when the couple decided. The emphasis was therefore placed on the advantage of birth control for increasing the birth rate, aligning the article with the familialist policy in France. In Medawar's view, deliberate planning merely encouraged married couples to want several children since spacing the children prevented the wife's feelings of exhaustion and anxiety.[56] The journalist also emphasised the human dimension of the work carried out at the clinic. She interviewed Dr Rosalie Taylor, a psychosexual counsellor, who worked at the FPA and took an 'interest in the patient's personality'. Taylor tried to understand why some patients did not return for follow-up appointments and why some gave up the recommended methods. By emphasising how Taylor dealt with sexual difficulties within marriage, the journalist showed that the work of an FPA clinic was not restricted to prescribing contraception mechanically but entailed the treatment of sexual disorders and fears that could affect a happy marriage. The British experience was therefore put forward as a positive model that increased the birth rate – as the baby boom testified – and helped the stability of the marital relationship.

Besides the explicit example that Britain offered for the MFPF, letter exchanges between French and British doctors suggest that French doctors, Dalsace in particular, asked female British doctors for information on contraception. In December 1954, Vera Houghton, executive secretary of the IPPF, sent him leaflets explaining the aims of the federation and its first annual report. The same letter also testifies to a meeting between Dalsace and Cecily Mure in Paris. While the content of the meeting is not mentioned, this meeting without doubt provided the latter with practical insights into the running of family planning clinics. Leaflets on family planning were sent to Lagroua Weill-Hallé upon request in 1956.[57] Arlette Fribourg from Paris also wrote to Eleanor Mears asking for information about the contraceptive pill in 1961: 'I wish to know if they are now obtainable in your department of the FPA and experience you have already in England about this method. In case you can send contraceptive pills, can you tell me if they are the same (same product or pharmaceutical product) as in the USA?'[58] The same year, the FPA granted permission to Catherine Valabrègue, secretary of the French association, to make a French version of the 24-minute film *Birthright* made by the FPA in 1958.[59] This film presented the work of the British clinics and advocated for the need to develop birth control in developing countries as a means to fight poverty. It was divided into six sections: 'wanted' children, infertility, pre-marital counselling, gynaecological problems, contraception and concern for global population growth. The film was made available for members of the association and was screened during training sessions. Therefore, the film provided the French audience with all the necessary information to understand family planning and the initiatives developed in Britain to help couples have a child when they wanted one.

Training and visits to Britain by many French doctors, as individuals or members of the Mouvement Français pour le Planning Familial, also demonstrate the influence of British doctors on French doctors. In 1947, Dr Suzanne Képès, a gynaecologist who was well versed in psychiatry, undertook a trip to London and received training in contraception at one of the family planning clinics. Following this trip, convinced of the necessity of contraception, she started to import caps and diaphragms clandestinely to France and made numerous trips between the two countries for this purpose.[60] She would later explain that, similarly to the reason behind the creation of family planning clinics in Britain, the solution to unwanted pregnancy and the high level of illegal abortions was contraception: 'I threw myself into this fight with my own motivations. Something needed to be done, doing what was fair and right for women and men.'[61] In 1955, she met Lagroua Weill-Hallé and joined the association in 1956.

In 1957, the IPPF report for the region of Europe recognised the decisive role of the British FPA in helping the French medical body to develop family planning: 'The number of doctors from France who have called at the regional office, visited the headquarters of the FPA and seen over a Clinic is most encouraging. It indicates growing concern at the present situation in France where the 1920 law forbids any propaganda for birth control or the giving of advice on contraception.'[62] The same report stated that both Lagroua Weill-Hallé and Evelyne Sullerot had embarked on study trips to London.[63] According to letters exchanged between British members, Lagroua Weill-Hallé visited the headquarters and shared her main problem with the French situation: 'to convince the doctors in France that family planning has positive aspects and is not designed to limit the population.'[64] Lagroua Weill-Hallé met with Helena Wright, whom she described as 'the champion of contraception in Britain', and learnt about the insertion and the placing of the occlusive pessary.[65] In addition, she took back with her to France the books written by Helena Wright and Joan Malleson. She later wrote back to the headquarters, thanking them for having given a wide range of documentation to Evelyne Sullerot.

During the first decade after the creation of the Mouvement Français pour le Planning Familial, such a trip seemed to be an initiation ritual for new doctors joining the movement. In 1959, Yvonne Dornes and Catherine Valabrègue spent forty-eight hours in London and met Helena Wright, Joan Rettie and Cecily Mure. They were taught at the FPA headquarters in 'a room adjacent to a laboratory where toads frolicked in a small tub'. Toads were used by the FPA to detect pregnancy, while in France rabbits were used for the same purpose.[66] French doctors were being instructed alongside a diverse audience of foreign doctors and nurses. Doctors were asked to train in the fitting of contraceptive devices by practising on the body model designed by Helena Wright.[67] According to the testimony of Catherine Valabrègue, published in the journal of *Maternité Heureuse*, 'Helena Wright displayed great human empathy in her speech, which made her particularly fascinating.'[68] She regularly checked that her audience had followed her demonstration by asking whether they had any questions. She urged the doctors to be especially sensitive to the issues of 'adjustment of the patient to the contraceptive methods recommended' and of the follow-up appointment, usually one week after the initial fitting, during which the doctor ensured that the patient understood the functioning of the method and that she was satisfied with it.[69]

The French women doctors Le Sueur-Capelle, Boutet de Montvel and Kahn-Nathan made their way to London to take a practical internship at the family planning clinic in 1961 and 1962,[70] as did four French doctors in 1963.[71] Dr Elisabeth Aubény, a gynaecologist who would later become the president of the French Association of Contraception, reflected on her experience in London. In 1963, as a medical student in gynaecology, she did an internship at the Broca Hospital in Paris, where both Jean Dalsace and Raoul Palmer worked, specialising in issues around sterility. There, she discovered the idea of family planning. While she encountered deaths in her practice due to backstreet abortions, the condom was the only method she would recommend to her patients since it was permitted in France as a means to fight venereal disease. At Broca, Dalsace shared his interest in family planning and suggested that she should take a training course in London. Aubény, along with her two female gynaecologist interns, went to London and were received by the IPPF. As she later recalled, they were very impressed by the efficiency of the organisation. They were sent to visit birth control clinics and were amazed by the large number of patients that were seen in a short period.[72] They learnt how to insert a cap along with contraceptive jelly and practised on Helena Wright's pelvic body model. They bought caps and diaphragms and clandestinely brought them back to Paris. They also noticed that some birth control clinics prescribed the pill to their patients for a trial period. Aubény was shocked, as she recalled that when the pill arrived on the French market, she was unwilling to prescribe it, explaining that 'it was not how medicine was taught to us during our study years. The duty of the doctor is to treat diseases that endanger life. The doctor offered a diagnosis, established a treatment. In the case of contraception, all the classical schemes were shattered.'[73] Having had the opportunity to be trained in contraception and in how to insert a diaphragm, these women doctors knew they were part of a broader movement. They travelled back from London 'satisfied and proud, conscious of bringing to their female patients a contraceptive technique, admittedly restrictive and not entirely reliable, but a technique that they would own and practise themselves', as Aubény recalled *a posteriori*.[74] In France, they would follow the exact procedures they had learnt in Britain to teach their private patients, applying the knowledge they gained in their own daily practice.

The inspiration and training provided by the British model was not limited to contraception but also extended to psychosexual counselling. Suzanne Képès, who was in charge of the training of doctors at the MFPF from 1965, suggested in 1968 that doctors working with the MFPF should be trained in psychology, based on the seminar training that the FPA offered to its doctors – the Balint seminar.[75] Képès had attended a training seminar at the Tavistock Clinic under the supervision of Balint in 1966. In 1968, she contacted Dr Sara Abel, a FPA trainee in Balint's technique, to offer a report on her work. The idea was to share her experience with members of the MFPF to provide basic information on the method. The FPA doctors who underwent this training were handling a wide range of issues, including sexual disorders such as vaginismus, frigidity and non-consummation, which were issues familiar to French doctors. She suggested setting up similar seminars in which MFPF doctors could share and analyse their cases and gain input from each other. The Balint seminar, she suggested, could be delivered under the supervision of Dr Michel Sapir, a well-known psychiatrist and a follower of Balint with whom she collaborated regularly, Dr Main from London, and even, periodically, Balint himself. Suzanne Képès would be a loyal follower of Balint and apply his method for her entire career. In 1972, she wrote that in her view, Balint's legacy in the way medicine was practised would be greater than Freud's contribution.[76]

The Family Planning Association also provided French doctors with contraceptive products. Many letters from private doctors to the secretary of the FPA testify to this mailing of devices. By 1960, the FPA had noticed a dramatic increase in the numbers of French requests for contraceptive devices, as shown by a letter from the medical secretary of the FPA to Nelson-Barette:

> During the past two years orders from patients in France for contraceptives have increased from the occasional one about every six months to an average of ten a day. During 1960, the total value of the orders was approximately 1000 (which includes an estimate for the last two weeks of December). The orders are largely for Durex Dutch caps (on which the profit on the cost prices is 71.4%) and duracreme on which the profit on cost price is 50%.[77]

Finally, presentations by British members at conferences organised by the French body and contributions to French publications also support the hypothesis of a decisive British influence. As early as 1955, in the special issue of *Gynécologie Pratique* on birth control, Horder, president of the FPA, was asked by Dalsace to write an article on family planning in the UK. In June 1960, Cecily Mure was invited by Maternité Heureuse to take part in a publicity weekend in Paris in favour of family planning. She spoke at two meetings about the work done by the FPA in Britain.[78] In November 1963, Eleanor Mears gave a paper at a conference organised by Dalsace and Palmer on contraception. She also spent some time with them and with Lagroua Weill-Hallé while she was in Paris.[79]

Conclusion

From the mid-1930s, British women doctors actively campaigned to add birth control and contraception to the list of legitimate medical specialties. This important work, carried out on a national scale, was also pursued on an international one. They were instrumental in recreating a transnational movement for birth control, changing to calling it planned parenthood at the dawn of the Second World War, and continuing afterwards. While male scientists were highly visible at the first postwar international conference (1948) dedicated to this subject – mirroring the stratification of the field of medicine and the fact that men seemingly held the positions of prestige – British women doctors were nevertheless very influential. Working behind the scenes, they took up the practical and organisational tasks of running the event and liaised with different individuals to build a transnational movement for planned parenthood. While often overlooked, this type of work was essential and significant in shaping the aims of this new alliance. During this international conference and those that followed, contraception became increasingly defined as a human right.

Women doctors' new position within medical circles at both national and international levels made their knowledge particularly attractive to foreign doctors seeking accurate knowledge on contraception. It is thus unsurprising that French doctors turned to their British counterparts to gain insight into family planning issues. In the French national context, where the advertisement of and recourse to birth control methods were prohibited, the experience of British doctors and their expertise on contraception constituted a useful and significant example to rely upon. By writing letters, attending training sessions and inviting British women doctors to meetings, French medical circles found the perfect example of a well-organised, efficient family planning movement where scientific considerations replaced moral arguments. Therefore, British women doctors played a pivotal role in the creation of the family planning movement in France and the transfer of knowledge was a decisive tool for implementing family planning services in France.

Notes

1. Parts of this chapter appeared in *Medical History*: see Rusterholz, 'English women doctors'.
2. Bashford, *Global Population*.
3. Wellcome Collection, London, PP/CPB/C.2, 'Birth Control International Information Centre'.
4. Butler Library, University of Columbia, New York, Margaret Sanger papers, microfilm, Series III, Collected Document Series, Subseries II, Organisation and Conference, 'Birth Control International Information Centre'.
5. Wellcome Collection, London, PP/EPR/F.1/1:Box 5, 'World-wide birth control an appeal'.
6. Wellcome Collection, London, PP/EPR/F.1/1:Box 5, 'List of correspondents'.
7. M. Fielding (ed.), *Birth Control in Asia: A Report of a Conference Held at the London School of Hygiene & Tropical Medicine, November 24–5, 1933* (London: Birth Control International Information Centre, 1935), p. 11.
8. On the relationship between India and BCIIC see chapter 2 in S. Hodges, *Contraception, Colonialism and Commerce: Birth Control in South India, 1920–1940* (Aldershot: Ashgate, 2008), pp. 47–75.
9. Fielding, *Birth Control in Asia*, p. 79.
10. Ibid., p. 80.
11. Wellcome Collection, London, PP/CPB/C.2, 'Birth Control International Information Centre, 1936'.
12. Ibid.
13. Ibid.
14. Ibid.
15. For the rhetoric of rationalisation see Marks, *Sexual Chemistry*, p. 21.
16. On the subject of population explosion and its connected fears see Bashford, *Global Population*; Connelly, *Fatal Misconception*.

17 S. Kling, 'Reproductive health, birth control and fertility change in Sweden, circa 1900–40', *The History of the Family*, 15:2 (2010), pp. 161–73.
18 Wellcome Collection, London, SA/FPA/A10/10, IPPF Conferences 1946–66, 'Letter from Elise Ottesen-Jensen to Joan Malleson, 10 July 1946'.
19 Women's Library, London School of Economics, London, 8SUF/B/130, 'Interview with Helena Wright'.
20 Women's Library, London School of Economics, London, 8SUF/B/149, 'Interview with Helena Wright'.
21 Wellcome Collection, London, PP/EFG/A.46 Griffith: Publication on NBCA/FPA 1930s–40s, 'Proceedings of the International Congress on Population and World Resources in relation to the Family, August 1948, Cheltenham England', p. 8.
22 The London eugenics leader Carlos Paton Blacker and the president of the British FPA Thomas Jeeves Horder, who presided over the Asian conference in 1933, were also both present.
23 Women's Library, London School of Economics, London, 8SUF/B/149, 'Interview with Helena Wright'.
24 Wellcome Collection, London, PP/EFG/A.46 Griffith: Publication on NBCA/FPA 1930s–40s, 'Proceedings of the International Congress on Population and World Resources in relation to the Family, August 1948, Cheltenham England', p. 109.
25 *Ibid.*, p. 111.
26 *Ibid.*, p. 111.
27 Women's Library, London School of Economics, London, 8SUF/B/149, 'Interview with Helena Wright'.
28 Wellcome Collection, London, PP/EFG/A.46 Griffith: Publication on NBCA/FPA 1930s–40s, 'Proceedings of the International Congress on Population and World Resources in relation to the Family, August 1948, Cheltenham England', p. 244.
29 Women's Library, London School of Economics, London, 8SUF/B/130, 'Interview with Helena Wright'.
30 Butler Library, University of Columbia, New York, Margaret Sanger papers, microfilm, Series III, subseries 1 correspondence, 'Letter from Helen Donington to Margaret Sanger, 10th November 1948'.
31 Butler Library, University of Columbia, New York, Margaret Sanger papers, microfilm, Series III, subseries 1 correspondence, 'Letter from Margaret Sanger to Helen Donington, 13th January 1949'.
32 Butler Library, University of Columbia, New York, Margaret Sanger papers, microfilm, Series III, subseries 1 correspondence, 'Letter from Helen Donington to Margaret Sanger, 28th January 1949'.

33 On these tensions see D. H. Linder, *'Crusader for Sex Education'*: *Elise Ottesen-Jensen (1886–1973) in Scandinavia and on the International Scene* (Lanham, MD: University Press of America, 1996), pp. 175–82.
34 V. Houghton, 'Report of meeting of International Committee on Planned Parenthood', *The Eugenics Review*, 43:3 (1951), p. 141.
35 Wellcome Collection, London, SA/FPA/A10/8, 1955–66 IPPF, 'Letter from Helena Wright to medical members of the IPPF's governing body, 3 March 1955': 'I proposed the setting-up of a medical sub-committee of doctors only, for the purposes outlined in IPPF 35(L). The governing body gave its sanction and at the second meeting of the Medical Sub-Committee I was appointed Chairman.'
36 Bibliothèque interuniversitaire de Santé, Paris, Fonds Dalsace–Vellay, Vellay 9.5 IPPF, 'The IPPF Medical Committee', in *News of Population and Birth Control*, CXVII (1963).
37 Bibliothèque interuniversitaire de Santé, Paris, Fonds Dalsace–Vellay, Vellay 9.5 IPPF, 'First annual report, 29 November 1952/31 August 1953'.
38 Wellcome Collection, London, SA/FPA/A10/8, 1955–66 IPPF, 'International Planned Parenthood Federation region for Europe near East and Africa, Minutes of the Fifth Meeting of the Regional Council, November 1960'.
39 Wellcome Collection, London, SA/FPA/A10/8, 1955–66 IPPF, 'Letter from Elstone Secretary of the IPPF to Helena Wright, 8 November 1963'; 'Letter from Elstone Secretary of the IPPF to Mary Pollock, 20 April 1966'.
40 Wellcome Collection, London, PP/EFG/A.46 Griffith: Publication on NBCA/FPA 1930s–40s, 'Proceedings of the International Congress on Population and World Resources in relation to the Family, August 1948, Cheltenham, England'.
41 Bibliothèque interuniversitaire de Santé, Paris, Fonds Dalsace–Vellay, Vellay 9.5, 'First annual report, 29 November 1952/31 August 1953, IPPF'.
42 *Ibid.*
43 Wellcome Collection, London, SA/MWF/K.8/12, 'Report on the 11th Congress Vienna, 24–25 June 1968'.
44 Bashford, *Global Population*, p. 330.
45 See Pavard, *'Si je veux, quand je veux'*; Bard and Mossuz-Lavau, *Le planning familial*.
46 B. Pavard, 'Du birth control au planning familial (1955–60): un transfert militant', *Histoire@Politique*, 18:3 (2012), pp. 162–78.
47 See T. Ortiz-Gómez and A. Ignaciuk, 'The fight for family planning in Spain during late Francoism and the transition to democracy, 1965–79', *Journal of Women's History*, 30:2 (2018), pp. 38–62.
48 Bibliothèque interuniversitaire de Santé, Paris, Fonds Dalsace–Vellay, Dalsace 11.1.

49 Ibid.
50 Author's own translation: 'L'incursion de l'Etat, du docteur ou de tout autre personne dans l'intimité du couple', in Bibliothèque interuniversitaire de Santé, Paris, Fonds Dalsace–Vellay, Dalsace 13, '"Birth control", paper presented at the Groupe d'études philosophiques et scientifiques pour l'examen des tendances nouvelles, 15 février 1934'.
51 Author's own translation: 'le birth control y est officiellement reconnu et perçu comme nécessaire d'un point de vue humanitaire et charitable', in Bibliothèque interuniversitaire de Santé, Paris, Fonds Dalsace–Vellay, Dalsace 13, '"Birth control", paper presented at the Groupe d'études philosophiques et scientifiques pour l'examen des tendances nouvelles, 15 février 1934'.
52 Author's own translation: 'n'est pas incompatible avec une politique nataliste', in Bibliothèque interuniversitaire de Santé, Paris, Fonds Dalsace–Vellay, Dalsace 11.1. M.-A. Lagroua Weill-Hallé, 'Le contrôle des naissances et la loi française de 1920', *La semaine médicale, supplément de la semaine des hôpitaux* (22 mars 1953).
53 Author's own translation: 'L'opposition au contrôle des naissance est injustifiable dans un pays qui se flatte de permettre le libre exercice de la conscience. Dans d'autres pays comme les Etats-Unis, l'Angleterre, la Hollande ou la Suède, le contrôle des naissances est accepté comme une mesure sociale', in Bibliothèque interuniversitaire de Santé, Paris, Fonds Dalsace–Vellay, Dalsace 11.1. Lagroua Weill-Hallé, 'Considération sur la maternité volontaire, 15 December 1954'.
54 Wellcome Collection, London, SA/FPA/A21/8 France 1951–67, 'Letter from *La maternité Heureuse*, MFPF, 31 October 1961 to Mrs Pyke'.
55 Wellcome Collection, London, SA/FPA/A21/8 France 1951–67, M. Franck, 'Contrôles de naissances oui ou non?' in *France Soir* (March 1961).
56 Ibid.
57 For exchange of information between Britain and France see Bibliothèque interuniversitaire de Santé, Paris, Fonds Dalsace–Vellay, Vellay 9.5 IPPF. 'Letter from Vera Houghton'.
58 Wellcome Collection, London, SA/FPA/A21/8 France 1951–67, 'Letter from Arlette Fribourg to Eleanor Mears, 25 April 1961'.
59 Wellcome Collection, London, SA/FPA/A21/8 France 1951–67, 'Letter from Freda Parker to Mademoiselle D. Jeanson, January 20th 1961'.
60 B. Philippe, 'Suzanne Képès, une femme d'exception', *Le Carnet PSY*, 6:101 (2005), p. 36.
61 Author's own translation: 'Je me suis jetée dans cette bataille avec mes propres motivations. Quelque chose devait être fait. Je voulais faire quelque

chose de juste pour les femmes et les hommes'. S. Képès, *Du corps à l'âme, entretiens avec Danielle M. Lévy* (Paris: L'Harmattan, 1996), p. 102.
62 Wellcome Collection, London, SA/FPA/A10/8 1955–66 IPPF, 'Report of International Planned Parenthood Federation and accounts for the region for Europe, March 1957'.
63 They were not alone. According to a report from the FPA, Dr Pierre Bertrand, Dr Geneviève Hall, Dr Mato Medeau, Dr Elizabeth Palmer, Mrs Pechabrier (Ministry of Health and Education), Dr Yves Peninou, Evelyne Sullerot and Dr and Mrs Lagroua Weill-Hallé were all trained in 1956. See Wellcome Collection, London, SA/FPA/A10/8 1955–66 IPPF.
64 Wellcome Collection, London, SA/FPA/A10/8 1955–66 IPPF, '5th September 1956, Visit of Dr Weill-Hallé to headquarters'.
65 M.-A. Lagroua Weill-Hallé, *La prescription contraceptive* (Paris: Librairie Maloine, 1968), 11.
66 On pregnancy testing see J. Olszynko-Gryn, 'The demand for pregnancy testing: the Aschheim–Zondek reaction, diagnostic versatility, and laboratory services in 1930s Britain', *Studies in History and Philosophy of Science Part C: Studies in History and Philosophy of Biological and Biomedical Sciences*, 47 (2014), pp. 233–47.
67 On the body model see Chapter 1.
68 Author's own translation: 'Le Docteur Wright témoigne dans ses propos d'un sens humain qui la rend particulièrement captivante'. C. Valabrègue, '48 heures à Londres', in *La Maternité Heureuse, Bulletin trimestriel d'information*, 9 (1959), p. 11.
69 Ibid.
70 Wellcome Collection, London, SA/FPA/A21/8 France 1951–67, 'Letter from S. Le Sueur Cappel to E. Mears, 11 November 1961': 'I came back to Versailles very happy from my too short sejour in England. I thank you very much for the charming welcome I have found wherever I have been received and all the centres I have seen, [they] were very interesting for me.'
71 Wellcome Collection, London, SA/FPA/A10/8 1955–66 IPPF, 'Letter to Joan Rettie, 8 November 1963': 'Herewith the usual forms and literature for the four who will be attending the lectures and demonstration session in London on Tuesday 12 November: Dr Chatelin [male doctor] Dr Houdville [male doctor], Dr Jacqueline Cahen-Wolff, Dr Branle.'
72 Private phone interview with Dr E. Aubény, 25 September 2017.
73 'Ce n'était pas comme ça qu'on nous enseignait la médecine durant nos années d'études. Le devoir du médecin est de traiter les maladies qui mettent en danger la vie humaine. Le médecin offre un diagnostique, établit un traitement. Dans le cas de la contraception, tous les schémas

classiques étaient bouleversés' in E. Aubény, 'La contraception à l'hôpital December 1988', private archive. I would like to thank Dr Aubény for having kindly shared her material with me.

74 'satisfaites et fières, conscientes de ramener à leurs patientes une techniques de contraception, certes contraignante et pas entièrement fiable, mais une technique qu'elles allaient pouvoir posséder et utiliser elles-mêmes' in E. Aubény, 'La contraception, Histoire d'une liberté pour les femmes. Principes et Réalités', paper presented at Assises Nationales des Sages-Femmes, Nantes, 20 May 2011, private archive.

75 Bibliothèque interuniversitaire de Santé, Paris, Fonds Dalsace–Vellay, Dalsace 11.5, 'Formation psychologique des médecins en Angleterre, 30 September 1968'.

76 Archives du féminisme, Anger, Fond Képès 19AF28: 'S. Képès, Aspects relationnels de la consultation de contraception, 14 January 1972'. Many thanks to Fabrice Cahen who kindly collected the requested documentation for me.

77 Wellcome Collection, London, SA/FPA/A10/8 1955–66 IPPF, 'Letter from Mrs Wintersgill to Mrs Nelson-Barette, 13 December 1960'.

78 Wellcome Collection, London, SA/FPA/A13/85B, 'The FPA Walworth Women's Welfare Centre, annual report 1960'.

79 Wellcome Collection, London, SA/FPA/A10/8 1955–66 IPPF, 'Letter from medical secretary Mears to Mr and Mrs Dalsace, 15 November 1963' and 'Letter from Mears to Raoul Palmer, 15 November 1963'; 'Letter from Mears to Lagroua Weill-Hallé, 15 November 1963'.

5

Testing IUDs: a transnational journey of expertise

> Failures do not occur Douglas. There is not a single case on record of a woman fitted with the Gräfenberg ring becoming pregnant.[1]
>
> Ethel Mannin, 1930s

The excerpt above is reproduced from the correspondence between Ethel Mannin and Douglas Goldring – two literary figures of the interwar years. Ethel Mannin, a British novelist, recommended the Gräfenberg ring, an early version of what later became known as an intrauterine device (IUD), to her friend Douglas Goldring as an effective method of contraception for his wife, Malin Goldring.[2] Mannin had been fitted by Norman Haire, a Jewish-Australian gynaecologist and sexologist and a well-known, if eccentric, figure within London's elite medical community; he had an exclusive, private clinical practice on Harley Street. Norman Haire was not alone in experimenting with the ring. The female gynaecologist Helena Wright, with the backup of the Birth Control Investigation Committee (BCIC), was testing the ring in her private practice, while Dr Margaret Jackson also fitted her patients with the device in her private practice in Devonshire up until the 1960s, at which point she started testing other new intrauterine devices as well.

The last chapter of this book takes the testing of the Gräfenberg ring and later forms of intrauterine devices as a case study through which to explore the crucial contributions of Helena Wright and Margaret Jackson to the assessment of new contraceptive technologies, from a transnational perspective. Despite its short-lived use in the 1930s, the success of the ring constituted evidence that new contraceptive technologies were much needed. As I have shown in Chapter 1, female doctors became increasingly engaged with the testing of contraceptive devices and the broader production of medical contraceptive knowledge from the 1930s onwards. Finding an efficient, reliable and easy-to-use contraceptive method was one of the key goals of birth control activists in the interwar years and onwards.[3] Indeed, birth control advocates agreed that contraceptives prescribed in birth control clinics remained unsatisfactory in terms of reliability, and difficult to use for certain clients. The Gräfenberg ring was seen as a promising reliable method; it only needed to be re-inserted once a year, and therefore was less constraining than the cap or the diaphragm. It had the particular appeal of preventing pregnancy without interfering overtly with the sexual act. In addition, the ring had to be inserted by a physician, preferably a gynaecologist, giving it greater medical credibility.

However, before being endorsed and widely prescribed in birth control clinics, the ring had to be tested and approved. Drawing on the archives of the National Medical Birth Control Committee, articles published in medical journals, proceedings of international conferences and reports on contraceptive tests and trials, this chapter explores these clinical trials in detail, and places them within the wider British and international medical and professional context. It examines the criteria deemed essential for the assessment of a new contraceptive technology and therefore the ways that medical authority and expertise were obtained and secured.[4] Wright, Haire and Jackson had divergent medical authority and visions of expertise, evident in the networks that supported them and the criteria they used to assess the ring. Wright tested the device with the support of the research-driven elite of the BCIC and adopted the standardised clinical assessments and laboratory-based evidence promoted by the BCIC; she also provided a careful statistical analysis of her patients' records. Haire, on the other hand, was well connected and respected internationally, but had difficulties in being accepted by the BCIC. He did use statistical analysis, but did not provide a careful analysis of his patients' records, and his clinical expertise seems to have been based on accumulated experience and expert observation rather than sound statistical analysis. From the mid-1930s, Jackson fitted her patients with the device in her own private practice and collected information on these patients' experiences. In the mid-1960s, her clinic was one of the four international centres of the Cooperative Statistical Programme, a large-scale study on the safety and efficacy of IUDs directed by Austrian-American physician Christopher Tietze and funded by the Population Council.⁵

This chapter first focuses on the ways the Gräfenberg ring became internationally debated before turning to its testing in Britain in the interwar years, and the testing of new forms of intrauterine devices in the postwar era.

Transnational experts on the Gräfenberg ring

Invented by Dr Ernst Gräfenberg, a German gynaecologist who owned a private practice in Berlin and started experimenting with intrauterine contraceptives in the early 1920s, the Gräfenberg ring was made of silver or gold wire, twisted and inserted in the uterus.⁶ Gräfenberg presented this new device at the Third International Congress of the World League for Sexual Reform (WLSR), which took place in London in 1929. He started by stressing that the assessment of a good contraceptive method rested not only on medical and hygienic considerations but also on women's 'subjective experience'.⁷ The ring answered a demand from female patients, since it required no preparation or touching of the genitals – what Gräfenberg qualified as common 'psychological repugnance'.⁸ He first differentiated the ring from other intrauterine pessaries available at the time, such as the stem pessary, the Put's pessary, and various silkworm guts held together by silver wire. These intrauterine pessaries lay in the uterus but maintained contact with the vagina, and as such 'provide[d] a path whereby germs from the vagina might enter the uterus'.⁹ The Gräfenberg ring, by contrast, was a 'genuinely intra-uterine method'¹⁰ with no open path between the uterine cavity and the vagina or cervical canal. Gräfenberg then reported on his first attempts at developing the intrauterine device: he had tested star-shaped devices with coils of silkworm gut, but faced a high number of failures due to their expulsion from the uterus. He eventually settled for a ring of coiled silver wire, trialled on 150 patients; he estimated the failure rate at 0.66 per cent, since only one ring was expelled, resulting in a pregnancy.¹¹ Gräfenberg vigorously emphasised the contraindications of the ring: any infections were identified through a thorough examination of genital secretions, inflammation of the pelvis and menorrhagia. Finally, he provided a detailed step-by-step guide for inserting the ring under careful aseptic conditions. The procedure relied on sterilised specialised surgical equipment including a uterine sound, a vaginal speculum, volsellum and tenaculum forceps, and Hagar's dilator (a series of cylindrical bougies of graduated sizes used to dilate the cervical canal). These instruments were all in routine use by gynaecologists from the turn of the twentieth century.[12] The position of the patient during the fitting – lying on her back with knees bent, legs spread apart and feet in stirrups – also marked the use of the Gräfenberg ring as an ordinary part of gynaecology. While Gräfenberg claimed that 'the operation involved only the slightest pain'[13] and that anaesthetic was unnecessary, he nevertheless acknowledged that slight pain and slight bloody discharge 'invariably' followed the insertion of the ring. If these side effects lasted more than a couple of days and the pain increased, the ring had to be removed.

Members of the BCIC attended the conference and were impressed by the method. As a result, they decided to finance a study trip to Berlin for Wright to obtain training and information on the method from Gräfenberg directly.[14] At that time, Wright was chief medical officer of the North Kensington Women's Welfare Centre.[15] She was therefore in a position where she could travel internationally and learn new skills that she could bring back to Britain. Upon her return, she started fitting her patients with the rings at her private clinic in London. The BCIC devised a questionnaire that centred on the medical and technical aspects of the ring, with the idea of setting out a practical guide for inserting and removing it. The first questions referred to the number of cases where the method had been tried, its potential side effects, as well as its contraindications and ways to identify them. Wright covered issues around the length of time that the ring could be left in situ, whether it might become embedded in the endometrium, and the extent to which a follow-up system had been in use. Questions focused also on the attitude of the medical profession in Germany, experience of the patients and available literature on the subject. These questions reflected the scientific approach of the BCIC, namely 'to establish facts and to publish these facts as a basis on which a sound public and scientific opinion can be built'.[16]

Wright added questions related to her own personal interest in the physiological effects of the ring on the endometrium and the uterus, and whether its insertion was painful for the patient.[17] This interest in the patient's experience was illustrative of Wright's understanding of what mattered when assessing the ring: side effects, efficiency and potential pain. She wrote that 'overall, patients were enthusiastic about the method'. Regarding the potential pain induced by the ring, she seemed to be extremely cautious, as she underlined that the insertion of the ring only seemed to be painful when Gräfenberg placed the ring with the help of the volsellum forceps. Yet, she underscored that speed and comfort when placing the ring might greatly depend on the dexterity, gentleness and skill of the doctor.[18] She compared the smooth experience of Gräfenberg's patients with one patient in England, 'who found the insertion of the ring so painful that it had to be stopped and was not finished'.[19] The patient was most probably Norman Haire's. Haire had discovered the Gräfenberg ring while attending the Congress of the International Society for Sex Research in 1926 in Berlin, and attended a course of lectures on birth control given by Gräfenberg himself in 1928.[20] In July 1929, Haire started fitting the ring for his patients in his own private practice and at his Cromer Welfare and Sunlight Centre, and he gave a talk on his preliminary results at the 1929 WLSR congress.

As Ivan Crozier has argued, his advocacy of the new device offered Haire a strategy for positioning himself as a British specialist in a novel and promising scientific method. Haire was 'stamping out a territory for himself'.[21] A gynaecologist by training, Norman Haire was nevertheless an outsider in interwar London as a Jew, an Australian and a homosexual. He struggled to be accepted among the members of the birth control movement, due partly to his difficult personality. He argued with many figures in the movement such as the leaders of the Malthusian League, Dr Charles Vickery Drysdale and his wife Bessie Drysdale.[22] He was appointed as the Medical Advisor to the Walworth Women's Welfare Centre, set up by the Malthusian League, but after a few months he resigned or was forced to resign, 'leaving bad feelings behind him'.[23] Haire opened his own birth control clinic in 1927, and the Cromer Welfare and Sunlight Centre in St Pancras, which was not, however, part of the established Society for the Provision of Birth Control Clinics. Further, Haire had a problematic relationship with the feminist Stella Browne, a leading figure in the birth control movement. Therefore, when he started fitting the ring, he did it on his own terms, without the financial support of the BCIC. He did try to apply for funding from the BCIC, but his request was flatly refused, possibly due to his conflictual relationship with several birth control advocates and because Wright was already carrying out a clinical trial with the method.[24] At the 1929 conference, Haire basically replicated Gräfenberg's talk by flagging up the differences between the ring and other intra-cervical pessaries. In particular, he described the wishbone pessary as very dangerous, since it involved a v-shaped spring that was held against the cervix by a metal plate, with the spring extending into the uterus.[25] Haire had some previous involvement with this method in 1922 when he was asked by the famous birth control activist Marie Stopes to accept two patients who wanted to be fitted. He declined, warning Stopes that it could act as an abortifacient by inducing miscarriage.[26] The Gräfenberg ring, by contrast, did not induce miscarriage, Haire explained, but he still recommended inserting the ring during a menstrual period. He also detailed the instruments used during the insertion of the ring and its contra-indications. He presented the ring as a modern medical method that required a sound understanding of gynaecology for its use. The medical office was the appropriate place for the fitting procedure, placing the ring under the responsibility of the medical profession and, he suggested, 'the gynaecologist only'.[27] Having tested the ring in his private clinic but recognising its limited experience, he nevertheless shared his enthusiasm for the method he deemed 'superior to any previously available'.

Assessing the ring

By the end of 1929, both Haire and Wright were fitting clients with the Gräfenberg ring in their medical practices. Eager to assert his mastery of the device, Haire wrote a letter to the *British Medical Journal* to draw attention to the ring. The choice of the *BMJ* was not arbitrary; the journal was highly respected both nationally and internationally. By using the *BMJ* as a platform, Haire presented himself as the expert on the device. In his 1929 letter, referencing an article on the 'revocable sterilisation of the female', Haire took the opportunity to present the ring as a means of temporary sterilisation.[28] The choice of vocabulary is relevant; by emphasising the reversibility or temporary effect of the ring, Haire was trying to bypass the potential contemporary criticisms of contraception as leading to sterility.[29] Haire advocated the use of the device based on both Gräfenberg's and his own personal experiences, at this point limited to 100 cases in his private practice and in the Cromer Welfare and Sunlight Centre. He attributed the reliability of the method to 'the skill of the medical attendant, and not (as in most other contraceptives) on the skill or care of the patients'.[30] In addition, he emphasised the safety of the ring in the right hands: 'the procedure appears to be harmless in the absence of genital infection, provided it is carried out with strict aseptic precautions. The absence of harmful irritative effects is apparently due to the fact that the uterine mucosa is cast off at each menstrual period'.[31] His hands-on professional experience, coupled with reports of positive results, highlighted his position as the major clinical advocate for the device.

Not all doctors, however, agreed with Haire's positive assessment of the ring. Another letter in the *BMJ* from one Dr Richard Fawcitt, for instance, described a patient who had experienced 'nasty discharge' following the insertion of the ring by a colleague in London – plausibly targeting Haire, who identified himself so closely with the device.[32] Fawcitt asked whether other practitioners had experienced difficulty with the method. In his letter of reply to Fawcitt, Haire did not yield much ground, although his tone softened somewhat in underlining the precautions to follow before and after inserting the ring to 'avoid such a condition [nasty discharge]'. He argued that neither the ring nor the process of insertion were necessarily responsible for the discharge, since 'it must be remembered that pelvic disturbances which occur subsequent to the introduction of the ring are not necessarily caused by the ring'.[33] Haire nonetheless acknowledged that if the risk of 'such complication [pelvic disturbances] is too great to compensate for the advantages of the method it must be abandoned'.

Alongside Haire's response, the *BMJ* also published a letter in response to the doctor's concerns from Wright. By taking part in the debate on the ring, Wright positioned herself as an alternative interlocutor. She made sure to mention her travels to Berlin to visit the inventor of the ring, relying on her international expertise: 'The letters of Haire and Fawcitt … raise points which need emphasis, in view of the possibility that the method may become widely used in this country. I have just returned from a visit to Dr Gräfenberg in Berlin.'[34] Wright emphasised the contra-indications established by Gräfenberg and the care with which he selected his cases. Furthermore, she explained that patients were closely followed up by Gräfenberg after insertion of the device, insinuating that the culprit doctor did not do his job properly and had put his patient's safety at risk. Further debate took place between Haire and Wright. The 1930 Zurich international conference on contraception provided an initial forum for discussing their results, positioning both of them as international experts of the ring and bringing their different views on the subject into the international sphere.

A focal point in these debates was the use of statistical data and the determination of what considerations had priority in assessing the method. In the 1920s the BCIC joined the International Medical Group for the Investigation of Contraception in leading the quest for careful trials with laboratory support and detailed statistical assessment for contraceptive methods.[35] For these two organisations, developing a scientific birth control method through sound clinical trials was an important step toward establishing birth control as a legitimate endeavour of medicine. Their work took place at a time when the Medical Research Council (MRC) – set up in 1913 as a single research organisation for the whole of the UK, with funds provided under the National Insurance Act for medical research – increasingly defined the laboratory as indispensable to the work of medical trials, and progressively made statistical analysis a major consideration.[36] The BCIC financed much of the research on fertility carried out in laboratories by physiologists, thus helping to promote the new vision adopted by the MRC. Trials with the same methods were also carried out in birth control clinics or private practice headed by women doctors. These methods met with resistance, however, from a segment of the medical profession, who called for a more 'individualised conception of illness and its treatment', made possible by the critical eye of individual doctors acquired through long experience at the bedside.[37] In such struggles, rhetoric was especially valuable in negotiating boundaries, particularly among the circle of people working on the contentious topic of physician-controlled contraception.[38] Haire and Wright drew from different visions of medicine in their efforts to take ownership of the processes for evaluating the Gräfenberg ring.

A primary difference between Haire's and Wright's approaches to evaluation lay in how they presented their results. At the 1930 Zurich conference, Haire relied heavily on his first-hand experience with the method. He introduced himself as the follower of Gräfenberg and as the only other expert physician working on the subject. Illustrating his priority, he pointed out that, apart from Gräfenberg, he was the only doctor contributing to the compilation of sound data: 'There are few statistics yet available about this method. The only ones I have been able to find in the literature are those of Gräfenberg ... I am offering a preliminary report of my own cases.'[39] Noting with restrained modesty that 'my own cases are only 270 in numbers', he pronounced himself 'very pleased with the method'.[40] He then outlined the results, in a fashion that served to diminish the failure rates. He explained that in 13 per cent of the 270 cases, the ring had fallen out. However, he added, after reinserting the ring, he obtained a final figure that looked much better, since 'the actual failure rate was 1 in 270'.[41] It is unclear to what extent Haire's rhetorical turns with the numbers supported his case, but this probably gave the report a more promotional character. Presenting alongside Haire, in her discussion of substantially fewer cases, Wright adopted a cooler tone, although without rejecting the potential value of the ring. She emphasised contraindications to the use of the method and noted Gräfenberg's careful attention to the process of selecting appropriate cases for use of the ring. She took special care to underscore the precautions that had to be taken to avoid complications. She offered a more critical perspective on the efficacy of the device, which was in part unavoidable given the high rate of failures she had witnessed, with the expulsion of the ring in four cases out of fifteen. What was problematic for Wright was the potential for the expulsion of the ring to lead to an unwanted pregnancy. She discussed the unreliability of the method, explaining that in one case of expulsion the ring was of the correct size and perfectly in place: 'I have both the X-ray and the ring, and anyone can see it was not the fault of the size or the position ... The ring is sitting there in its perfectly round position.'[42] In another case, the ring broke inside the uterus: 'that may have been due to faulty construction in England.'[43] These rings were made by Down Bros Ltd., surgical instrument makers, and were copied from those supplied by Gräfenberg, but were cheaper. Having collected detailed accounts of individual experiences, she offered to share her reports with 'anyone interested'. She continued to support the cautious use of the ring. As shown in the previous chapter, the Zurich conference had helped to make women doctors legitimate experts on birth control. Alongside other interventions on the cap and pessary and on the work carried out at the North Kensington Women's Welfare Centre, Wright contributed to the debate on the ring, therefore strengthening her credentials not only as an international expert on birth control in general but more specifically on the Gräfenberg ring; she challenged Haire's results through her careful presentation of her own results.

The acknowledgement of Wright's expertise and her sound approach to contraceptive methods on the international scale was not limited to the Zurich conference. In 1931, the International Medical Group for the Investigation of Contraception published a report compiling three articles on the Gräfenberg ring by Wright, Leunbach (a Danish general practitioner who tested the ring in his own private practice on 178 patients) and Haire. This report, as well as the correspondence between Haire and the report's editor, Blacker, shows how the issue of reliable results, and the handling of statistical and numerical evidence, worked in favour of Wright. In the foreword to the report, Blacker underlined contradictory results between Haire, on the one hand, and Wright and Leunbach on the other. Haire submitted, Blacker noted, 'in general terms a favourable account of his findings ... [but] abstains from giving any but the vaguest figures'.[44] In comparison, Wright and Leunbach presented 'detailed and exact figures' that conveyed a 'less favourable impression of the ring'.[45] Furthermore, Blacker expressed his gratitude to them for 'the trouble they have taken in submitting their material to such searching scrutiny and for presenting it with such candidness'.[46]

Indeed, Wright provided a detailed account of the thirty-eight patients she fitted with the ring in her private practice in London. She laid out her cautious assessment of the methods in a thorough appraisal of individual cases. She was careful to emphasise the recurring problem of ejection of the ring out of the cervix, since only nine of the thirty-eight patients she had fitted still had the ring in place at the time of publication. Despite these unconvincing preliminary results, she laid considerable stress on the satisfaction felt by the nine patients who still had the ring, which encouraged her to 'persevere'. She called for the systematic collection of data on the subject: 'large numbers of accurate, detailed records will have to be collected before the laws of behaviours of the ring could be deduced'.[47] This request offered a stark contrast to the methods of Haire, who had referred to his results in vague terms, using words such as 'a few' or 'many' to describe his experience with the use of the ring in more than 400 cases.[48]

Haire wrote to Blacker to express his disapproval. Arguing defensively that his results should not be compared to work by inexperienced clinicians, he took a backhand swipe at Wright's record: 'I think that you and your committee or sub-committee are putting yourselves in a ridiculous position when you adopt this omniscient attitude about birth control methods. When I look through the list of names I still fail to see anybody who has any considerable knowledge about contraceptive techniques at all.'[49] Haire spoke with the backing of extensive experience in the use of the ring, as well as a notable clinical position as a medical officer-in-charge at the Walworth Women's Welfare Centre and a physician who operated his own birth control clinic. Haire also referred to an unnamed colleague who fitted 'rings of inferior quality' that broke within the cervix.[50] It is worth noting that in the original letter that he submitted to the editor, Haire identified the culprit as a 'woman doctor', targeting Wright specifically. The editor altered the text and suggested the word 'colleague' instead of woman doctor, which reveals how Blacker was protecting Wright.[51] Haire went on to announce that he was buying rings from a Dutch firm, since he found the rings supplied by the German and English firms 'far from satisfactory'. Moreover, he implied that clinical experience provided the gynaecologist with a certain ease in recognising 'the sort of uterus from which the ring is likely to escape', implying that his good results with the ring were a result in part of greater expertise and superior judgement. Haire adhered to a traditional vision of medical expertise that was grounded in experience and in cultivated observational skills.[52] Indeed, he valued his own experience with patients as his main source of knowledge and authority.

However, Blacker had a different vision of what he considered to be good research practices, consistent with the more straightforward and restrained character of laboratory-based medicine.[53] In his letter in reply to Haire, this conception was implicit:

> I wrote what I did because I did not wish the report to be construed as an advertisement for you which at the same time would injure the other two contributors on the Gräfenberg ring [Wright and Leunbach] who submitted detailed statistical reports which reflected somewhat unfavourably on their results and present them impartially in my contribution. I did not want them to suffer for it. I am myself persuaded that the results of all birth control methods, including the Gräfenberg ring, turn

out to be less favourable when they are carefully analysed than when they are judged by general impression.[54]

Given the strong disapproval of medical advertisement at the time, Haire had to read Blacker's note as a subtle criticism against his promotional uses of the data he had collected in experience with the ring.[55] The doctor was supposed to show a less self-interested commitment to medical research.[56]

Haire replied and 'was forced' to acknowledge the downsides of the method: 'I quite agree that careful analysis reveals less favourable results for all birth control methods than one would think from general impressions.'[57] However, as a defence, he strongly emphasised that he privileged the care of his patients as his main concern: 'It seems to me that there is a fundamental difference in the emphasis we place on two aspects of birth control work – you are primarily concerned with collecting reliable statistical data about the efficacy of various methods, and only secondary is the individual woman who is in need of advice. I am primarily concerned with the urgent need of individual women.'[58] Indeed, according to Haire, the main advantages of the ring were that it was 'free from the aesthetic disadvantages of all the other methods of birth control … does not interfere at all with the spontaneity of intercourse and requires no preparation before intercourse'.[59] Such concerns were likely to be central to the choice of birth control methods among the middle-class women who constituted the clientele of private practices such as those of Wright and Haire. The oral history study by Szreter and Fisher on birth control practices in Britain between 1918 and 1963 demonstrates this point convincingly. Middle-class women found that barrier methods were at odds with the spontaneity that they valued so deeply, and was offered by natural methods of birth control. Szreter and Fisher also found that barrier methods went against the 'expectation that women should play a relatively passive role in sex'.[60] Wright was no less deeply concerned with the quality of her patients' sex lives, as she made evident in the several sex manuals that she had authored. But her allegiance to the BCIC, and the associated desire to make birth control work a 'scientific' enterprise, restrained her attention to the aesthetic qualities of sex. She underscored, instead, efficacy and a lack of side effects as the major criteria for judging a good birth control method. These requirements were the utilitarian criteria developed by the BCIC: a good contraceptive method needed to be effective, harmless, easy to use and cheap. Haire found himself under attack by members of the BCIC for a lack of scientific rigour and a lack of attention to the requirements for statistical evidence.

Side effects and risks of pregnancy

The debates over the ring also shed light on the significance of side effects as a key element in assessing the contraceptive method. Here again, Haire's and Wright's results differed. In his 1931 report, Haire vigorously, but in general terms, supported the reliability of the ring: 'Of the catastrophic complications which are supposed by many critics to be an inevitable consequence of the use of this method, I have had no experience ... Many of my patients have been wearing the ring for over two years, and the greater my experience with the method the more I am convinced of its value in suitable cases.'[61] At that time, Gräfenberg was still recommending that the device should be replaced once a year. Without mentioning this admonition, Haire did note that 'in a few cases he removed the ring as its presence cause[d] pain or discomfort'. Importantly, he did not consider these side effects as 'catastrophic complications', although pain might well be considered a legitimate motive for advising against the method.

In comparison, Wright presented a detailed assessment of the full range of specific side effects. Among her patients, many had experienced bleeding and menstrual irregularity. She also scrupulously followed the guidance offered by Gräfenberg on contraindications, and noted that in one case a patient who seemed to have a healthy pelvis at the first medical examination did not inform her of her history of pelvis sepsis, a contraindication to use of the ring. As a result, an infection occurred and the patient had to undergo a hysterectomy, a risky operation before the widespread availability of antibiotics.[62] The fact that Wright shared this negative experience was typical of her commitment to systematic disclosure of results. As she had done at the 1930 Zurich conference, she again stressed the unreliability of the method: 'the great obstacle to the spread of the method is obviously the uncertain protection against pregnancy which it affords.'[63] In an attempt to address the defects of the method, Wright devised two strategies. First, she designed her own ring and asked Dr H. M. Carleton, a physiologist from Oxford University, to test it. This experiment was funded by the BCIC. Carleton was tasked with investigating the 'effects of foreign bodies in the uterine cavities of animals, with a view to ascertaining the possible effect of the much discussed Gräfenberg ring'.[64] Using animals and carrying out trials in laboratories became common in the 1930s under the influence of the MRC. Carleton presented his results in the *British Journal of Obstetrics and Gynaecology* in 1933. The ring devised by Wright was made of a silver ring, the coils of which were covered by India rubber, which should ease the process of insertion owing to its smoothness and avoid the ring breaking in situ. The downside of the smoothness of the material was that it facilitated the expulsion of the ring. Apart from this expulsion, the ring was as efficient as the Gräfenberg ring, with the advantage that it seemed to avoid the creation of histological changes in the cells of the uterine lining. The second strategy devised by Wright was to fit the patients with the ring on the condition that they would practise other forms of contraception (such as spermicide) continuously during the first, trial year. Then, if after one year it was still in situ, the patient could rely solely on the ring.

Regarding the expulsion of the ring from the uterus, Haire also briefly alluded to this in vague terms: 'in a certain number of cases'. Nevertheless, Haire also engaged with the risk of pregnancy, since he mentioned his previous accident with one patient who had delivered a baby despite the presence of the ring. According to Haire, the ring did not provoke a miscarriage and, as such, should not be considered an abortifacient, a recurring accusation against intrauterine devices.

This incident was used again by Haire in a debate in the *British Medical Journal* in 1932. Colonel Green-Armytage, professor of obstetrics and gynaecology at the Medical College in Calcutta, wrote a letter to the journal complaining about a 'London physician who is a protagonist of birth control' who had fitted the ring and assured his patient of its reliability. The patient became pregnant.[65] In his reply, Haire avoided any acknowledgement of involvement in the case. However, he once more used the occasion to position himself as a 'reliable' expert on the ring. Using the case to air his own experience, Haire presented himself as a pioneer in handling such complications: 'until August, 1930, no such case was reported in the literature, but in that month I read a paper before the International Society for Sexual Research at the B.M.A. in London, in which I reported a case of pregnancy in one of my own patients while wearing a Gräfenberg ring.'[66] Haire then added that the pregnancy, under careful observation, went well: 'The normal nature of this pregnancy would appear to be a reply to Colonel Green-Armytage's speculation whether pregnancy could continue to full term without damage for the mother or the foetus.'[67] Clearly, a failure of the ring was perceived not only as a threat to the woman but also to the foetus in cases of pregnancy. As criticisms against the method began to appear, Haire sought to rectify claims, putting his own expertise at the centre of the discussions. Nevertheless, increasing concern about side effects and efficacy made this tactic difficult. The ardour on Haire's part to defend a method that seemed less promising than previously began to weaken his position. Haire gradually became ostracised by the medical birth control establishment in Britain due to his lack of adherence to careful statistical analysis and his difficult personality; plausibly, this may also have been due to bias against his Jewishness and homosexuality.

His absence from the programme of the 1932 conference on medical contraception testified to his colleagues' hesitations. In July 1932, the National Birth Control Association held a conference in London on Medical Problems of Contraception. Among the speakers was Wright. The correspondence between Blacker, leading organiser of the conference and honorary secretary of the Birth Control Investigation Committee, and Wright is instructive. Due to her national and international recognition, Wright was gaining a position as the expert on the value of the ring, and she began to employ her growing reputation to the detriment of Haire. Wright was invited to the conference to present her latest results on the Gräfenberg ring. She wrote back to share concerns about the possible presence of Haire, pointing out that 'last time we met by accident at a public meeting, at which he was only a member of the audience, he took the opportunity to be personally and publicly offensive, to such an extent that the audience protested.'[68] After hearing her concerns, Blacker made the necessary arrangements to remove Haire's name from the programme, reassuring Wright of the BCIC's opinion: 'the general feeling is that official speakers at the Conference whose names appear on the program should be people in whom the committee has confidence and whose report they regard as trustworthy.'[69] The subsequent review of the conference published in the *British Medical Journal* added insult to injury. The article emphasised growing disillusionment about the method:

> Every new method in medicine passed through three stages: first, being new, it was scoffed at, then there followed a phase in which it received passionate support of the suggestible elements in the community, who, very naturally, were disillusioned by the immediate results; and finally there came the time when critical intelligences went to work and assessed the method as its true value.[70]

It presented the research carried out by Wright and Dr Carleton of the Department of Physiology at the University of Oxford. The latter outlined his main results based on over 100 experiments with rabbits. Both researchers shared their concerns around the efficacy of the method. Haire was mentioned, but only as an 'enthusiastic follower' of Gräfenberg and as the only doctor who 'applied extensively' the ring in a birth control clinic. Haire had been pushed outside the bounds of that third category described in the introduction, where 'critical intelligences went to work'.

Haire was fully excluded by 1933, when the BCIC and the NBCA held a second conference at British Medical Association House on medical problems with contraception. His name did not appear on the programme, and no mention was made of his work in the published reports. Wright was present and chaired a session. Carleton presented a paper on the after-effects of using the Gräfenberg ring, and Wright was named as the other expert working on the subject.[71] In addition, the conference ended with a call to stop fitting patients with a contraception method that was deemed unreliable and harmful: 'it could hardly be doubted that there was a potential danger in introducing into the uterine cavity a foreign body which was apt to undergo both chemical changes and physical fragmentation'.[72] In 1932, Haire had fitted more than 400 patients and this number had extended to 1,000 by 1939.[73] However, in his book, published in 1936, he was less enthusiastic about the ring, emphasising its lack of reliability. This led him to recommend the combination of the ring with a spermicide jelly. Hence, in his view, the ring lost one of its main advantages, namely the absence of preparation before intercourse that guaranteed the spontaneity of the sexual act.

Legacy of the ring and new IUD clinical trials

Despite medical warnings and data on side effects and unreliability, the Gräfenberg ring retained its appeal for a number of patients. Wright asserted in a 1936 letter to the physician and birth control advocate, Gladys Cox, that she would insert the ring 'only if the patient insists in spite of knowing the disadvantages of the method'.[74] This shows a demand on the part of patients, and suggests that Wright's patients occasionally insisted on being fitted with the ring – with interesting hints at the concerns about proper informed consent that would stir a decade later.[75]

Similarly, Margaret Jackson explained that, in spite of being taught as a student that 'the Gräfenberg ring was [the] devil's work'[76] and that its insertion was 'unethical', she returned to this method 'in desperation as long ago as 1939' and prescribed it for 'cases where orthodox methods had failed, sometimes repeatedly, because of non-use or misuse'. In her view, the method was best suited for 'feckless and hyperfertile couples' since it was the only method 'free of patient error'.[77] This assertion was based on eugenic considerations towards the fertility of specific women.

After the Second World War and with the fear of global population growth, intrauterine devices regained their popularity. Feminist scholars have provided accounts of IUDs as an oppressive technology and a means for coercive population policy in the 1960s, targeting the Global South especially.[78] IUDs were presented as a potential solution for slowing population growth. In 1959, two key publications, by Oppenheimer in Israel and Ishihama in Japan about their positive experience with the Gräfenberg ring or a modified version of it, put intrauterine devices back under the spotlight. By the 1960s, two new plastic intrauterine devices had been designed in the US and proved reliable: the Lippes Loop and Margulies Spiral, named after their inventors.

As was the case with the Gräfenberg ring, these new devices found their way to Britain by way of international conferences. In 1961, Alan Guttmacher, Chief of the Department of Obstetrics and Gynaecology at Mount Sinai Hospital in New York and the new president of the Planned Parenthood Federation of America's World Population Emergency Campaign, was tasked by the Population Council in tandem with the International Planned Parenthood Federation to undertake a study trip to review 'efforts at conception control around the world'.[79] Created in 1952 by John D. Rockefeller III, the Population Council, which still exists today, is an international non-governmental organisation that conducts biomedical research on contraceptives and social science research on decision-making for contraception.[80] Guttmacher toured India and Southeast Asia and came back convinced that 'the reason the restraint of population growth in these areas is moving so slowly is the fact that the methods which we offer are Western methods, methods poorly suited to their culture and to the control of mass-population growth. Our methods are largely birth control for the individual, not for a nation.'[81] As a result, he recommended intrauterine devices as promising methods for the so-called 'war on population' and urged the Population Council to invest money in developing knowledge on the subject in order to ascertain their efficacy and harmlessness. Following this recommendation, the First International Conference on Intra-Uterine Contraception was held in New York under the auspices of the Population Council to analyse the 'effectiveness, the safety and the possibility of widespread use of intra-uterine contraceptives as a method of regulating fertility'.[82] The organisers of the conference, Guttmacher, Warren O. Nelson (medical director of the Population Council) and Dr Christopher Tietze (director of research at the National Committee on Maternal Health), invited only forty participants from eleven countries. Jackson was one of them, and presented her experience with the Gräfenberg ring. Between 1939 and 1962, she had fitted 192 patients with the ring for a total of 10,711 menstrual cycles. The average patient fitted with the ring was a woman of 34 with six children; many of them 'were problem patients and mothers of problem families'. While at first the ring had been advocated and tested for middle-class patients in interwar Britain, its demographic had evolved over time to be, as flagged up by Jackson, almost exclusively what were called 'problem families'. The term 'problem families' had been popularised by the Eugenics Society in the late 1940s through its Problem Families Committee. Problem families were perceived as a threat to society due to their 'intractable ineducability', 'squalid homes', 'multiple social problems', and mental and physical deficiencies. Their fertility was a particular concern.[83]

Jackson provided a careful description of her experience based on statistics and the assessment of side effects. She found the degree of protection offered by the method 'quite high': eighteen unwanted pregnancies had occurred and twenty-four patients did not tolerate the ring. Calculated using the Pearl Index, a technique used in clinical trials for assessing the effectiveness of a birth control method, the pregnancy rate was 2.[84] The method was harmless as long as strict obedience to 'Gräfenberg's meticulous criteria' was respected, in particular the need for a normal, healthy pelvis. Furthermore, Jackson insisted on close follow-up of patients since the ring had to be removed and replaced once a year. She recommended fitting and changing the ring during the first half of the menstrual cycle. Nevertheless, she reckoned that there were side effects, such as painful insertion, strong pelvic disturbances, menorrhagia, discharge and pain, which would lead to the removal of the ring. Other patients found the insertion and removal so painful that they went back to their previous methods of birth control. All in all, Jackson emphasised that 'the woman's fertility was not disturbed by this method' and that no 'pelvic inflammatory conditions had developed'.[85]

At the conference, Jackson also learnt of the existence of the two new plastic devices and was impressed by their seemingly good results. When she returned to Britain, she started fitting her patients with these new plastic devices. In 1963, she published a paper in *Family Planning* that reviewed her experience with the Gräfenberg ring and the new plastic IUDs. She experimented with 116 patients, over 504 cycles, who were from the same social milieu as her Gräfenberg ring patients. She praised the new IUDs' flexible material, which made insertion less painful for the patient since it reduced the need for dilatation. In addition, discharge and menorrhagia seemed to have reduced. She explained that she had removed five devices, and four others had slipped out. She also emphasised that there was no infection introduced, due to the nylon thread which extended through the external os.

Jackson's support from the FPA, the IPPF and the Population Council reinforced her expertise and gave her credentials to the extent that her clinic served as one of the four international centres (the others being Puerto Rico, Fiji and Sweden) of the Cooperative Statistical Program, a study of the safety and efficacy of IUDs funded by the Population Council and headed by Austrian-American physician Christopher Tietze.[86] Jackson carefully collected data on her patients and gathered information on 3,600 IUD users in southwest England. Therefore, she played a key role in popularising IUDs in Britain and advancing knowledge on their reliability and safety. In July 1965, the *BMJ* published a lead article about the new IUDs, claiming that 'evidence is growing that in skilled hands the method is safe, giving rise to relatively few and trivial complications'.[87]

Meanwhile, the FPA-affiliated Council for the Investigation of Fertility Control (CIFC), of which Jackson was a member, had quietly begun a trial, fitting the Lippes Loop, Margulies Spiral, and a new model, the Birnberg Bow, in 341 women in order to assess their suitability for use in FPA clinics in Birmingham.[88] The North Kensington Women's Welfare Centre also hosted a trial of intrauterine contraceptive devices under the joint supervision of Dr Blair and Dr Sara Field-Richards.[89] The method 'had a great success with the extreme ends of the social scale: the desperate ladies brought by Health Visitors who think this is an acceptable alternative to sterilisation, and the highly sophisticated ladies who have read about this in the *Guardian* and are determined to have the newest wear in contraception'.[90] In spring 1965, the Medical Advisory Council of the FPA recognised the safety and reliability of IUDs and agreed to recommend the method in FPA centres.[91] Therefore, while immediately after the Second World War IUDs had originally been perceived as acceptable for women who could not use other contraceptive methods, or who could not be trusted to use them correctly, their users eventually expanded to include women from a wide range of backgrounds. By 1970, IUDs were used by 5 per cent of British female contraceptive users, including middle-class mothers and childless professionals.[92]

Conclusion

By contextualising and tracing the evolution of a device from its appearance in limited medical circles to its testing, its brief championing, and progressive condemnation, and its resurfacing after the Second World War, this chapter outlines broader issues in the diverging means for judging the value of new medical devices, in a period that saw the consolidation of accepted mechanisms for clinical assessment.[93] This chapter identifies the key forebears of IUDs in Britain: Norman Haire, Helena Wright and Margaret Jackson. Identifying their respective positions within the national and international medical landscape – where networks, alliances and interpersonal relationships took shape – helps to explain whose voice was heard and legitimated within the medical circles. Haire built up an exclusive private clinical practice on Harley Street, but he seems to have been out of touch with the research-driven elites of the BCIC, to which Helena Wright belonged. Indeed, the BCIC declined to finance Haire's research and gradually ostracised him. Wright, instead, became the trusted voice on questions about the Gräfenberg ring within this influential community as well as the international birth control group. After the war, Jackson was influential in popularising new IUDs in Britain.

Haire's and Wright's different positions of power within the medical establishment and birth control movement were reinforced in part by divergent visions of medical expertise, perceptible in the criteria they used to assess the ring. While Wright embraced the clinical and laboratory-based evidence promoted by the BCIC, Haire adhered to traditional criteria based on accumulated experience and expert observation, but also heavily invested in an individual understanding of clients' needs. The predominance in scientific publications of the issue of the efficacy of the ring heightened the latent tension between Wright and Haire. Wright provided a detailed, objective account of results and adopted a cautious approach to the new method, presenting her negative results alongside positive ones. Haire, on the other hand, generalised from his experience, providing only imprecise numerical results, relying on the strength of his clinical reputation to carry his points. He expressed little interest in statistical analysis, instead privileging his extensive experience with the method and advocating for the needs of his patients. There was evidence of such a demand among patients for contraceptives that did not interfere with the spontaneity of the sexual act. Haire proved reluctant to give up on a method that was drawing increasing criticism, but he sustained a busy practice, testified to by the numbers of procedures he could report. Despite the potential appeal of this strategy, however, Haire gradually lost professional credibility in favour of Wright, who developed a transparent approach to assessing the use of the ring that was based on the critical and judicious interpretation of clinical evidence. After the Second World War, Jackson became a central figure in the testing of new IUDs in Britain. She had the backup of the powerful Population Council and provided a thorough assessment of her experience with the new devices.

This chapter thus offers a fresh look at the successes and failures of the Gräfenberg ring, showing how evolving scientific criteria for evaluation impacted the device's reception among the medical community, internationally and in Britain. A division emerged among members of the birth control movement who prescribed and assessed contraception, between the circle of doctors and scientists that welcomed Helena Wright (and her fellow female colleagues) and her developing command of scientific clinical assessments, and individuals such as Norman Haire and Marie Stopes who, although popular with clients, came to be treated as eccentrics, poorly versed in proper scientific method. In addition, the tensions between Haire and Wright revealed professional dynamics whereby some individuals were marginalised in order to assert medical authority and professional power. The impersonal approach towards collecting scientific data seems to have won out in this instance, with the publication by the BCIC in 1937 of a list of approved contraceptives, which ratified the required methods for use in assessing contraceptive methods as shown in Chapter 1. Jackson followed these recommendations when she evaluated the potential of new IUDs in the 1960s.

Notes

1 See University of Victoria, British Columbia, Douglas Goldring papers, Acc 95–012: Series 1, files 78–9 correspondence from Ethel Mannin c.1920s–1930s. 'Letter from Mannin to Douglas Goldring, undated'. I am very grateful to Lesley Hall who kindly transmitted these letters to me. In the same correspondence Mannin complained about the price that Haire charged patients for fitting the ring. She had used to be fitted by him for £33, but was once fitted by Gräfenberg himself in Berlin for £7 with anaesthetic.
2 Parts of this chapter have been published in the *Journal of the History of Medicine and Allied Sciences*. See C. Rusterholz, 'Testing the Gräfenberg ring in interwar Britain: Norman Haire, Helena Wright, and the debate over statistical evidence, side effects, and intra-uterine contraception', *Journal of the History of Medicine and Allied Sciences*, 72:4 (2017), pp. 448–67.
3 Löwy, '"Sexual chemistry" before the pill'; Soloway, 'The "perfect contraceptive"'.
4 On these elements see S. Sturdy, 'Looking for trouble: medical science and clinical practice in the historiography of modern medicine', *Social History of Medicine*, 24:3 (2011), pp. 739–57.

5 A. Gurel, 'The Demand for IUDs: Making a "Respectable" Alternative to Oral Contraception in Britain'. MPhil dissertation, History and Philosophy of Science, University of Cambridge, 2016, p. 22.
6 A. Dugdale, 'Devices and Desires: Constructing the Intrauterine Device, 1908–1988'. PhD thesis, Department of Science and Technology Studies, University of Wollongong, 1995. On Gräfenberg see R. J. Thomsen, 'Historical: Ernst Gräfenberg and the golden year of the silver ring' in E. S. Hafez and W. A. van Os (eds), *Medicated Intrauterine Devices: Physiological and Clinical Aspects* (The Hague: Springer Netherlands, 1980), pp. 3–8.
7 E. Gräfenberg, 'The intra uterine method of contraception' in N. Haire (ed.), *World League for Sexual Reform: Proceedings of the Third Congress, London, 1929* (London: Paul, Trench, Trübner, 1930), p. 611.
8 Ibid.
9 Ibid.
10 Ibid.
11 Ibid., p. 616.
12 Although their initial use met with medical opposition, especially the speculum. See Moscucci, *The Science of Woman*, pp. 112–30.
13 Gräfenberg, 'The intra uterine method of contraception', p. 615.
14 Wellcome Collection, London, SA/FPA/A13/5/2, 'Birth control investigation committee, summary of activity 1930'.
15 Wellcome Collection, London, SA/FPA/A13/5/2, 'Minutes of the Eighth meeting of the BCIC, 23 November 1927'.
16 Rolleston, 'Birth Control Investigation Committee', p. 805.
17 Wellcome Collection, London, SA/FPA/A13/5/2, 'Helena Wright, Report of visit to Berlin to investigate Dr Gräfenberg's silver ring contraceptive'.
18 For more information about the issue of skills see the special issue N. Whitfield and T. Schlich (eds), 'Skills through history', *Medical History*, 59:3 (2015), pp. 349–85.
19 This patient was probably Malin Goldring, the wife of Douglas Goldring. See University of Victoria, British Columbia, Douglas Goldring papers, Acc 95-012: Series 1, files 78–9 correspondence from Ethel Mannin c.1920s–1930s, 'Letter from Mannin to Douglas Goldring, undated'.
20 Sanger and Stone, *The Practice of Contraception*, p. 47; N. Haire, 'Sterilisation, birth control and abortion', in Haire, *Proceedings of the Third Congress*, p. 111.
21 I. Crozier, 'Becoming a sexologist: Norman Haire, the 1929 London World League for Sexual Reform Congress, and organising medical knowledge about sex in interwar England', *History of Science*, 39:3 (2001), p. 300.

22 On the difficulties Haire faced in establishing a name for himself in London see Crozier, 'Becoming a sexologist', p. 309. See also Crozier, '"All the world's a stage"'. On the idea of the gentleman doctor see C. Lawrence, 'A tale of two sciences: bedside and bench in twentieth-century Britain', *Medical History*, 43:4 (1999), pp. 421–49. His expertise in sexology constituted an added obstacle. Sexual medicine was a topic strongly associated with the Continent, which English doctors engaged with reluctantly: see L. Hall, '"The English have hot-water bottles": The Morganatic marriage between sexology and medicine in Britain since William Acton', in R. Porter and M. Teich (eds), *Sexual Knowledge, Sexual Science: The History of Attitudes to Sexuality* (Cambridge: Cambridge University Press, 1994), pp. 350–66.
23 Crozier, 'Becoming a sexologist', p. 309.
24 'Minutes of the meeting of the Birth Control Investigation Committee January 16th 1930', in SA/EUG/ L/6/6/6, Wellcome Collection, London.
25 Fisher, *Birth Control*, p. 36.
26 For more information see J. Rose, *Marie Stopes and the Sexual Revolution* (London: Faber and Faber, 1992), 161–2; Wyndham, *Norman Haire*, pp. 84–6.
27 N. Haire, 'Sterilisation, birth control and abortion', p. 111.
28 N. Haire, 'Revocable sterilisation of the female', *British Medical Journal*, 2:3597 (1929), p. 1134.
29 The idea that contraception led to sterility was common in medical circles at that time. See the debate in the *British Medical Journal* in 1938 (Chapter 1).
30 Haire, 'Revocable sterilisation of the female' (1929).
31 *Ibid.*
32 R. Fawcitt, 'Revocable sterilisation of the female', *British Medical Journal*, 1:3600 (1930), p. 45.
33 N. Haire, 'Revocable sterilisation of the female', *British Medical Journal*, 1:3602 (1930), pp. 129–30.
34 H. Wright, 'Revocable sterilisation of the female', *British Medical Journal*, 1:3602 (1930) pp. 129–30.
35 Clinical trials as a form of objective knowledge have a long-contested history. The resort to clinical trials as a way of acquiring objective medical knowledge first appeared in the second half of the nineteenth century, when doctors, through the British Medical Association, tried to fight secret remedies prescribed and sold by charlatans, quack doctors and patent medicine manufacturers, in order to assert their power over this domain and hence reinforce their professional credentials and position. To do this, they promoted clinics as the best place in which to judge

therapeutic efficacy. Many authors have emphasised the resistance from elite doctors to the laboratory expansions: see Cox-Maksimov, 'The Making of the Clinical Trial in Britain'; Toth, 'Clinical Trials in British Medicine'.
36 J. Austoker, and L. Bryder, *Historical Perspectives on the Role of the MRC* (Oxford: Oxford University Press, 1989).
37 On these elements, see C. Lawrence, 'Still incommunicable: clinical holists and medical knowledge in interwar Britain' in C. Lawrence and G. Weisz (eds), *Greater than the Parts: Holism in Biomedicine 1920–50* (Oxford: Oxford University Press, 1998), pp. 94–111; C. Timmerman, 'Clinical research in postwar Britain, the role of the Medical Research Council' in C. Hannaway (ed.), *Biomedicine in the 20th Century: Practices, Policies and Politics* (Amsterdam: IOS Press, 2008), pp. 231–54; S. Sturdy and R. Cooter, 'Science, scientific management, and the transformation of medicine in Britain c.1870–1950', *History of Science*, 36:114 (1998), pp. 421–66; S. Sturdy, 'The political economy of scientific medicine: science, education and the transformation of medical practice in Sheffield, 1890–1922', *Medical History*, 36:2 (1992), pp. 125–59.
38 Crozier convincingly argued that rhetoric, social power and symbolic capital are key elements in understanding the construction of medical knowledge. See his excellent article: I. Crozier, 'Social construction in a cold climate: a response to David Harley, "Rhetoric and the Social Construction of Sickness and Healing" and to Paolo Palladino's comment on Harley', *Social History of Medicine*, 13:3 (2000), pp. 535–46.
39 Sanger and Stone, *The Practice of Contraception*, p. 50.
40 *Ibid*.
41 N. Haire, 'A preliminary note on the intrauterine silver ring' in Sanger and Stone, *The Practice of Contraception*, p. 55.
42 *Ibid*.
43 *Ibid*.
44 C. P. Blacker, 'Foreword', *International Medical Group for the Investigation of Contraception*, 4th issue (1931), p. 3.
45 *Ibid*.
46 *Ibid*.
47 H. Wright, 'Notes on the 38 cases fitted with Gräfenberg ring', *International Medical Group for the Investigation of Contraception*, 4th issue (1931), p. 65.
48 N. Haire, 'Clinical experience of the past year', *International Medical Group for the Investigation of Contraception*, 4th issue (1931), p. 68.
49 Wellcome Collection, London, SA/FPA/A22/1, 'Letter from Norman Haire to Blacker, 29.03.32'.
50 Haire, 'Clinical experience of the past year', p. 69.

51 Wellcome Collection, London, SA/FPA/A22/1, 'Letter from Norman Haire to Blacker, 29.03.32'.
52 S. E. D. Shortt, 'Physicians, science, and status: issues in the professionalisation of Anglo-American medicine in the nineteenth century', *Medical History*, 27:1 (1983), pp. 51–68; M. W. Weatherall, 'Making medicine scientific: empiricism, rationality, and quackery in mid-Victorian Britain', *Social History of Medicine*, 9:2 (1996), pp. 175–94.
53 Cunningham and Williams, *The Laboratory Revolution in Medicine*.
54 Wellcome Collection, London, SA/FPA/A22/1, 'Letter from Blacker to Norman Haire, 07.04.1932'.
55 Loeb underlines the difficult negotiation between gentility and financial interests within the British medical profession since 1870. See L. Loeb, 'Doctors and patent medicines in modern Britain: professionalism and consumerism', *Albion*, 33:3 (2001), pp. 404–25.
56 Toth, 'Clinical Trials in British Medicine'.
57 *Ibid*.
58 Wellcome Collection, London, SA/FPA/A22/1, 'Letter from Norman Haire to Blacker, 09.04.1932'.
59 Norman Haire, 'A preliminary note on the intrauterine silver ring', p. 50.
60 Szreter and Fisher, *Sex before the Sexual Revolution*, p. 256. See, in particular, chapter 6 on this issue.
61 Haire, 'Clinical experience of the past year', p. 69.
62 On the history of hysterectomy see C. Sutton, 'Hysterectomy: a historical perspective', *Baillière's Clinical Obstetrics and Gynaecology*, 11:1 (1997), pp. 1–22.
63 Wright, 'Notes on the 38 cases fitted with Gräfenberg ring', p. 65.
64 Wellcome Collection, London, SA/ FPA/A13/5, 'Memorandum on work of the Birth Control Investigation committee, 1931'.
65 C. Green-Armytage, 'Contraceptive', *British Medical Journal*, 1:3704 (1932), pp. 13–14.
66 N. Haire, 'The Gräfenberg ring', *British Medical Journal*, 1:3705 (1932), pp. 76–7.
67 *Ibid*.
68 Wellcome Collection, London, PPCPB/C/1/16, 'Letter from Wright to Blacker, 18 March 1932'.
69 Wellcome Collection, London, PPCPB/C/1/16, 'Letter from Blacker to Wright, 14 April 1932'.
70 'Medical problems of contraception', *British Medical Journal*, 1:3726 (1932), pp. 1047–8.
71 'Medical problems of contraception', *British Medical Journal*, 2:3784 (1933), pp. 118–20.

72 *Ibid.*, p. 120.
73 N. Haire, *Birth Control Methods (Contraception, Abortion, Sterilisation)* (London: George Allen & Unwin, 1936).
74 Quoted from a private letter exchange between Gladys Cox and Helena Wright, in Cox, *Clinical Contraception*, p. 118.
75 On the history of informed consent in medicine, see T. L. Beauchamp, 'Informed consent: its history, meaning, and present challenges', *Cambridge Quarterly of Healthcare Ethics*, 20:4 (2011), pp. 515–23.
76 M. Jackson, 'Silver ring and plastic loops, a comparison of intrauterine devices for problem cases', *Family Planning*, 12:1 (1963), p. 12.
77 M. Jackson, 'England: family planning in England and India', *The Journal of Sex Research*, 3:4 (1967), p. 270.
78 A. Dugdale, 'Intrauterine contraceptive devices, situated knowledges, and the making of women's bodies', *Australian Feminist Studies*, 15:32 (2000), pp. 165–76; A. Dugdale, 'Inserting Gräfenberg's IUD into the sex reform movement' in D. MacKenzie and J. Wajcman (eds), *The Social Shaping of Technology* (Buckingham: Open University Press, 1999); Takeshita, *The Global Biopolitics of the IUD*; A. Tone, *Devices and Desires: A History of Contraceptives in America* (New York: Farrar, Straus and Giroux, 2001); Clarke, *Disciplining Reproduction*; N. Grant, *The Selling of Contraception: The Dalkon Shield Case, Sexuality, and Women's Autonomy* (Columbus: Ohio State University Press, 1992).
79 A. Guttmacher, 'Intra-uterine contraceptive device', *Family Planning*, 13:14 (1965), p. 94.
80 On the Population Council and its role in the international campaign for family planning see Connelly, *Fatal Misconception*, pp. 159–220.
81 A. Guttmacher (ed.), 'Introduction', *Intra-Uterine Contraceptive Devices: Proceedings of the Conference, April 30–May 1, 1962, New York City* (New York: Excerpta Medica Foundation, 1962), p. 7.
82 *Ibid.*
83 J. Welshman, 'In search of the "problem family": public health and social work in England and Wales 1940–70', *Social History of Medicine*, 9:3 (1996), pp. 447–65.
84 M. Jackson, 'The Gräfenberg silver ring in a series of patients who had failed with other methods' in Guttmacher, *Intra-Uterine Contraceptive Devices*, pp. 37–40.
85 *Ibid.*
86 Guttmacher, 'Intra-uterine contraceptive device', pp. 91–5. See also Takeshita, *The Global Biopolitics of the IUD*.
87 'Intrauterine contraceptive devices', *British Medical Journal*, 2:5456 (1965), p. 249.

88 'Intra-uterine contraceptive device', *Family Planning*, 15:1 (1966), p. 26.
89 Wellcome Collection, London, SA/FPA/SR7, 'Minutes of the meetings of the Executive Committee held 9.12.1964'.
90 Wellcome Collection, London, SA/FPA/SR7, 'Letter to Margaret Spring Rice, 10.11.1965'.
91 'Intra-uterine contraceptive device', *Family Planning*, 15:1 (1966), p. 26.
92 'Evaluating the I.U.D', *Lancet*, 1:7854 (1974), pp. 394–5.
93 S. Clarke, 'Pure science with a practical aim: the meanings of fundamental research in Britain, circa 1916–1950', *Isis*, 101:2 (2010), pp. 285–311; A. Hull, 'Teamwork, clinical research, and the development of scientific medicines in interwar Britain: the "Glasgow School" revisited', *Bulletin of the History of Medicine*, 81:3 (2007), pp. 569–93.

Conclusion

I am writing about an important uncertainty affecting many women doctors working in family planning. As you will no doubt be aware many of us have acquired over the years considerable expertise in this field and there seems to be a strong possibility in light of the government proposals that this work will largely be taken over by General Practitioners of very varied training in family planning and of course mostly male.

It is also true that some hospitals are opening Birth Control Clinics but in many instances these are staffed by registrars who are birds of passage and incidentally again mainly male.

One outcome of these changes is that an important source of work for women doctors, and one ... which they are ideally qualified to undertake, many being wives and mothers, will be closed. I feel it is important that the MWF should approach the British Medical Association and also make representations to the department of Health and Social Security about the uncertain future many of us now face.

There are about 1,900 doctors, mostly women, in the FPA and one suspects that if there were to be any suggestions of the work of a similar number of male doctors being in jeopardy, very strong representations would be made. I would be grateful if you could place this letter before the next committee meeting of the MWF.[1]

In 1967, Labour MP Edwin Brook's Family Planning Act allowed local authorities to provide birth control to all women, married or single; in the same year, the Abortion Act legalised abortion by registered practitioners in Britain. On the other side of the channel, French authorities revoked the 1920 law and authorised the provision of contraceptives. In 1974, contraception became free under the NHS in Britain. These new laws were the culmination of long battles fought by British women doctors in Britain, and indirectly in France. But they nevertheless opened up a new front on struggles for control of female bodies that would later be denounced by feminists: the increasing burden on women to control their own fertility, the extensive power given to the predominantly male doctors in reproductive health, and the threat this power posed to the women doctors who staffed family planning clinics. The letter of a female doctor and member of the Medical Women's Federation reproduced at the beginning of this conclusion vividly illustrates the concerns that this power provoked among organised female doctors.

Women doctors played a key role in the provision of contraception and family planning advice in the decades preceding the introduction of these new laws. Highlighting their role, and the social context, networks, opportunities and constraints faced by women doctors, helps to challenge two types of narratives: the negative narrative of medicalisation as an oppressive process and the celebratory narrative of progress and scientific discovery underpinning the idea of sexual liberalisation. In so doing, this book adds to a growing body of research that has cast doubt on the notion of a linear process of emancipation or liberalisation.[2] Moreover, this study is part of a burgeoning field of research on the history of birth control practices and sexuality, and on the leading international role of women during the twentieth century.[3] It has shed light on the lived experiences of women doctors and their scientific contributions to birth control and family planning, as well as the many ways through which women doctors developed knowledge on this subject and shaped the national and international debates around it.

Most feminist historical analyses have depicted the medicalisation of the female body during the twentieth century as an exercise of the power of male doctors over their female patients. The medicalisation process in England only partially matches this description. Women doctors actively contributed to it. They did so with a view to empowering women to avoid pregnancies and adopt female-oriented methods of birth control. But they also aspired to take these issues away from the moralists; instead, birth control, contraception and family planning were to be regarded as medical fields of research and practice in which female doctors would be central actors. By engaging medically with this topic and entering the field in large numbers, women doctors were trying to secure territory for themselves. Despite a feminist sensitivity to and awareness of their patients' needs, they were nevertheless wielding authority over the female body.

At the national level, women doctors tirelessly advocated for access to contraception and reliable methods of birth control. They did so despite the opposition of the majority of the medical profession. In addition, they harnessed the public and specialised discourses around the quality and quantity of the population by bringing to the fore the medical side of birth control. Furthermore, women doctors were instrumental in challenging the moral arguments against birth control. By participating actively in debates at national conferences and in scientific publications, a small group of vocal women doctors developed arguments running counter to common assumptions about the negative effects of contraceptives on women's fertility and the state of the nation. Drawing on their own experience in birth control clinics, which they used to assert their professional authority, women doctors presented data that established contraception as a cornerstone of preventive medicine, and a driver of women's health and the well-being of the family. They produced scientific knowledge on contraceptive methods that were tested in laboratories based on well-defined scientific criteria. In so doing, women doctors collaborated with eminent scientists who lent their work an air of respectability and gave them the financial support they required, as shown by the example of the testing of the Gräfenberg ring by Helena Wright. British women doctors also forged alliances with famous individuals such as Lord Horder or with scientific bodies they helped to create such as the Birth Control Investigation Committee. This generated support and legitimacy for a field of medicine hitherto considered inferior or marginal. Women doctors were able to exploit opportunities in this area partly because of its low status. They disseminated contraceptive knowledge to a wider audience via books, manuals and scientific articles, as well as training sessions on birth control for medical students and their fellow colleagues. In this way they developed a specific form of communication that favoured technical language when addressing their colleagues; the development of this technical language contributed to medicalising family planning and securing job opportunities by increasing the value of this new field of medicine.

In addition to this active role in the production of contraceptive knowledge and expertise, British women doctors also expanded the

Conclusion

notion of family planning and gave it a new meaning. From the mid-1930s onwards, family planning no longer encompassed solely the provision of contraceptive advice, but also advice on sexual disorders and infertility, two new subjects born out of patients' needs and demands. Helena Wright and Joan Malleson were the forerunners of sexual counselling – compared to their colleagues who wrote and engaged with the issue of sexual pleasure in the 1930s, their approach was nothing short of radical. Wright and Malleson set up sexual counselling sessions centred on female sexual pleasure. They put forward a strong narrative of female emancipation from traditional norms in that they encouraged women to take an active role during sexual intercourse, breaking with the expected passive role of women in sexual relations. Wright called for a revision of gender roles and focused on the importance of the clitoris as the locus for pleasure; Malleson put her patients' demands at the centre of her work. She used psychological theory to help patients overcome their sexual disorders. Overall, the period between 1935 and 1956 saw women doctors undermining traditional notions of gender roles based on the patriarchal order. However, this radical period proved short-lived: women doctors taking over after Malleson's death in 1956 turned to the formal training available at the Tavistock Clinic, reverting to the traditional vision of sexual roles in the process.

Birth control became a topic intensively debated at the international level in a context where the state of the world's population created many anxieties, between fears of overpopulation and degeneration. Furthermore, population was coming to be framed in terms of struggles for world resources and issues of peace and war. Birth control was therefore presented as a possible solution and a way of maintaining peace. British women doctors participated in debates about the medicalisation of birth control at conferences in the 1920s and 1930s, alongside other famous international figures such as Margaret Sanger. They contributed to positioning birth control as an international health issue. Several British women doctors were able to use the experience they gained from working in birth control clinics as a tool for advancing the cause of birth control at the international level. This book has used international conferences as a lens through which to assess the respective positions of British and French women doctors within their national medical fields and the extent to which divergent political contexts impacted their stances. British and French women doctors were a minority in the male-dominated field of medicine, and while British women doctors became agents of the medicalisation of birth control, French women doctors remained constrained by their political and social contexts and were highly familialist. The experiences of British women doctors and the connections they established in the interwar years were useful elements when it came to reactivating the international movement of birth control after the Second World War and shaping it into planned parenthood. Finally, they also had an influence at the transnational level; for instance, they helped establish family planning centres in France. Britain seems to have been seen as an acceptable and legitimate model on which to base the French family planning movement. By drawing on the experience of a well-organised movement, French doctors found an efficient model and adapted a debate that came from abroad to the French context. In addition, Britain functioned as a hub for training French doctors and as a channel for importing contraceptives into France.

This book has challenged the idea of a progressive liberalisation of birth control. Indeed, women's journey to advance and medicalise the cause of birth control has not been an entirely successful one. Women doctors pressed for the integration of contraception within the medical curriculum, without much success. At the international level, their role in setting up and organising conferences on birth control and family planning was too often obscured by the famous male scientists who chaired these conferences. Thus, women remained in a marginal position within medical hierarchies; family planning centres provided opportunities for women doctors who were married with children to work part-time, but their work conditions were very poor. 'Sub-fertility' and sexual counselling were slow to develop, and no formal or compulsory training was instituted until 1974. Furthermore, in the 1960s, sexual counselling was increasingly framed through traditional and gendered roles.

With the advent of the 'second wave' of feminism, the widespread adoption of male-controlled forms of contraception was increasingly criticised, as was the medicalisation of women's bodies.[4] What was at first perceived by female doctors as an essential step for women's emancipation would, with the advent of the contraceptive pill and the legalisation of contraception, be increasingly seen as oppressive since general practitioners and gynaecologists, the majority of them male, became the main providers of both mechanical and hormonal contraceptives, i.e. the contraceptive pill, IUDs and sterilisation. In addition, fears arose due to the potentially fatal adverse effects of these new forms of contraception.[5] In this context, feminist health activists denounced the medicalisation of the female body and found alternative forms of medical practices; some were also pressuring the National Health Service to improve the quality of its service for women.[6] Psychiatry and psychology, too, would be called into question by feminists who perceived them as intrinsically misogynist.[7] While there is no doubt that psychology was a powerful tool for controlling and spreading the normative vision of sexual behaviours, this book nevertheless shows that psychological tools could also be used with another agenda in mind: that of giving women control over their sexuality and sexual pleasure, at least in the early form of sexual counselling. But with the advent of the medicalisation of sexuality, through Viagra and other medicines designed to improve sexual performance, a new form of domination has been taking place that no longer denies women the right to pleasure, but on the contrary has made sexual pleasure an imperative that needs to be monitored.[8] As a result, lack of sexual pleasure has become a pathological problem that needs to be addressed through medicine and magic pills; female sexual dysfunctions are today the object of aggressive pharmaceutical campaigns and marketing.[9] Joan Malleson might well have been ahead of her time when she warned against the 'fallacy' of over-emphasis on orgasms.

By placing women centre stage in the history of birth control, this research has shed light on the centrality of characters who had until now remained overshadowed by more famous and prestigious advocates of birth control. Precisely because they were marginalised in the medical field, women doctors colonised birth control and developed expertise in a field that was until then deemed illegitimate. This book has argued for the integration of women into histories, be they doctors, nurses or social workers, as active agents in the medicalisation of reproduction. This focus allows for the reconciliation of contradictory narratives of oppression and emancipation. Paying attention to broader national and international political and social contexts, as well as the structural stratification of the field of medicine, makes it possible to rethink a history that has too often lacked nuance.

The story of these women doctors did not end in 1967. Helena Wright retained her fighting spirit and remained a strong voice within reproductive health organisations. She was especially active at the international level with the IPPF; she travelled around the world to teach birth control and visited Sri Lanka in 1974, at the age of 87. She semi-retired in 1975 and died in 1982. Margaret Jackson remains a famous figure in the field of infertility. She practised as a doctor for fifty-three years and continued treating patients until she was 83, helping many infertile couples to have babies. She died in 1987. In honour of her work, a Margaret Jackson Centre was opened in Exeter, in the premises of her private clinic. The centre provides counselling for individuals facing personal difficulties. Sylvia Dawkins pursued her career in the FPA clinic and acted as a sexual counselling group leader. When she retired from the FPA, she continued to lead groups in London and Cambridge.[10] She died in 1996. Prudence Tunnadine continued her engagement in psychosexual counselling and was a founding member of the Institute of Psychosexual Medicine in 1974. She also started her own private practice on Harley Street in 1974.

Today, as I write these concluding remarks, the FPA has been placed into liquidation. These pioneers would have been very sad to see this organisation, for which they relentlessly fought, being closed. Its disappearance means that an important page of the history of reproductive health has now been turned. This closure reminds us how important activism is when it comes to sexual health and how precious and vulnerable our reproductive rights are. This book is dedicated to all the wonderful women doctors who created and worked in this organisation. I hope this book contributes to keeping their spirit alive.

Notes

1 Wellcome Collection, London, SA/MWF/H.41/6, 'Letter from Erpys Christopher to Jean Lawrie 25th June 1973'.
2 Cook, *The Long Sexual Revolution*; Szreter and Fisher, *Sex Before the Sexual Revolution*.
3 Brock, *English Women Surgeons and their Patients*; McCarthy, *Women of the World*; Crowther and Dupree, *Medical Lives in the Age of Surgical Revolution*; Kelly, *Irish Women in Medicine*.
4 See in particular M. Daly, *Gyn/Ecology: The Metaethics of Radical Feminism* (Boston, MA: Beacon Press, 1978); see also R. Pringle, *Sex and Medicine: Gender, Power and Authority in the Medical Profession* (Cambridge: Cambridge University Press, 1998); Pfeffer, *The Stork and the Syringe*.

Conclusion   231

5 Takeshita, *The Global Biopolitics of the IUD*; Clarke, *Disciplining Reproduction*, pp. 197–200; Grant, *The Selling of Contraception*.
6 Kline, *Bodies of Knowledge*; M. Wandor (ed.), *The Body Politic: Writings from the Women's Liberation Movement in Britain 1969–1972* (London: Stage, 1972); J. Olszynko-Gryn, 'The feminist appropriation of pregnancy testing in 1970s Britain', *Women's History Review*, 28:6 (2019), pp. 869–94.
7 S. Firestone, *The Dialectic of Sex: The Case for Feminist Revolution* (London: Jonathan Cape, 1971); J. Irvine, 'From difference to sameness: gender ideology in sexual science', *The Journal of Sex Research*, 27:1 (1990), pp. 7–24.
8 M. Loe, *The Rise of Viagra: How the Little Blue Pill Changed Sex in America* (New York: New York University Press, 2004); J. R. Fishman, 'Making Viagra: from impotence to erectile dysfunction' in A. Tone and E. Siegel Watkins (eds), *Medicating Modern America* (New York: New York University Press, 2007), pp. 229–52; J. Fishman and L. Mamo, 'Potency in all the right places: Viagra as a technology of the gendered body', *Body & Society*, 7 (2001), pp. 13–35; A. Giami, 'De l'impuissance à la dysfonction érectile. Destins de la médicalisation de la sexualité' *in* D. Fassin and D. Memmi (eds), *Le Gouvernement des Corps* (Paris: Editions de l'EHESS, 2004), pp. 77–108; N. Bajos and M. Bozon (eds), 'La sexualité à l'épreuve de la médicalisation: le cas du Viagra', *Actes de la Recherche en Sciences Sociales*, 128 (1999), pp. 34–7.
9 J. R. Fishman, 'The biomedicalisation of female sexual dysfunction' in A. Clarke et al. (eds), *Biomedicalisation: Theorising Technoscientific Transformation in the United States* (Durham, NC: Duke University Press, 2010), pp. 289–306; J. R. Fishman, 'Manufacturing desire: the commodification of female sexual dysfunction' in S. Sismondo and J. Greene (eds), *The Pharmaceutical Studies Reader* (Hoboken: Wiley-Blackwell, 2015), pp. 106–20; D. Gardey and I. Hasdeu, 'Cet obscur sujet du désir', *Travail, genre et sociétés*, 2:34 (2015), pp. 73–92; R. Moynihan, 'The making of a disease: female sexual dysfunction', *British Medical Journal*, 326:7379 (2003), pp. 45–7; M. Vuille, 'Le désir sexuel des femmes, du DSM à la nouvelle médecine sexuelle', *Genre, sexualité & société* [online], 2014, available at: http://gss.revues.org/3240 (accessed 25 June 2020).
10 J. Barnes, 'Sylvia Dawkins', *British Medical Journal*, 312:7041 (1996), p. 1295.

References

Archives

Archives du féminisme, Anger
Fond Képès

Bibliothèque interuniversitaire de Santé, Paris
Fonds Dalsace-Dellay

Butler Library, University of Columbia, New York
Margaret Sanger papers

Manchester Medical Collection, Manchester
Biographical files

University of Victoria, British Columbia
Douglas Goldring papers

Wellcome Library, London
GC/105   In the club, interview
PP/HRW   Helena Rosa Wright Collection
PP/MAL   Joan Malleson
SA/EUG   Eugenics Society Collection
SA/FPA   Family Planning Association Collection
SA/MWF   Medical Women's Federation Collection

Women's Library, London School of Economics, London

Medical journals

British Medical Journal
Family Planning

Gynécologie pratique
Journal of Hygiene
Lancet
Medical Women's Federation Newsletter
Post-Graduate Medical Journal
The Eugenics Review
The Medical Press
The Practitioner

Handbooks

Charles, E., *The Practice of Birth Control: An Analysis of the Birth-Control Experiences of Nine Hundred Women* (London: Williams & Norgate, 1932).
Cox, G., *Clinical Contraception* (London: Heinemann, 1933).
Cox, G. M., *Clinical Contraception*, 2nd edition (London: Butterworth-Heinemann, 1937).
Dawkins, S., *Planning Your Family* (London: Foyles Health Handbooks, 1959).
Fielding, M. (ed.), *Birth Control in Asia: A Report of a Conference Held at the London School of Hygiene & Tropical Medicine, November 24–25, 1933* (London: Birth Control International Information Centre, 1935).
Friedman, L. J., *Virgin Wives: A Study of Unconsummated Marriages* (London: Tavistock Publications, 1962).
Hart, D. B., and A. H. Freeland Barbour, *Manual of Gynaecology* (Edinburgh: W. & A. K. Johnston, 1890).
Haire, N. (ed.), *World League for Sexual Reform: Proceedings of the Third Congress, London, 1929* (London: Paul, Trench, Trübner, 1930).
Haire, N., *Birth Control Methods (Contraception, Abortion, Sterilisation)* (London: George Allen & Unwin, 1936).
Lagroua Weill-Hallé, M.-A., *La prescription contraceptive* (Paris: Librairie Maloine, 1968).
Macaulay, M., *The Art of Marriage* (London: Delisle, 1952).
Malleson, J., *The Principles of Contraception: A Handbook for General Practitioners* (London: V. Gollancz Limited, 1935).
Malleson, J., *Any Wife or Any Husband: A Book for Couples Who Have Met Sexual Difficulties and for Doctors* (London: Penguin Handbook, 1950).
Moore White, M., *Womanhood* (London: Cassell, 1947).
Pierpoint, R., *Report of the Fifth International Neo-Malthusian and Birth Control Conference: Kingsway Hall, London, July 11th to 14th, 1922* (London: William Heinemann Medical Books, 1922).
Pollock, M. (ed.), *Family Planning: A Handbook for the Doctor* (London: Tindall & Cassell, 1966).

Sanger, M. (ed.), *Medical and Eugenic Aspects of Birth Control: The Sixth International Neo-Malthusian and Birth Control Conference, Volume III* (New York: American Birth Control League, 1926).
Sanger, M. and H. Stone (eds), *The Practice of Contraception: An International Symposium and Survey* (Baltimore: Williams & Wilkins, 1931).
Secor Florence, L., *Birth Control on Trial* (London: George Allen and Unwin Ltd., 1932).
Tunnadine, P., *Contraception and Sexual Life: A Therapeutic Approach* (London: Tavistock Publications, 1970).
Tunnadine, P. and J. Pasmore, 'Sexual problems in marriage in women' in M. Pollock (ed.), *Family Planning* (London: Tindall & Cassell, 1966).
Wright, H., *The Sex Factor in Marriage: A Book for Those who Are, or are About to Be, Married* (London: Noel Douglas, 1930).
Wright, H., *Birth Control: Advice on Family Spacing and Healthy Sex Life* (London: Cassell, 1935).
Wright, H., *More about the Sex Factor in Marriage* (London: Williams and Norgate, 1947).
Wright, H., *Contraceptive Technique: A Handbook of Practical Instruction*, 3rd edition (London: Churchill, 1968).
Wright, H. and H. B. Wright, *Contraceptive Technique: A Handbook for Medical Practitioners and Senior Students* (London: J&A Churchill Ltd., 1951).

Articles

Alabaster, G. H., 'Contraception and fertility', *Lancet*, 231:5973 (1938), p. 462.
Anchel-Bach, M., 'La mortalité maternelle et l'avortement', *Bulletin de l'Association français des femmes médecins*, 18 (1937), p. 29.
Baker, J. R., 'The spermicidal powers of chemical contraceptives: II. Pure substances', *Journal of Hygiene*, 31:2 (1931), p. 211.
Balint, M., 'Training general practitioners in psychotherapy', *British Medical Journal*, 1:4854 (1954), pp. 115–20.
Balint, M., 'Psychotherapy and the general practitioner: I', *British Medical Journal*, 1:5011 (1957), p. 157.
Balint, M., 'The marital problem clinic – a problem child of the FPA', *Family Planning*, 9:1 (1960), pp. 18–20.
Barnes, J., 'Sylvia Dawkins', *British Medical Journal*, 312:7041 (1996), p. 1295.
Barton, M. and B. P. Wiesner, 'The receptivity of cervical mucus to spermatozoea', *British Medical Journal*, 2:4477 (1946), pp. 606–10.
Blacker, C. P., 'Foreword', *International Medical Group for the Investigation of Contraception*, 4th issue (1931), p. 3.

Blacker, C. P., 'The choice of a contraceptive', *The Practitioner*, 131:3 (1933), p. 256.
Blanchier, D., 'Compte-rendu de l'enquête faite à propos du 'Birth control'!', *Bulletin de l'Association française des femmes médecins*, 15 (1933), p. 24.
Campbell, J., 'Abortion in relation to maternal mortality', *Journal of the Medical Women's Federation*, (May 1936), p. 27.
'Contraception', *The Practitioner*, 111 (1923), p. 5.
E. H., 'Margaret Moore White, Womanhood', *Medical Women's Federation Quarterly Review* (1959), p. 37.
Eckstein, P. et al., 'The Birmingham Oral Contraceptive Trial', *British Medical Journal*, 2:5261 (1961), pp. 1172–9.
'Evaluating the I.U.D', *Lancet*, 1:7854 (1974), pp. 394–5.
Fawcitt, R., 'Revocable sterilisation of the female', *British Medical Journal*, 1:3600 (1930), p. 45.
Gräfenberg, E., 'The intra uterine method of contraception' in N. Haire (ed.), *World League for Sexual Reform: Proceedings of the Third Congress, London, 1929* (London: Paul, Trench, Trübner, 1930), p. 611.
Green-Armytage, C., 'Contraceptive', *British Medical Journal*, 1:3704 (1932), pp. 13–14.
Guttmacher, A. (ed.), *Intra-Uterine Contraceptive Devices: Proceedings of the Conference, April 30–May 1, 1962, New York City* (New York: Excerpta Medica Foundation, 1962).
Guttmacher, A., 'Intra-uterine contraceptive device', *Family Planning*, 13:14 (1965), pp. 91–5.
Haire, N., 'Health aspects of birth control' in M. Sanger (ed.), *Medical and Eugenic Aspects of Birth Control: The Sixth International Neo-Malthusian and Birth Control Conference, Volume III* (New York: American Birth Control League, 1926), p. 95.
Haire, N., 'Revocable sterilisation of the female', *British Medical Journal*, 2:3597 (1929), p. 1134.
Haire, N., 'Revocable sterilisation of the female', *British Medical Journal*, 1:3602 (1930), pp. 129–30.
Haire, N., 'Clinical experience of the past year', *International Medical Group for the Investigation of Contraception*, 4th issue (1931), p. 68.
Haire, N., 'The Gräfenberg ring', *British Medical Journal*, 1:3705 (1932), pp. 76–7.
Harding, K., 'Sterility in the female', *The Medical Press* (29 April 1953).
Harding, K., 'Management of infertility', *The Medical Press* (November 1960), p. 436.
Hick, R. H. P., 'Advice on sterility', *British Medical Journal*, 1:4300 (1943), p. 707.

Horder, L., 'Sterility', *Lancet*, 241:6247 (1943), p. 664.
Houghton, V., 'Report of meeting of International Committee on Planned Parenthood', *The Eugenics Review*, 43:3 (1951), p. 141.
Huxley, F., 'The clinical study of fertility cases with notes and treatments', *Medical Women's Federation Journal* (1 July 1935), pp. 28–37.
'Intrauterine contraceptive devices', *British Medical Journal*, 2:5456 (1965), p. 249.
'Intra-uterine contraceptive device', *Family Planning*, 15:1 (1966), p. 26.
Jackson, M., 'Birth control and the medical profession', *British Medical Journal*, 1:3621 (1930), p. 1022–3.
Jackson, M. C. N., 'Contraceptives and fertility', *British Medical Journal*, 1:4026 (1938), p. 539.
Jackson, M., 'Advice on sterility', *British Medical Journal*, 1:4303 (1943), p. 803.
Jackson, M., 'The organisation of a sterility service within a Family Planning Association clinic', *Post-Graduate Medical Journal*, 20:225 (1944), p. 237.
Jackson, M., 'A medical service for the treatment of involuntary infertility', *The Eugenics Review*, 36:4 (1945), p. 117.
Jackson, M., 'Artificial insemination', *British Medical Journal*, 1:4512 (1947), p. 945.
Jackson, M., 'Human artificial insemination', *Family Planning*, 9:3 (1960), p. 6.
Jackson, M., 'The Gräfenberg silver ring in a series of patients who had failed with other methods', in A. Guttmacher (ed.), *Intra-Uterine Contraceptive Devices: Proceedings of the Conference, April 30–May 1, 1962, New York City* (New York: Excerpta Medica Foundation, 1962), pp. 37–40.
Jackson, M., 'Oral contraception in practice', *Journal of Reproduction and Fertility*, 6:1 (1963), pp. 153–73.
Jackson, M., 'Silver ring and plastic loops, a comparison of intrauterine devices for problem cases', *Family Planning*, 12:1 (1963), p. 12.
Jackson, M., 'England: family planning in England and India', *The Journal of Sex Research*, 3:4 (1967), p. 270.
Jex-Blake, S. (1874), 'The medical education of women', a paper read at the Social Science Congress, Norwich, October 1873 (London), p. 3, quoted in L. Kelly, '"The turning point in the whole struggle": the admission of women to the King and Queen's College of Physicians in Ireland', *Women's History Review*, 22:1 (2013), pp. 97–125.
Lewis-Faning, E., 'Report of an enquiry into family limitation and its influence on human fertility during the past fifty years' in *The Royal Commission on Population*, Papers Vol. 1 (London: HM Stationery Office, 1949).
Malleson, J., 'Contraceptives and fertility', *British Medical Journal*, 1:4025 (1938), p. 484.

Malleson, J., 'Vaginismus: its management and psychogenesis', *British Medical Journal*, 2:4259 (1942), pp. 213–16.
Malleson, J., 'Contraception and sterility', *British Medical Journal*, 2:4317 (1943), p. 434.
Malleson, J., 'Contraception and sterility', *British Medical Journal*, 2:4322 (1943), p. 587.
Malleson, J., 'Contraception and sterility', *British Medical Journal*, 2:4328 (1943), pp. 796–7.
Malleson, J., 'Sexual disorders in women, their medical significance', *British Medical Journal*, 2:4746 (1951), p. 1480.
McIlroy, A. L., 'The harmful effects of artificial contraceptive methods', *The Practitioner* (July 1923), pp. 25–35.
Mears, E., 'Clinical trials of oral contraceptives', *British Medical Journal*, 2:5261 (1961), pp. 1179–83.
Mears, E., 'Oral contraception: the results', *Family Planning*, 10:4 (1962), p. 4.
'Medical problems of contraception', *British Medical Journal*, 1:3726 (1932), pp. 1047–8.
'Medical problems of contraception', *British Medical Journal*, 2:3784 (1933), pp. 118–20.
Montreuil-Strauss, G., 'Le Birth control: exposé historique par Montreuil-Strauss', *Bulletin de l'Association française des femmes médecins*, 12 (1933), pp. 3–22.
Moore White, M., 'The endocrine treatment of sterility', *Post-Graduate Medical Journal*, 20:225 (1944), pp. 215–22.
Moore White, M., 'The problem of sterility, its investigation and treatment', *The Practitioner*, 158:946 (1947), p. 279.
Moore White, M. and M. Barton, 'Conception in spite of extreme oligozoospermia', *British Medical Journal*, 1:4709 (1951), p. 741.
Murphy, K., 'Joan Malleson, the principles of contraception', *Medical Women's Federation Quarterly Review* (1935–6), p. 65.
Nixon, W. C. W., 'Joan Malleson', *British Medical Journal*, 1:4978 (1956), p. 1304.
'Obituary', *British Medical Journal*, 1:4977 (1956), p. 1242.
'Obituary', *Lancet*, 267:6926 (1956), p. 810.
Pyke, M. A., 'Contraception and fertility', *Lancet*, 231:5972 (1938), p. 405.
'Reports of societies', *British Medical Journal*, 2:3157 (1921), p. 11.
Rolleston, H., 'Birth Control Investigation Committee', *British Medical Journal*, 2:3486 (1927), p. 805.
Valabrègue, C., '48 heures à Londres', *La Maternité Heureuse, Bulletin trimestriel d'information*, 9 (1959), p. 11.

Wright, H., 'Revocable sterilisation of the female', *British Medical Journal*, 1:3602 (1930), pp. 129–30.

Wright, H., 'Notes on the 38 cases fitted with Gräfenberg ring', *International Medical Group for the Investigation of Contraception*, 4th issue (1931), p. 65.

Secondary literature

Accampo, E., *Blessed Motherhood, Bitter Fruit: Nelly Roussel and the Politics of Female Pain in Third Republic France* (Baltimore: Johns Hopkins University Press, 2006).

Akira, I. and P. I. Saunier (eds), *The Palgrave Dictionary of Transnational History* (Basingstoke: Palgrave Macmillan, 2009).

Al-Gailani, S., '"The mothers of England object": public health, privacy and professional ethics in the early twentieth-century debate over the notification of pregnancy', *Social History of Medicine*, 33:1 (2020), pp. 18–40.

Allen, A. T., 'Feminism and eugenics in Germany and Britain, 1900–40: a comparative perspective', *German Studies Review*, 23:3 (2000), pp. 477–505.

Allen, A. T., *Feminism and Motherhood in Western Europe, 1890–1970: The Maternal Dilemma* (New York: Palgrave Macmillan, 2005).

Andrew, H., '"The Reluctant Stork": Science, Fertility and the Family in Britain, 1943–60'. PhD dissertation, York University Toronto, 2016.

Austoker, J. and L. Bryder, *Historical Perspectives on the Role of the MRC* (Oxford: Oxford University Press, 1989).

Bajos, N. and M. Bozon (eds), 'La sexualité à l'épreuve de la médicalisation: le cas du Viagra', *Actes de la Recherche en Sciences Sociales*, 128 (1999), pp. 34–7.

Bard, C., *Les filles de Marianne: Histoire des féminismes; 1914–40* (Paris: Fayard, 1995).

Bard, C. and J. Mossuz-Lavau, *Le planning familial: histoire et mémoire, 1956–2006* (Rennes: Presses Universitaires de Rennes, 2007).

Bashford, A., *Purity and Pollution: Gender, Embodiment and Victorian Medicine* (Basingstoke: Macmillan Press Ltd., 1998).

Bashford, A., 'Nation, empire, globe: the spaces of population debate in the interwar years', *Comparative Studies in Society and History*, 49:1 (2007), pp. 170–201.

Bashford, A., *Global Population: History, Geopolitics, and Life on Earth* (New York: Columbia University Press, 2014).

Bashford, A. and P. Levine (eds), *The Oxford Handbook of the History of Eugenics* (Oxford: Oxford University Press, 2010).

Beachy, R., 'The German invention of homosexuality', *The Journal of Modern History*, 82:4 (2010), pp. 801–38.

Beauchamp, T. L., 'Informed consent: its history, meaning, and present challenges', *Cambridge Quarterly of Healthcare Ethics*, 20:4 (2011), pp. 515–23.

Beccalossi, C., 'Nineteenth-century European psychiatry on same-sex desires: pathology, abnormality, normality and the blurring of boundaries', *Psychology & Sexuality*, 1:3 (2010), pp. 226–38.

Benninghaus, C., 'Beyond constructivism?: Gender, medicine and the early history of sperm analysis, Germany 1870–1900', *Gender & History*, 24:3 (2012), pp. 647–76.

Bland, L. and L. Hall, 'Eugenics in Britain: the view from the metropole', in A. Bashford and P. Levine (eds), *The Oxford Handbook of the History of Eugenics* (Oxford: Oxford University Press, 2010), pp. 213–27.

Borge, J., 'The Psychosexual Counselling Tapes of Dr Joan Malleson: New Theories'. Unpublished MA thesis, Institute of Historical Research, School of Advanced Study, University of London, 2012.

Borowy, I., *Coming to Terms with World Health: The League of Nations Health Organisation 1921–1946* (Frankfurt am Main: Peter Lang, 2009).

Brock, C., *English Women Surgeons and their Patients (1860–1918)* (Cambridge: Cambridge University Press, 2017).

Brooke, S., '"A new world for women?" Abortion law reform in Britain during the 1930s', *The American Historical Review*, 106:2 (2001), pp. 431–59.

Brooke, S., *Sexual Politics: Sexuality, Family Planning and the British Left from the 1880s to the Present Day* (Oxford: Oxford University Press, 2011).

Brookes, B., *Abortion in England 1900–67* (Beckenham: Croom Helm, 1988).

Busfield, J., 'Restructuring mental health services in twentieth century Britain' in M. Gijswijt-Hofstra and R. Porter (eds), *Cultures of Psychiatry*, Clio Medica 49 (Amsterdam: Rodopi, 1998), pp. 9–28.

Cahen, F., *Gouverner les moeurs: la lutte contre l'avortement en France, 1890–1950* (Paris: Institut National d'Etudes Démographiques, 2016).

Cahen, F. and C. Capuano, 'La poursuite de la répression anti-avortement après Vichy', *Vingtième Siècle Revue d'Histoire*, 111:3 (2011), pp. 119–31.

Cahen, F. and A. Minard, 'Les mobilisations pour "la vie" et contre les "fléaux sociaux" dans l'entre-deux-guerres: essai de cartographie sociale', *Histoire et Mesure*, 31:2 (2016), pp. 141–70.

Carey, J., 'The racial imperatives of sex: birth control and eugenics in Britain, the United States and Australia in the interwar years', *Women's History Review*, 21:5 (2012), pp. 733–52.

Carol, A., *Histoire de l'eugénisme en France: Les médecins et la procréation, XIXe–XXe Siècle* (Paris: Le Seuil, 1998).

Carribon, C. and A. Duetto, '*Le Bulletin de l'Association française des femmes médecins* (1929–40). Un discours médical spécifique aux femmes?', *Le Temps des médias*, 23:2 (2014), pp. 46–8.

Chesler, E., *Woman of Valor: Margaret Sanger and the Birth Control Movement in America* (New York: Simon and Schuster, 2007).

Chettiar, T., 'The Psychiatric Family: Citizenship, Private Life, and Emotional Health in Welfare-State Britain, 1945–79'. PhD dissertation, University of Evanston, Illinois, 2013.

Chorev, N., *The World Health Organization between North and South* (Ithaca, NY: Cornell University Press, 2012).

Clarke, A., *Disciplining Reproduction: Modernity, American Life Sciences, and 'the Problems of Sex'* (Berkeley: University of California Press, 1998).

Clarke, S., 'Pure science with a practical aim: the meanings of fundamental research in Britain, circa 1916–1950', *Isis*, 101:2 (2010), pp. 285–311.

Cohen, D. A., 'Private lives in public spaces: Marie Stopes, the mothers' clinics and the practice of contraception', *History Workshop Journal*, 35:1 (1993), pp. 95–116.

Cole, J., *The Power of Large Numbers: Population, Politics, and Gender in Nineteenth-Century France* (Ithaca, NY: Cornell University Press, 2000).

Collins, M., *Modern Love: An Intimate History of Men and Women in Twentieth-Century Britain* (London: Atlantic Books, 2003).

Connelly, M., *Fatal Misconception: The Struggle to Control World Population* (Cambridge: The Belknap Press of Harvard University Press, 2009).

Conrad, P., 'Medicalization and social control', *Annual Review of Sociology*, 18:1 (1992), pp. 209–32.

Conrad, P., *The Medicalization of Society: On the Transformation of Human Conditions into Treatable Disorders* (Baltimore: Johns Hopkins University Press, 2007).

Cook, M., *London and the Culture of Homosexuality* (Cambridge: Cambridge University Press, 2003).

Cook, H., *The Long Sexual Revolution: English Women, Sex, and Contraception 1800–1975* (Oxford: Oxford University Press, 2004).

Cook, H., 'Sex and the doctors: the medicalisation of sexuality as a two-way process in early to mid-twentieth-century Britain', in W. de Blécourt and C. Usborne (eds), *Cultural Approaches to the History of Medicine* (Basingstoke: Palgrave Macmillan, 2004), pp. 192–211.

Cook, H., 'The English sexual revolution: technology and social change', *History Workshop Journal*, 59:1 (2005), pp. 109–28.

Cova, A., *Au service de l'Eglise, de la patrie et de la famille: femmes catholiques et maternité sous la III République* (Paris: L'Harmattan, 2000).

Cox-Maksimov, D., 'The Making of the Clinical Trial in Britain, 1910–45: Expertise, the State and the Public'. PhD thesis, University of Cambridge, 1997.

Crowther, A. and M. Dupree, *Medical Lives in the Age of Surgical Revolution* (Cambridge: Cambridge University Press, 2010).

Crozier, I., 'Social construction in a cold climate: a response to David Harley, "Rhetoric and the Social Construction of Sickness and Healing" and to Paolo Palladino's comment on Harley', *Social History of Medicine*, 13:3 (2000), pp. 535–46.

Crozier, I., 'Becoming a sexologist: Norman Haire, the 1929 London World League for Sexual Reform Congress, and organising medical knowledge about sex in interwar England', *History of Science*, 39:3 (2001), pp. 299–329.

Crozier, I., 'The medical construction of homosexuality and its relation to the law in nineteenth-century England', *Medical History*, 45:1 (2001), pp. 61–82.

Crozier, I., '"All the world's a stage": Dora Russell, Norman Haire, and the 1929 London World League for Sexual Reform Congress', *Journal of the History of Sexuality*, 12:1 (2003), pp. 16–37.

Cryle, P. and A. Moore, *Frigidity: An Intellectual History* (Basingstoke: Palgrave Macmillan, 2011).

Cunningham, A. and P. Williams, *The Laboratory Revolution in Medicine* (Cambridge: Cambridge University Press, 2002).

Dale, P. and K. Fisher, 'Contrasting municipal responses to the provision of birth control services in Halifax and Exeter before 1948', *Social History of Medicine*, 23:3 (2010), pp. 567–85

Daly, M., *Gyn/Ecology: The Metaethics of Radical Feminism* (Boston, MA: Beacon Press, 1978).

Davey, C., 'Birth control in Britain during the interwar years: evidence from the Stopes correspondence', *Journal of Family History*, 13:3 (1988), pp. 329–45.

Davidoff, L. et al., *The Family Story: Blood, Contract and Intimacy* (London: Longman, 1998).

Davin, A., 'Imperialism and motherhood', *History Workshop Journal*, 5:1 (1978), pp. 9–65.

Davis, G., 'Health and sexuality' in Mark Jackson (ed.), *Oxford Handbook on the History of Medicine* (Oxford: Oxford University Press, 2011), pp. 504–23.

Davis, G., 'A tragedy as old as history, medical response to infertility in Britain' in G. Davis and T. Loughran (eds), *The Palgrave Handbook of Infertility in History: Approaches, Contexts and Perspectives* (London: Palgrave Macmillan, 2017), pp. 359–81.

Davis, G. and T. Loughran (eds), *The Palgrave Handbook of Infertility in History: Approaches, Contexts and Perspectives* (London: Palgrave Macmillan, 2017).

De Luca Barrusse, V., *Les familles nombreuses: une question démographique, un enjeu politique: France, 1880–1940* (Rennes: Presses Universitaires de Rennes, 2008).

De Luca Barrusse, V., 'Pro-natalism and hygienism in France, 1900–40. The example of the fight against venereal disease', *Population*, 64:3 (2009), pp. 477–506.

De Luca Barrusse, V. and A.-F. Praz, 'Les Politiques de Population: Resituer L'objet de Recherche', *Annales de Démographie Historique*, 1:129 (2016), pp. 149–64.

Debenham, C., *Birth Control and the Rights of Women: Post-Suffrage Feminism in the Early Twentieth Century* (London: I. B. Tauris, 2014).

deVries, J. R., 'A moralist *and* moderniser: Mary Scharlieb and the creation of gynecological knowledge, ca. 1880–1914', *Social Politics*, 22:3 (2015), pp. 298–318.

Digby, A., *Making a Medical Living: Doctors and Patients in the English Market for Medicine, 1720–1911* (Cambridge: Cambridge University Press, 1994).

Digby, A., *The Evolution of British General Practice 1850–1948* (Oxford: Oxford University Press, 1999).

Dose, R., 'The World League for Sexual Reform: some possible approaches', *Journal of the History of Sexuality*, 12:1 (2003), pp. 1–15.

Drouard, A., 'Aux origines de l'eugénisme en France: le néo-malthusianisme (1896–1914)', *Population*, 47:2 (1992), pp. 435–59.

Duden, B., *The Woman Beneath the Skin: A Doctor's Patients in Eighteenth-Century Germany* (New Haven: Harvard University Press, 1991).

Dugdale, A., 'Devices and Desires: Constructing the Intrauterine Device, 1908–1988'. PhD thesis, Department of Science and Technology Studies, University of Wollongong, 1995.

Dugdale, A., 'Inserting Gräfenberg's IUD into the sex reform movement', in D. MacKenzie and J. Wajcman (eds), *The Social Shaping of Technology* (Buckingham: Open University Press, 1999).

Dugdale, A., 'Intrauterine contraceptive devices, situated knowledges, and the making of women's bodies', *Australian Feminist Studies*, 15:32 (2000), pp. 165–76.

Dyhouse, C., 'Driving ambitions: women in pursuit of a medical education, 1890–1939', *Women's History Review*, 7:3 (1998), pp. 321–43.

Dyhouse, C., 'Women students and the London medical schools, 1914–39: the anatomy of a masculine culture', *Gender & History*, 10:1 (1998), pp. 110–32.

Ehrenreich, B. and D. English, *Witches, Midwives and Nurses: A History of Women Healers* (New York: The Feminist Press, 1973).

Elston, M. A. C., 'Women Doctors in the British Health Services: A Sociological Study of Their Careers and Opportunities'. PhD dissertation, University of Leeds, 1986.

Elston, M. A., '"Run by women, (mainly) for women": medical women's hospitals in Britain, 1866–1948' in A. Hardy and L. Conrad (eds), *Women and Modern Medicine*, Clio Medica 61 (Leiden: Brill Rodopi, 2001), pp. 73–107.

Evans, B., *Freedom to Choose: The Life and Work of Dr Helena Wright, Pioneer of Contraception* (London: The Bodley Head, 1984).

Featherstone, L., 'The science of pleasure: medicine and sex therapy in mid-twentieth-century Australia', *Social History of Medicine*, 31:3 (2018), pp. 445–61.
Fette, J., 'Pride and prejudice in the professions: women doctors and lawyers in Third Republic France', *Journal of Women's History*, 19:3 (2007), pp. 60–86.
Finch, J. and P. Summerfield, 'Social reconstruction and the emergence of companionate marriage, 1945–59', D. Clarke (ed.), *Marriage, Domestic Life and Social Change: Writings for Jacqueline Burgoyne (1944–88)* (London: Routledge, 1991), pp. 7–32.
Firestone, S., *The Dialectic of Sex: The Case for Feminist Revolution* (London: Jonathan Cape, 1971).
Fisher, K., 'Contrasting cultures of contraception: birth control clinics and the working-classes between the wars' in M. Gijswijt-Hofstra, G. M. van Heteren and T. Tansey (eds), *Biographies of Remedies: Drugs, Medicines and Contraceptives in Dutch and Anglo-American Healing Cultures*, Clio Medica 66 (Amsterdam: Rodopi, 2002), pp. 141–57.
Fisher, K., *Birth Control, Sex and Marriage in Britain, 1918–60* (Oxford: Oxford University Press, 2006).
Fishman, J. R., 'Making viagra: from impotence to erectile dysfunction' in A. Tone and E. Siegel Watkins (eds), *Medicating Modern America* (New York: New York University Press, 2007), pp. 229–52.
Fishman, J. R., 'The biomedicalisation of female sexual dysfunction' in A. Clarke et al. (eds), *Biomedicalisation: Theorising Technoscientific Transformation in the United States* (Durham: Duke University Press, 2010), pp. 289–306.
Fishman, J. R., 'Manufacturing desire: the commodification of female sexual dysfunction', in S. Sismondo and J. Greene (eds), *The Pharmaceutical Studies Reader* (Hoboken: Wiley-Blackwell, 2015), pp. 106–20.
Foucault, M., *La volonté de savoir: histoire de la sexualité 1* (Paris: Gallimard, 1976).
Franklin, S. and H. Ragoné (eds), *Reproducing Reproduction: Kinship, Power, and Technological Innovation* (Philadelphia: University of Pennsylvania Press, 1998).
Freeden, M., 'Eugenics and progressive thought: a study in ideological affinity', *The Historical Journal*, 22:3 (1979), pp. 645–71.
Freud, S., *Three Essays on the Theory of Sexuality: The 1905 Edition* (New York: Verso, 2017).
Gardey, D. and I. Hasdeu, 'Cet obscur sujet du désir', *Travail, genre et sociétés*, 2:34 (2015), pp. 73–92.
Gelly, M., *Avortement et contraception dans les études médicales: une formation inadaptée* (Paris: Editions l'Harmattan, 2006).

Giami, A., 'De l'impuissance à la dysfonction érectile. Destins de la médicalisation de la sexualité', in D. Fassin and D. Memmi (eds), *Le Gouvernement des Corps* (Paris: Éditions de l'EHESS, 2004), pp. 77–108.

Gillis, R., L. A. Tilly and D. Levine (eds), *The European Experience of Declining Fertility: A Quiet Revolution 1850–1970* (Cambridge: Blackwell, 1992).

Gordon, F., *The Integral Feminist: Madeleine Pelletier, 1874–1939* (Minneapolis: University of Minnesota Press, 1991).

Gordon, L., *The Moral Property of Women: A History of Birth Control Politics in America* (Urbana: University of Illinois Press, 2002).

Gowing, L., *Common Bodies: Women, Touch and Power in Seventeenth-Century England* (New Haven: Yale University Press, 2003).

Grant, N., *The Selling of Contraception: The Dalkon Shield Case, Sexuality, and Women's Autonomy* (Columbus: Ohio State University Press, 1992).

Grier, J., 'Eugenics and birth control: contraceptive provision in North Wales, 1918–1939', *Social History of Medicine*, 11:3 (1998), pp. 443–8.

Grossman, A., *Reforming Sex: The German Movement for Birth Control and Abortion Reform, 1920–50* (Oxford: Oxford University Press, 1995).

Gruber, H., 'French women in the crossfire of class, sex, maternity and citizenship', in H. Gruber and P. Graves (eds), *Women and Socialism, Socialism and Women: Europe between the Two World Wars* (New York: Berghahn Books, 1998), pp. 279–320.

Hall, L., '"The English have hot-water bottles": The Morganatic marriage between sexology and medicine in Britain since William Acton', in R. Porter and M. Teich (eds), *Sexual Knowledge, Sexual Science: The History of Attitudes to Sexuality* (Cambridge: Cambridge University Press, 1994), pp. 350–66.

Hall, L. A., 'Marie Stopes and her correspondents: personalising population decline in an era of demographic change', in R. Peel (ed.), *Marie Stopes, Eugenics and the English Birth Control Movement* (London: Galton Institute, 1997), pp. 27–48.

Hall, L. A., 'Malthusian mutations: the changing politics and moral meanings of birth control in Britain' in B. Dolan, *Malthus, Medicine and Morality*, Clio Medica 59 (Leiden: Brill Rodopi, 2000), pp. 141–63.

Hall, L. A., 'A suitable job for a woman: women doctors and birth control to the inception of the NHS' in A. Hardy and L. Conrad (eds), *Women and Modern Medicine*, Clio Medica 61 (Leiden: Brill Rodopi, 2001), pp. 127–47.

Hall, L. A., 'In ignorance and in knowledge: reflections on the history of sex education in Britain', in L. D. H. Sauerteig and R. Davidson (eds), *Shaping Sexual Knowledge: A Cultural History of Sex Education in Twentieth Century Europe* (London: Routledge, 2009), pp. 19–36.

Hall, L. A., *The Life and Times of Stella Browne: Feminist and Free Spirit* (London: I. B. Tauris, 2011).

Hall, L., *Sex, Gender and Social Change in Britain since 1880*, 2nd edition (Basingstoke: Palgrave Macmillan, 2012).
Hall, L. A., *Outspoken Women: An Anthology of Women's Writing on Sex, 1870–1969*. (London: Routledge, 2014).
Hanley, A. R., *Medicine, Knowledge and Venereal Diseases in England, 1886–1916* (London: Palgrave Macmillan, 2017).
Herzog, D., *Sexuality in Europe: A Twentieth-Century History* (Cambridge: Cambridge University Press, 2011).
Hilevych, Y., 'Abortion and gender relationships in Ukraine, 1955–1970', *The History of the Family*, 20:1 (2015), pp. 86–105.
Hodder, J., S. Legg and M. Heffernan, 'Introduction: historical geographies of internationalism, 1900–1950', *Political Geography*, 49 (2015), pp. 1–6.
Hodges, S., *Contraception, Colonialism and Commerce: Birth Control in South India, 1920–1940* (Aldershot: Ashgate, 2008).
Hodgson, D. and S. Watkins, 'Feminists and neo-Malthusians: past and present alliances', *Population and Development Review*, 23:3 (1997), pp. 469–523.
Hoggart, L., 'The campaign for birth control in Britain in the 1920s' in A. Digby and J. Stewart (eds), *Gender, Health and Welfare* (London: Routledge, 1996), pp. 143–66.
Hoggart, L., 'Socialist feminism, reproductive rights and political action', *Capital and Class*, 24:1 (2012), pp. 95–125.
Houlbrook, M., *Queer London: Perils and Pleasures in the Sexual Metropolis, 1918–57* (Chicago: University of Chicago Press, 2005).
Hull, A., 'Teamwork, clinical research, and the development of scientific medicines in interwar Britain: the 'Glasgow School' revisited', *Bulletin of the History of Medicine*, 81:3 (2007), pp. 569–93.
Huss, M.-M., 'Pronatalism in the inter-war period in France', *Journal of Contemporary History*, 25:1 (1990), pp. 39–68.
Ignaciuk, A., 'No Man's Land? Gendering contraception in family planning advice literature in state-Socialist Poland (1950s–80s)', *Social History of Medicine*, hkz007, available at: https://doi.org/10.1093/shm/hkz007 (accessed 25 June 2020).
Irvine, J., 'From difference to sameness: gender ideology in sexual science', *The Journal of Sex Research*, 27:1 (1990), pp. 7–24.
Irwin, R., '"To try and find out what is being done to whom, by whom and with what results": the creation of psychosexual counselling policy in England, 1972–79', *Twentieth Century British History*, 20:2 (2009), pp. 173–97.
Irwin, R., 'Recalling the early years of psychosexual nursing', *Oral History*, 39:1 (2011), pp. 43–52.
Jackson, M., *The Real Facts of Life: Feminism and the Politics of Sexuality, c.1850–1940* (London: Taylor & Francis, 1994).

Janz, O. and D. Schönpflug (eds), *Gender and History in a Transnational Perspective: Biographies, Networks, Gender Orders* (Oxford: Berghahn, 2014).

Jones, C. L., 'Under the covers? Commerce, contraceptives and consumers in England and Wales, 1880–1960', *Social History of Medicine*, 29:4 (2016), pp. 734–56.

Jones, E. L., 'The establishment of voluntary family planning clinics in Liverpool and Bradford, 1926–60: A comparative study', *Social History of Medicine*, 24:2 (2011), pp. 352–69.

Jones, G., *Social Hygiene in Twentieth Century Britain* (London: Croom Helm, 1986).

Jones, G., 'Marie Stopes in Ireland. The mother's clinic in Belfast, 1936–47', *Social History of Medicine*, 5:2 (1992), pp. 255–77.

Jones, G., 'Women and eugenics in Britain: the case of Mary Scharlieb, Elizabeth Sloan Chesser, and Stella Browne', *Annals of Science*, 52:5 (1995), pp. 481–502.

Kelly, L., '"Fascinating scalpel-wielders and fair dissectors": women's experience of Irish medical education c.1880s–1920s', *Medical History*, 54:4 (2010), p. 506.

Kelly, L., *Irish Women in Medicine, c.1880s–1920s* (Manchester: Manchester University Press, 2013).

Képès, S., *Du corps à l'âme, entretiens avec Danielle M. Lévy* (Paris: L'Harmattan, 1996).

Kevles, D. J., *In the Name of Eugenics: Genetics and the Uses of Human Heredity* (Berkeley: University of California Press, 1986).

King, H., *The Disease of Virgins: Green Sickness, Chlorosis and the Problems of Puberty* (London: Routledge, 2004).

Klausen, S. and A. Bashford, 'Fertility control: eugenics, neo-Malthusianism, and feminism' in A. Bashford and P. Levine (eds), *The Oxford Handbook of the History of Eugenics* (Oxford: Oxford University Press, 2010), pp. 98–115.

Kline, W., *Bodies of Knowledge: Sexuality, Reproduction, and Women's Health in the Second Wave* (Chicago: University of Chicago Press, 2010).

Kling, S., 'Reproductive health, birth control and fertility change in Sweden, circa 1900–40', *The History of the Family*, 15:2 (2010), pp. 161–73.

Knibiehler, Y., 'L'éducation sexuelle des filles au XXe siècle', *Clio: Femmes, Genre, Histoire*, 4 (1996), pp. 419–82.

Knibiehler, Y., *Accoucher: Femmes, sages-femmes et médecins depuis le milieu du 20e siècle* (Rennes: Editions de l'Ecole des Hautes Etudes en Santé Publique, 2007).

Koos, C. A., 'Gender, anti-individualism, and nationalism: the Alliance Nationale and the pronatalist backlash against the femme moderne, 1933–40', *French Historical Studies*, 19:3 (1996), pp. 699–723.

Kościańska, A., 'Sex on equal terms? Polish sexology on women's emancipation and "good sex" from the 1970s to the present', *Sexualities*, 19:1–2 (2016), pp. 236–56.
Langhamer, C., *The English in Love: The Intimate Story of an Emotional Revolution* (Oxford: Oxford University Press, 2013).
Laqueur, T., *Making Sex: Body and Gender from the Greeks to Freud* (Cambridge, MA: Harvard University Press, 1990).
Latham, M., *Regulating Reproduction: A Century of Conflict in Britain and France* (Manchester: Manchester University Press, 2002).
Lawrence, C., 'Still incommunicable: clinical holists and medical knowledge in interwar Britain' in C. Lawrence and G. Weisz (eds), *Greater than the Parts: Holism in Biomedicine 1920–50* (Oxford: Oxford University Press, 1998), pp. 94–111.
Lawrence, C., 'A tale of two sciences: bedside and bench in twentieth-century Britain', *Medical History*, 43:4 (1999), pp. 421–49.
Leathard, A., *The Fight for Family Planning: The Development of Family Planning Services in Britain, 1921–1974* (London: Macmillan Press, 1980).
Ledbetter, R., *A History of the Malthusian League, 1877–1927* (Columbia: Ohio State University Press, 1986).
Lewis, J., *The Politics of Motherhood: Child and Maternal Welfare in England, 1900–1939* (London: Croom Helm, 1980).
Lewis, J., 'The working-class wife and mother and state intervention, 1870–1918' in J. Lewis (ed.), *Women's Experience of Home and Family, 1850–1940* (Oxford: Blackwell, 1986).
Lewis, J., D. Clark and D. Morgan, *Whom God Hath Joined Together: Work of Marriage Guidance* (London: Routledge, 1992).
Linder, D. H., *'Crusader for Sex Education': Elise Ottesen-Jensen (1886–1973) in Scandinavia and on the International Scene* (Lanham, MD: University Press of America, 1996).
Lišková, K., *Sexual Liberation, Socialist Style: Communist Czechoslovakia and the Science of Desire, 1945–89* (Cambridge: Cambridge University Press, 2018).
Loe, M., *The rise of Viagra: How the Little Blue Pill changed Sex in America* (New York: New York University Press, 2004).
Loeb, L., 'Doctors and patent medicines in modern Britain: professionalism and consumerism', *Albion*, 33:3 (2001), pp. 404–25.
Löwy, I., '"Sexual chemistry" before the pill: science, industry and chemical contraceptives, 1920–1960', *British Journal for the History of Science*, 44:2 (2011), pp. 245–74.
Löwy, I. and G. Weisz, 'French hormones: progestins and therapeutic variation in France', *Social Science & Medicine*, 60:11 (2005), pp. 2609–22.

Mackenzie, D., *Statistics in Britain, 1865–1930: The Social Construction of Scientific Knowledge* (Edinburgh: Edinburgh University Press, 1981).

Macnicol, J., 'Eugenics and the campaign for voluntary sterilization in Britain between the wars', *Social History of Medicine*, 2:2 (1989), pp. 147–69.

Makepeace, C., 'To what extent was the relationship between feminists and the eugenics movement a "marriage of convenience" in the interwar years?', *Journal of International Women's Studies*, 11:3 (2009), pp. 66–80.

Malleson, A., *Discovering the Family of Miles Malleson 1888–1969* (2012) [online], available at: https://books.google.co.uk/books?id=WBVhkj_JAJ8C&printsec=frontcover&dq=discovering+the+family+of+miles+malleson&hl=en&sa=X&ved=0ahUKEwib0bDQ6MPlAhX4RBUIHebwB1gQuwUILTAA#v=onepage&q=discovering%20the%20family%20of%20miles%20malleson&f=false (accessed 30 October 2019).

Marks, L., *Metropolitan Maternity: Maternal and Infant Welfare Services in Early Twentieth Century London* (Amsterdam: Rodopi, 1996).

Marks, L., *Sexual Chemistry: A History of the Contraceptive Pill* (New Haven: Yale University Press, 2001).

Marland, H., 'Women, health and medicine' in M. Jackson (ed.), *The Oxford Handbook on the History of Medicine* (Oxford: Oxford University Press, 2011), pp. 484–502.

Maynes, M. J., B. Søland and C. Benninghaus, *Secret Gardens, Satanic Mills: Placing Girls in European History, 1750–1960* (Bloomington: Indiana University Press, 2005).

Mazumdar, P., *Eugenics, Human Genetics and Human Failings: The Eugenics Society, Its Sources and Its Critics in Britain* (London: Routledge, 2005).

McCarthy, H., *Women of the World: The Rise of the Female Diplomat* (London: Bloomsbury, 2014).

McClive, C., 'The hidden truths of the belly: the uncertainties of pregnancy in early modern Europe', *Social History of Medicine*, 15:2 (2002), pp. 209–27.

McLaren, A., *Birth Control in Nineteenth-Century England* (London: Croom Helm, 1978).

McLaren, A., *Twentieth-Century Sexuality: A History* (Oxford: Oxford University Press, 1999).

McLaren, A., *Reproduction by Design: Sex, Robots, Trees, and Test-Tube Babies in Interwar Britain* (Chicago: University of Chicago Press, 2012).

Michaelsen, K., 'Union is strength: the Medical Women's Federation and the politics of professionalism, 1917–30' in K. Cowman and L. Jackson (eds), *Women and Work Culture, Britain c.1850–1950* (Aldershot: Ashgate, 2005), p. 165.

Mitchell, C., 'Madeleine Pelletier (1874–1939): the politics of sexual oppression', *Feminist Review*, 33 (1989), pp. 72–92.

Mold, A., 'Repositioning the patient: patient organisations, consumerism, and autonomy in Britain during the 1960s and 1970s', *Bulletin of the History of Medicine*, 87:2 (2013), pp. 225–49.
Moore, A., 'Relocating Marie Bonaparte's clitoris', *Australian Feminist Studies*, 24:60 (2009), pp. 149–65.
Morantz-Sanchez, R., *Sympathy and Science: Women Physicians in American Medicine* (Oxford: Oxford University Press, 1985).
More, E. S., E. Fee and M. Parry (eds), *Women Physicians and the Cultures of Medicine* (Baltimore: Johns Hopkins University Press, 2009).
Moscucci, O., *The Science of Woman: Gynaecology and Gender in England, 1800–1929* (Cambridge: Cambridge University Press, 1990).
Moulin, A. M., 'The Pasteur Institute's international network: scientific innovations and French tropisms' in C. Charle, J. Schriewer and P. Wagner (eds), *Transnational Intellectual Networks: Forms of Academic Knowledge and the Search for Cultural Identities* (Frankfurt: Campus Verlag, 2004), pp. 135–62.
Moynihan, R., 'The making of a disease: female sexual dysfunction', *British Medical Journal*, 326:7379 (2003), pp. 45–7.
Murphy, M., *Seizing the Means of Reproduction: Entanglements of Feminism, Health, and Technoscience* (Durham, NC: Duke University Press, 2012).
Neill, D., *Networks in Tropical Medicine: Internationalism, Colonialism, and the Rise of a Medical Specialty, 1890–1930* (Stanford: Stanford University Press, 2012).
Neuhaus, J., 'The importance of being orgasmic: sexuality, gender, and marital sex manuals in the United States, 1920–63', *Journal of the History of Sexuality*, 9:4 (2000), pp. 447–73.
Oakley, A., *The Captured Womb: A History of the Medical Care of Pregnant Women* (Oxford: Basil Blackwell Publisher Ltd., 1984).
Offen, K., 'Depopulation, nationalism, and feminism in fin-de-siècle France', *The American Historical Review*, 89:3 (1984), pp. 648–76.
Offen, K., *Les féminismes en Europe (1700–1950): une histoire politique* (Rennes: Presses Universitaires de Rennes, 2012).
Ogden, P. E. and M.-M. Huss, 'Demography and pronatalism in France in the nineteenth and twentieth centuries', *Journal of Historical Geography*, 8:3 (1982), pp. 283–98.
Olszynko-Gryn, J., 'The demand for pregnancy testing: the Aschheim–Zondek reaction, diagnostic versatility, and laboratory services in 1930s Britain', *Studies in History and Philosophy of Science Part C: Studies in History and Philosophy of Biological and Biomedical Sciences*, 47 (2014), pp. 233–47.
Olszynko-Gryn, J., 'Technologies of contraception and abortion' in N. Hopwood, R. Flemming and L. Kassell (eds), *Reproduction: Antiquity to the Present* (Cambridge: Cambridge University Press, 2018), pp. 535–51.

Olszynko-Gryn, J., 'The feminist appropriation of pregnancy testing in 1970s Britain', *Women's History Review*, 28:6 (2019), pp. 869–94.
Olszynko-Gryn, J. and C. Rusterholz (eds), 'Introduction: Reproductive Politics in Britain and France', *Medical History*, 63:2 (2019), pp. 117–33.
Ortiz-Gómez, T. and A. Ignaciuk, 'The fight for family planning in Spain during late Francoism and the transition to democracy, 1965–79', *Journal of Women's History*, 30:2 (2018), pp. 38–62.
Oudshoorn, N., *Beyond the Natural Body: An Archaeology of Sex Hormones* (London: Routledge, 1994).
Parry, M., *Broadcasting Birth Control: Mass Media and Family Planning* (New Brunswick: Rutgers University Press, 2013).
Pavard, B., 'Du birth control au planning familial (1955–60): un transfert militant', *Histoire@ Politique*, 18:3 (2012), pp. 162–78.
Pavard, B., *'Si je veux, quand je veux': Contraception et avortement dans la société française (1956–79)* (Rennes: Presses Universitaires de Rennes, 2012).
Pedersen, J. E., 'Regulating abortion and birth control: gender, medicine, and republican politics in France, 1870–1920', *French Historical Studies*, 19:3 (1996), pp. 673–98.
Pedersen, S., *Family, Dependence, and the Origins of the Welfare State: Britain and France, 1914–1945* (Cambridge: Cambridge University Press, 1995).
Peel, J., 'Contraception and the medical profession', *Population Studies*, 18:2 (1964), pp. 133–45.
Pfeffer, N., *The Stork and the Syringe: A Political History of Reproductive Medicine* (Cambridge: Polity Press, 1993).
Philippe, B., 'Suzanne Képès, une femme d'exception', *Le Carnet PSY*, 6:101 (2005), p. 36.
Pinell, P., 'Champ médical et processus de spécialisation', *Actes de la Recherche en Sciences Sociales*, 1 (2005), pp. 4–36.
Porter, R. and L. Hall, *The Facts of Life: The Creation of Sexual Knowledge in Britain, 1650–1950* (New Haven: Yale University Press, 1995).
Pringle, R., *Sex and Medicine: Gender, Power and Authority in the Medical Profession* (Cambridge: Cambridge University Press, 1998).
Ramsden, E., 'Social demography and eugenics in the interwar United States', *Population and Development Review*, 29:4 (2003), pp. 547–93.
Ratcliff, K., *Women and Health: Power, Technology, Inequality and Conflict in a Gendered World* (Boston, MA: Allyn and Bacon, 2002)
Rebreyend, A.-C., *Intimités amoureuses: France 1920–75* (Toulouse: Presses Universitaires du Mirail, 2008).
Reggiani, A. H., 'Procreating France: the politics of demography, 1919–45', *French Historical Studies*, 19:3 (1996), pp. 725–54.

Reinish, J. (ed.), 'Agents of internationalism', *Contemporary European History*, 25:2 (2016), pp. 195–205.
Roemer, M., 'Internationalism in medicine and public health' in D. Porter (ed.), *The History of Public Health and the Modern State* (Amsterdam: Rodopi, 1994), pp. 403–22.
Ronsin, F., *La grève des ventres: propagande néo-malthusienne et baisse de la natalité française, XIXe–XXe siècles* (Paris: Aubier Montaigne, 1980).
Rose, J., *Marie Stopes and the Sexual Revolution* (London: Faber and Faber, 1992).
Rose, N., 'Beyond medicalization', *Lancet*, 369:9562 (2007), pp. 700–2.
Rosental, P.-A., *L'Intelligence démographique: Sciences et politiques des populations en France (1930–1960)* (Paris: Odile Jacob, 2003).
Rusterholz, C., 'Testing the Gräfenberg ring in interwar Britain: Norman Haire, Helena Wright, and the debate over statistical evidence, side effects, and intra-uterine contraception', *Journal of the History of Medicine and Allied Sciences*, 72:4 (2017), pp. 448–67.
Rusterholz, C., 'English and French women doctors in international debates on contraception (1920–1935)', *Social History of Medicine*, 31:2 (2018), pp. 328–47.
Rusterholz, C., 'English women doctors, contraception and family planning in transnational perspective (1930s–70s)', *Medical History*, 63:2 (2019), pp. 153–72.
Rusterholz, C., '"You can't dismiss that as being less happy, you see it is different". Sexual therapy in 1950s England', *Twentieth Century British History*, 30:3 (2019), pp. 375–98.
Sauerteig, L. D. H. and R. Davidson (eds), *Shaping Sexual Knowledge: A Cultural History of Sex Education in Twentieth Century Europe* (London: Routledge, 2009).
Schneider, W. H., *Quality and Quantity: The Quest for Biological Regeneration in Twentieth-Century France* (Cambridge: Cambridge University Press, 2002).
Shortt, S. E. D., 'Physicians, science, and status: issues in the professionalisation of Anglo-American medicine in the nineteenth century', *Medical History*, 27:1 (1983), pp. 51–68.
Simmons, C., *Making Marriage Modern: Women's Sexuality from the Progressive Era to World War II* (Oxford: Oxford University Press, 2009).
Sohn, A.-M., *Du premier baiser à l'alcôve: La sexualité des Français au quotidien (1850–1950)* (Paris: Aubier, 1996).
Soloway, R. A., 'Neo-Malthusians, eugenists, and the declining birth-rate in England, 1900–1918' *Albion*, 10:3 (1978), pp. 264–86.
Soloway, R. A., *Birth Control and the Population Question in Britain, 1870–1930* (Chapel Hill: University of North Carolina Press, 1982).

Soloway, R. A., *Demography and Degeneration: Eugenics and the Declining Birthrate in Twentieth-Century Britain* (Chapel Hill: University of North Carolina Press, 1990).

Soloway, R. A., 'The "perfect contraceptive": eugenics and birth control research in Britain and America in the interwar years', *Journal of Contemporary History*, 30:4 (1995), pp. 637–64.

Soloway, R., 'The Galton Lecture 1996: Marie Stopes, eugenics, and the birth control movement' in R. Peel (ed.), *Marie Stopes: Eugenics and the English Birth Control Movement* (London: Galton Institute, 1997), pp. 49–76.

Sonn, R. D., '"Your body is yours": anarchism, birth control, and eugenics in interwar France', *Journal of the History of Sexuality*, 14:4 (2005), pp. 415–32.

Strange, J.-M., 'The assault on ignorance: teaching menstrual etiquette in England, c.1920s to 1960s', *Social History of Medicine*, 14:2 (2001), pp. 247–65.

Sturdy, S., 'The political economy of scientific medicine: science, education and the transformation of medical practice in Sheffield, 1890–1922', *Medical History*, 36:2 (1992), pp. 125–59.

Sturdy, S., 'Looking for trouble: medical science and clinical practice in the historiography of modern medicine', *Social History of Medicine*, 24:3 (2011), pp. 739–57.

Sturdy, S. and R. Cooter, 'Science, scientific management, and the transformation of medicine in Britain c.1870–1950', *History of Science*, 36:114 (1998), pp. 421–66.

Sutton, C., 'Hysterectomy: a historical perspective', *Baillière's Clinical Obstetrics and Gynaecology*, 11:1 (1997), pp. 1–22.

Sylvest, C., 'Continuity and change in British liberal internationalism, c.1900–1930', *Review of International Studies*, 31:2 (2005), pp. 263–83.

Szreter, S., 'The idea of demographic transition and the study of fertility change: a critical intellectual history', *Population and Development Review*, 19:4 (1993), pp. 659–701.

Szreter, S., *Fertility, Class and Gender in Britain, 1860–1940* (Cambridge: Cambridge University Press, 2002).

Szreter, S., *Health and Wealth: Studies in History and Policy* (Rochester, NY: University of Rochester Press, 2005).

Szreter, S. and K. Fisher, *Sex Before the Sexual Revolution* (Cambridge: Cambridge University Press, 2010).

Szuhan, N., 'Sex in the laboratory: the Family Planning Association and contraceptive science in Britain, 1929–1959', *The British Journal for the History of Science*, 51:3 (2018), pp. 1–24.

Takeshita, C., *The Global Biopolitics of the IUD: How Science Constructs Contraceptive Users and Women's Bodies* (Cambridge, MA: MIT Press, 2012).

Tamagne, F., *La Ligue Mondiale Pour La Réforme Sexuelle: La science au service de l'émancipation sexuelle?* (Paris: Editions Belin, 2005).

Tammeveski, P., 'Repression and incitement: a critical demographic, feminist, and transnational analysis of birth control in Estonia, 1920–39', *The History of the Family*, 16:1 (2011), pp. 13–29.

Teitelbaum, M. S., *The British Fertility Decline: Demographic Transition in the Crucible of the Industrial Revolution* (Princeton: Princeton University Press, 2014).

Thane, P., 'Visions of gender in the making of the British welfare state: the case of women in the British Labour Party and social policy, 1906–45' in G. Bock and P. Thane (eds), *Maternity and Gender Policies: Women and the Rise of the European Welfare States 1880s–1950s* (London: Routledge, 1991), pp. 93–118.

Thomsen, R. J., 'Historical: Ernst Gräfenberg and the golden year of the silver ring' in E. S. Hafez and W. A. van Os (eds), *Medicated Intrauterine Devices: Physiological and Clinical Aspects* (The Hague: Springer Netherlands, 1980), pp. 3–8.

Timmerman, C., 'Clinical research in postwar Britain, the role of the Medical Research Council' in C. Hannaway (ed.), *Biomedicine in the 20th Century: Practices, Policies and Politics* (Amsterdam: IOS Press, 2008), pp. 231–54.

Toms, J., *Mental Hygiene and Psychiatry in Modern Britain* (Basingstoke: Palgrave Macmillan, 2013).

Toms, J., 'MIND, Anti-Psychiatry, and the Case of the Mental Hygiene Movement's "Discursive Transformation"', *Social History of Medicine*, online, hky096, available at: https://doi.org/10.1093/shm/hky096 (accessed 25 June 2020).

Tone, A., *Devices and Desires: A History of Contraceptives in America* (New York: Farrar, Straus and Giroux, 2001).

Tong, R., *Feminist Approaches to Bioethics: Theoretical Reflections and Practical Applications* (Boulder: Westview Press, 1997).

Toth, B., 'Clinical Trials in British Medicine 1858–1948, with Special Reference to the Development of the Randomised Controlled Trial'. PhD thesis, University of Bristol, 1998.

Usborne, C., 'Women doctors and gender identity in Weimar Germany (1918–1933)' in A. Hardy and L. Conrad (eds), *Women and Modern Medicine*, Clio Medica 61 (Leiden: Brill Rodopi, 2001), pp. 109–26.

Vuille, M., 'Le désir sexuel des femmes, du DSM à la nouvelle médecine sexuelle', *Genre, sexualité & société*, online, 2014, available at: http://gss.revues.org/3240 (accessed 25 June 2020).

Walker, C. E. L., 'Making Birth Control Respectable: The Society for Constructive Birth Control and Racial Progress, and the American Birth Control

League, in Comparative Perspective, 1921–38'. PhD dissertation, University of Bristol, 2007.

Wandor, M. (ed.), *The Body Politic: Writings from the Women's Liberation Movement in Britain 1969–1972* (London: Stage, 1972).

Weatherall, M. W., 'Making medicine scientific: empiricism, rationality, and quackery in mid-Victorian Britain', *Social History of Medicine*, 9:2 (1996), pp. 175–94.

Weindling, P. (ed.), *International Health Organisations and Movements, 1918–39* (Cambridge: Cambridge University Press, 1995).

Welshman, J., 'In Search of the "Problem Family": Public Health and Social Work in England and Wales 1940–70', *Social History of Medicine*, 9:3 (1996), pp. 447–65.

Welshman, J., 'Eugenics and public health in Britain, 1900–40: scenes from provincial life', *Urban History*, 24:1 (1997), pp. 56–75.

Welshman, J., *Municipal Medicine: Public Health in Twentieth-Century Britain* (Oxford: Peter Lang, 2000).

Whitfield, N. and T. Schlich (eds), 'Skills through history', *Medical History*, 59:3 (2015), pp. 349–85.

Wyndham, D., *Norman Haire and the Study of Sex* (Sydney: Sydney University Press, 2012).

Index

Note: 'n.' after a page reference indicates the number of a note on that page

abortion 7–8, 12–3, 18, 30n.25 n.28, 31n.32, 32n.37, 35n.67, 40, 71, 73, 130n.12, 141, 148, 158, 160–2, 168nn.95–7, 180–1, 183, 185, 187, 218n.20, 219n.27, 222n.73
    Abortion Law Reform Association xii, 42, 73
    Abortion Act 8, 12, 224
    backstreet 180, 187
    conference on 141, 160–2
abstinence 18–9, 39, 42
activism 230
    birth control 4–5, 20–1, 40, 48, 124, 138–40, 142, 148, 150–1, 169–70, 180–1, 197, 201
    see also feminism
Adamson, R. H. 48
    Methods of Conception Control 48
Alabaster, G. 66
anxieties
    male doctor's 14
    population 9–10, 12, 45, 70, 73, 88, 121–2, 127, 137, 139–40, 157, 162, 169, 173, 175, 178–9, 185, 212–3, 227
    sexual 111, 118

artificial insemination xi, 105, 120, 125–6, 136n.144 n.147
Association Française des Femmes Médecins 23, 166n.68 n.70 n.76
Association Maternité Heureuse 13, 23, 180, 189
Aubény, E. 187–8, 194nn.72–3, 195n.74

Bac affair 180, 183
Baker, J. R. 21, 60, 68, 83n.107, 149, 153
Balint, M. 92, 115–20, 132n.38, 134nn.112–13, 135n.114, 188
Bard, C. 7, 28n.19, 30n.27, 167n.83
Barrett, F. 46–7
Barton, M. 105, 120, 123, 126–7, 135nn.133–4
Bashford, A. 26n.8, 29nn.21–3, 31n.32 n.34, 139–40, 164n.8, 169, 179, 190n.2 n.16, 192n.44
Besant, A. 10, 139
Bird, O. 70, 74
Birkett Committee 73

birth control
- as a medical responsibility 12, 40, 75, 146–54
- clinics 8, 11, 12, 16–23, 36–8, 40, 42–3, 45, 48–50, 55, 57, 59, 62, 66–8, 71, 75–6, 78 nn.26–7, 85, 87, 89, 93–4, 98, 144–5, 147–51, 153–5, 159, 165n.49, 170, 181–3, 187, 197, 200, 203, 206, 211, 224, 226–7
- husband's responsibility for 44
- methods *see* contraceptive methods
- opponents 39, 45, 63, 64, 67
- women's responsibility for 7, 145
- *see also* activism

Birth Control Investigation Committee xi, xii, 20–1, 35nn.75–6 n.78, 40, 42, 50, 63–4, 68–9, 149, 166n.53, 196–7, 199, 203, 208–11, 216–17, 218n.14 n.16, 219n.24, 221n.64, 226

Birth Control International Information Centre 21, 170–2, 181, 190nn.3–4 n.7 n.11

Bischoff, R. 117, 132n.38

Blacker, C. P. 20–1, 40, 42, 65, 78n.20, 88, 149, 165n.45, 174, 191n.22, 205–7, 210, 220n.44 n.49, 221n.51 n.54 n.58 nn.68–9

Blair, M. 70, 81n.71, 117, 132n.40, 215

Blanchier, D. 156–9, 166n.68 n.72, 167n.78 n.84 n.89

Blumberg, F. 150, 153

Booysen, C. 36n.80, 49, 69

Boyd Orr, J. 175–6

Bradlaugh, C. 10, 139

British Medical Women's Federation xi, 14, 23, 34n.55, 38, 45–9, 55, 79n.39, 124, 142, 150, 152, 155, 170, 178, 224, 225

British Postgraduate Medical School 48, 50, 80n.49

Brook, E. 12, 224

Brooke, S. 11, 33n.42, 78nn.21–2, 131n.21, 133n.60, 168n.95

Browne, S. 28n.20, 42, 77n.3, 78n.18

Butler, L. 152, 153, 155

Cambridge Birth Control Clinic 20, 64

Campbell, J. 161, 168n.97

cap *see under* contraceptive methods

Carleton, H. M. 60, 68, 209, 211

case cards 152
- clinic records 52, 66, 151, 197, 205
- case records 67

Catholic Church 48, 157
- Catholic doctor 156–7
- *Casti Connubii* 13

Charles, E. 63, 77n.7, 82n.86

circulation of knowledge 1, 5, 6, 140, 150, 153–4, 169, 171, 182–90

clinical trials xi, 21–3, 34n.65, 68–70, 76, 83n.111, 137, 197, 203, 209, 212–15, 219n.35, 221n.56

clitoris *see under* sexual pleasure

coitus interruptus *see under* contraceptive methods

community health 16, 41, 138

companionate marriage 86, 88, 125, 129n.5

Index

contraception
  criteria for good contraceptive methods 16–17, 20, 25, 44, 50, 64, 67–70, 76, 145, 147, 154, 160, 197–8, 202, 204, 207, 208, 210–14, 216, 226
  contraceptive culture 8, 18–22
  contraceptive failures 44, 65, 70, 148, 152–3, 196, 198, 204, 210
  as a human right 178–80
  legitimacy of 11, 24, 85, 144, 161, 226
  as a medical field and specialty 18, 22, 40, 47, 49–52, 57, 60, 62, 76, 85, 93, 151, 162
  memorandum on training in 52
  patients' experience with 2, 20, 22, 44, 50, 54, 68–9, 153, 197–200, 202, 204, 208–12, 214–15
  patients' education in 71, 99, 179
  side effects 23, 63, 69–70, 75, 199–200, 208–14, 217n.2
  step-by-step guide 62–3, 198
  training in 14, 25, 37, 40, 47–56, 63, 69, 76, 79n.42, 149, 156, 167n.82, 170–2, 177–9, 181, 185, 187, 199, 226, 228
  see also birth control
contraceptive methods
  caps and diaphragms 18, 20, 44, 48, 52–3, 56, 62–3, 68, 75–6, 151–2, 154, 159, 181, 185, 187–8, 197, 204
  coit interruptus and withdrawal 18–19, 42, 145
  condoms 12, 18, 144, 147, 159, 187
  intrauterine devices xi, 18, 25, 60, 151, Chapter 5
  pessaries 18, 20, 62, 146–7, 186, 198, 201, 204
  pill 12, 22, 30n.28, 35n.74, 44, 70, 74–7, 83n.107, 184–5, 187, 217n.3, 228–9
  spermicides 44, 68–9, 76, 149, 153–4, 209, 211
Cook, H. 26n.10, 30n.25, 31n.31, 35n.67, 38, 77n.4, 99, 129n.8, 130n.11, 230n.2
Council for the Investigation of Fertility Control 70, 83n.111, 215
Cova, A. 157, 167n.77
Cox, G. xi, 2, 36n.80, 49, 58–60, 62, 65, 81n.69, 82n.79, 154, 166n.63, 181, 212, 222n.74
  Clinical Contraception xi, 56, 81n.69, 82n.79, 166n.63, 222n.74
Crozier, I. 129n.2, 164n.12, 200, 218n.21, 219nn.22–3, 220n.38
Cullis, W. 40

Dalsace, J. 167n.90, 181–2, 184–5, 187, 189, 192nn.36–7 n.41 n.48, 193nn.50–3 n.57, 195n.75 n.79
Davidson, H. 122
Davis, G. 30n.28, 35n.68, 105, 133n.78, 135n.123, 136n.146
Dawkins, S. xi, 2, 47, 56, 68, 74–5, 79n.36, 81n.71 n.78, 83n.106, 90, 92, 98–9, 115, 117, 131n.29, 132n.38 n.58, 230, 231n.10
Dawson of Penn (Lord) 11, 39, 40

Debenham, C. 4, 27n.15, 28n.20, 32n.36, 36n.66, 42, 77n.12 n.16, 78n.19, 164n.14, 165n.49, 166n.66, 167n.92
degeneracy *see under* anxieties population
Dickinson, R. L. 59, 150
Donington, H. 176, 191nn.30–2
Drysdale, C. V. 142–3, 164n.18
Dunlop, B. 142–4, 164n.17

Eastbourne Family Planning Centre 92
education *see under* contraception; sexual pleasure
Ellis, H. 57, 115, 147
emotions and feelings 22, 112, 123, 128, 184
eugenics 9, 10, 23, 31n.35, 38, 43–4, 46, 78n.24 n.30, 82n.85, 140–4, 147, 164n.17, 174, 212–13
  Eugenics Society xii, 9, 20, 43, 58, 73, 85, 89, 142, 176, 213
  problem families 213
Exeter and District Women's Welfare Centre xi, 120, 124, 174
expertise 2, 8, 16, 18, 23–4, 56–61, 93, 197, 202, 216
  based on data and statistics 63–8, 144, 152–3, 197, 203–6
  based on professional experience 57–8, 61, 128, 145–6, 169–70, 172, 197, 203–5

familialism *see under* familial feminism
Family Planning Act 8, 12, 37, 75, 224
Family Planning Association xi, xii, 8, 12, 23, 36n.79, 37–8, 44, 49, 51, 56–9, 68, 70, 73–4, 80nn.56–7, 88–91, 97, 117–18, 120–6, 130n.13, 135n.124, 155, 170, 174, 176, 178, 183–6, 188–9, 214–15, 224, 230
Fawcitt, R. 202
female body 5, 53, 154, 159, 166n.52, 225, 229
  medicalisation of 2–3, 22, 128, 225–6
female patients' agency 3, 22, 86–7, 126, 128, 142
feminine fields of medicine 4, 15–7, 23, 41, 138
feminism
  activism 13, 42, 77, 229
  familial 157–62
  feminist health activism 2, 26n.3, 77, 229
  social purity 45
  welfare 17, 45–6, 142, 155–6, 160
fertility 2, 9, 12, 18, 31nn.29–30 n.32, 35n.70, 44, 57, 66, 69, 82nn.94–6 n.98, 86, 136nn.135–6, 143, 154, 176, 178–9, 203, 212, 214, 226
  control *see under* birth control
  decline 8–9, 18–19, 159, 172–3
  differential *see* eugenics
  infertility 7–8, 25, 30n.28, 85, 105, 120–8, 133n.78, 173, 181, 185
  see also natalism; sterility
Feversham Committee 126–7
Fifth International Neo-Malthusian and Birth Control Conference xi, 141–7
Fisher, K. 6, 19, 30n.26, 31n.28 n.31, 33n.44, 35n.66 n.69 n.72, 38, 44, 61, 77n.4, 78n.27,

Index

106, 130n.9 n.17, 134n.84, 165n.34, 207, 219n.25, 221n.60, 230n.2
Florence, L. S. 64–5, 82n.88
Birth Control on Trial 64–5, 82n.88
Foucault, M. 5, 28n.20
Franck, M. 183–4, 193n.55
Frankenburg, C. 42
French Association of Women Doctors 138
French Society for Sanitary and Moral Prophylaxis 158
Freud, S. 86–7, 100–1, 111, 118–19, 129n.7, 188
Fribourg, A. 185, 193n.58
Friedman, L. 117, 135n.115
frigidity *see under* sexual disorders
Fuller, E. 151–3

Galton, F. 9, 82n.85
gender roles
  feminine nature 15, 23
  femininity 64, 119
  in sexuality 19, 87, 92, 118–19, 125, 127, 227
  maternal nature 157, 159
  masculinity 103–5, 119
general practitioner 48–9, 63, 67, 74, 79n.43
Giles, A. 81n.71, 117
Gillie, A. 112, 155
Gimson, O. 36n.80, 45, 155
Goldring, D. and M. 196, 217n.1
Gräfenberg, E. 59, 151, 166n.52, 198–200, 202, 204, 208, 211, 214, 217n.1, 218nn.6–7 n.13 n.17
Graff, G. 49, 69, 83n.111
Grant, E. 69
Gray, A. H. 89

Green, S. 171
Green-Armytage V. 66–7, 209–10, 221n.65
Griffith, E. 36n.80, 89–90, 111, 130n.19, 131nn.26–7, 134n.99, 191n.21 n.24 n.28, 192n.40
Guttmacher, A. 74, 178, 212–13, 222n.79 n.81 n.84 n.86

Haire, N. 11, 16, 20, 35n.73, 40, 142, 144, 146–7, 164n.12 n.17, 165n.40, 196–8, 200–11, 215–17, 217nn.1–2, 218n.7 nn.20–1, 219n.22 nn.26–8 nn.30–1 n.33, 220n.41 nn.48–51, 221n.54 nn.58–9 n.61 n.66, 222n.73
Hall, L. 16, 25n.2, 27n.16, 28nn.19–20, 29n.21, 30n.35, 34n.61, 35n.66, 38, 77n.3 n.10, 78n.18 n.28 n.33, 79n.38, 81nn.67–8, 129n.8, 166n.50, 217n.1, 218n.19, 219n.22
Harding, K. 122–3, 125, 135n.131 n.133, 136n.140
Harvey, C. 121–2
Houghton, V. 89, 131n.25, 185, 192n.34, 193n.57
How-Martyn, E. 21, 140, 170, 172, 181
Hubback, E. 42, 71
Huxley, F. ix, 123, 136n.136, 142, 144–5, 147, 155, 164nn.15–16
Huxley, J. 20, 176
hymen 111, 114–15

impotence *see under* sexual disorders
infertility *see under* sexual disorders; sterility

International Birth Control Information Centre 140
International Committee on Planned Parenthood 90, 177, 192n.34
international conferences on birth control 6, 24, Chapter 3, 169–72, 197, 212, 227
International Medical Group for the Investigation of Contraception 21, 203, 205, 220n.44 nn.47–8
International Planned Parenthood Federation xii, 13, 23, 169–70, 173, 177–80, 182–3, 185–7, 191n.18, 192nn.35–9 n.41, 193n.57, 194nn.62–4 n.71, 195n.77 n.79, 212, 214, 230

Jackson, M. xi, 2, 25, 36n.80, 51, 60, 64–7, 69–70, 74, 82n.87 n.91 n.95 nn.98–9, 83n.104 n.111, 85, 92, 94, 120–4, 126–7, 135nn.124–5 n.133, 136n.137 n.144 n.147, 174, 177–9, 181, 196–7, 212–7, 222nn.76–7 nn.84–5, 230
Jeffries, L. 60, 155
Jex-Blake, S. 14–15, 34n.57

Kahn-Nathan, J. 187
Kelly, L. 15, 27n.14, 34n.52 n.54 n.57, 230n.3
Képès, S. 185, 188, 193n.60, 194n.61, 195n.76
Killick Millard, C. 39, 60, 71–2, 77n.7, 142–3, 164n.17
knowledge transfer *see under* circulation of knowledge
Knowles, F. I. 60
Knowlton, C. 139

laboratory-based medicine 18, 22, 63–71, 206
Labour Party xii, 11, 43, 71, 78n.21
Lagroua Weill-Hallé M.A. 13, 180, 182–3, 185–6, 189, 193nn.52–3, 194nn.63–5, 195n.79
Lambeth Conference 11, 72
Langhamer, C. 30n.25, 89, 131n.22 n.30
Le Sueur-Capelle, S. 187
Lewis-Faning Report 19

Macaulay, M. xii, 49, 81n.78, 89, 91–2, 155
  Art of Marriage 81n.78, 89
Mace, D. R. 89
Main, T. 118–19, 188
male-dominated medicine *see* medical hierarchy
Malleson, J. xii, 2, 38, 43–5, 49, 56–60, 62–3, 65–7, 69, 73, 80n.64, 82n.80 n.83 n.96 nn.100–1, 83n.102 n.105, 84nn.117–18, 85, 88–97, 99–107, 109–15, 119, 121–3, 126, 128, 128n.1, 130n.15, 131nn.32–3, 132n.41 nn.45–7 nn.50–1, 133n.62 n.66 nn.69–71, 134nn.96–9 nn.101–8, 150, 154, 174, 186, 191n.18, 227, 229
  Any Wife or Any Husband: A Book for Couples Who Have Met Sexual Difficulties and for Doctors (1950) 93, 95, 131n.32, 132n.41, 134n.97 n.102 n.107
  The Principles of Contraception: A Handbook for General Practitioners 57, 80n.64,

Index

82n.80, 132n.51, 133n.62 n.66, 134n.98
Malthus, T. R. 10
 La Ligue de la Régénération Humaine 10
Malthusianism and neo-Malthusianism 5, 6, 10, 24, 28n.19, 29n.21, 38, 137, 139–40, 142–4, 147, 162, 163n.6, 164n.18, 172, 182
Malthusian League 10, 20, 39, 139, 141–3, 164n.17
Mannin, E. 196, 217n.1, 218n.19
marital difficulties 88, 90–1, 94
 see also sexual disorders
Marriage Guidance Council 89, 130n.20, 131n.24
marriage guidance xii, 87, 89–90
marriage reformers 88–9
married women doctors 17, 91
Martindale, L. 46, 154, 159–60, 167n.87
maternity and child welfare centres 41, 43, 71
McIlroy, A. L. 155–6, 166n.65 n.67, 167n.87 n.91 n.93
Mears, E. 69–70, 80n.62, 81n.71, 83n.111, 105, 117, 126, 178, 185, 189, 193n.58, 194n.70, 195n.79
Medawar, J. 184
medical hierarchy 3, 14–15, 17, 23, 41, 72, 75, 85, 228
medical and scientific knowledge 3, 7, 8, 17–23, 26n.9, 37–8, 47, 51–2, 57, 61–71, 85–6, 110, 137, 151, 153, 169, 219n.35, 220n.38, 226
Medical Research Council 203, 209, 220nn.36–7

medical students 47–9, 52–3, 55–6, 62, 76, 79n.40 n.42, 138, 226
Medical Views on Birth Control 39–40
Medical Women's International Association 46, 141, 155–6, 166n.65
Memorandum 153/MCW 11–12, 39
menorrhagia 198, 214
Montreuil-Strauss, G. 156, 158, 166n.70
Moore White, M. 81n.71 n.78, 120, 122–4, 126, 135nn.133–4, 136n.139
motherhood 28nn.19–20, 32n.39, 43, 78n.24, 121, 133n.61, 155, 157–8, 166n.64, 182, 183
Mouvement Français pour le Planning Familial 13, 23, 170, 181–5, 188
Mure, C. 178, 185–6, 189

natalism and pronatalism 10, 13, 31n.32, 32n.39, 33n.46
National Birth Control Association xi, xii, 11, 21, 36n.80, 42, 48, 50, 57, 60, 68, 79n.47, 80n.50, 81n.69, 83n.108, 88–9, 155, 191n.21 n.24 n.28, 192n.40, 210–11
National Health Service 12, 15, 56, 229
Neal-Edwards, M. 81n.71, 91–2, 132n.38
Neuwirth Law 8, 13, 180
North Kensington Women's Welfare Centre xii, 20, 40, 47–9, 51, 59, 70–1, 79n.47, 83n.112, 88, 90–2, 96, 121–2, 135n.126, 151, 199, 204, 215

Odlum, D. 160
Ottesen-Jensen, E. 173–4, 176, 191n.18, 192n.33

Pasmore, J. 117, 119, 135n.119
Peberdy, M. 69
population issues *see under* anxieties
Pyke, M. 73, 81n.71, 82n.94, 176–7, 185

Sanger, M. 4, 21, 28n.20, 139–41, 147–8, 152, 169–70, 172, 174, 176–7, 227
Scharlieb, M. 45–6, 78n.30, 81n.67
sex education 139, 158, 178–9, 181
sexual counselling and therapy xi, xii, 2, 23–5, 45, 85–90, 92–120, 127–8
  training in 90, 94, 116–20, 188, 227
sexual disorders 1–2, 6–8, 13, 24, Chapter 2
  erectile dysfunction 104
  frigidity 24, 87, 94, 110–11, 114, 119, 129n.2, 188
  impotence 90
  vaginismus 92, 94, 104–5, 110, 112, 114, 132n.47 n.50, 133n.77 n.79, 134n.101 n.103 n.107, 188
sexual pleasure 24, 86–7, 89, 93–110, 113, 119, 127–8, 227, 229
  clitoris 87, 97, 100–2, 105, 107–10, 115, 119, 128
  education in 93, 99–100, 104–5
  penetration 89, 99, 101
  sexual ignorance 87, 96–8
  vaginal orgasm 87, 100–2, 119–20
  vaginal sensation 108–10
sterility 12, 39, 57, 66–7, 82n.91 n.100, 83nn.102–5, 88, 105, 120–7, 135n.124 n.127 n.133, 136n.137 n.139, 152, 155, 179, 181, 187, 201, 219n.29
Stopes, M. 4, 11, 19–20, 27n.16, 18n.19, 35n.66, 39, 41, 43, 46, 48, 65, 79n.38 n.42, 156, 182, 201, 217, 218n.26
speculum 51–2, 54, 63, 151, 199
statistics *see* expertise; medical and scientific knowledge
Stone, A. and H. 148, 152, 154, 175–6, 183
Sullerot, E. 180, 186
Szreter, S. 6, 9, 19, 30n.26, 31nn.29–32, 35n.69, 61, 106, 130n.9 n.17, 133n.61, 134n.84, 165n.34, 207, 221n.60, 230n.2

Tavistock Clinic 90–1, 115, 118, 188, 227
Taylor, R. 81n.71, 117, 132n.38, 184
Thuillier-Landry, M. 158
Tunnedine, P. xii, 17, 119

Valabrègue, C. 185–6
venereal diseases 10, 12, 31n.30, 73, 158
Voge, C. 21, 68, 149

Walworth Women's Welfare Centre xi, 20, 39, 48–9, 81n.69, 142, 144, 195n.78, 200, 206
women's health 41, 94, 140–1, 169, 226
Wright H. xii, 1, 2, 25, 36n.80, 37–8, 40–1, 47–53, 58–61, 63, 66, 69–72, 77n.1 n.13, 79n.49, 80n.49 n.52, 81n.66 n.71 n.72 n.77, 82n.81, 84n.116, 85, 88–2, 96–7, 99, 100,

107–9, 114–15, 119, 121, 126–8, 132n.49 nn.55–7, 133nn.64–5, 134n.85 n.88, 150–1, 153, 155, 170–2, 174–9, 186–7, 191n.19 n.20 n.23 n.27, 192n.35, 194n.68, 196–7, 199, 201–12, 215–17, 217n.2, 218n.17, 219n.34, 220n.47, 226–7, 229

Birth Control, Advice on Family Spacing and Healthy Sex Life 61

Contraceptive Technique 58, 59, 63, 81n.66 n.72, 82n.81

More about the Sex Factor in Marriage 132n.49 n.56, 134n.88

The Sex Factor in Marriage: A Book for Those Who Are, or Are About to Be, Married 61, 89, 132n.55, 133n.64

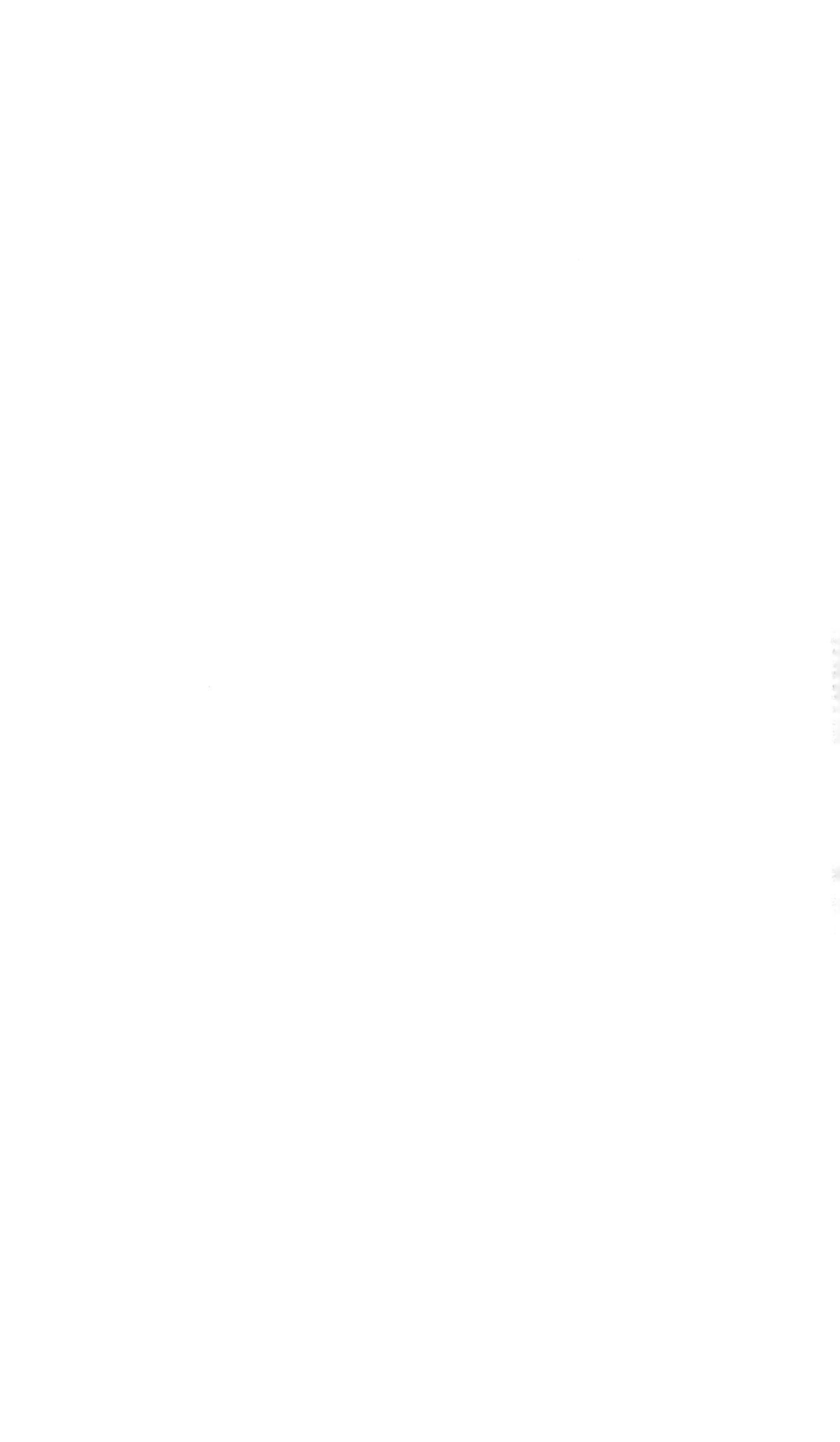

Lightning Source UK Ltd.
Milton Keynes UK
UKHW021836051220
374612UK00003B/161